Palpation and Assessment in Manual Therapy

Fourth edition

LEON CHAITOW

Palpation and Assessment in Manual Therapy

Learning the art and refining your skills

Foreword

Jerrilyn Cambron, LMT, DC, MPH, PhD

Chair, School of Allied Health Sciences and Distance Education;
Chair of the Massage Therapy Program; Professor, Department
of Research, National University of Health Sciences (NUHS), USA;
President, Massage Therapy Foundation, USA

Contributors

Sasha Chaitow

Whitney Lowe

Warrick McNeill

Sarah Mottram

Thomas W. Myers

Michael Seffinger

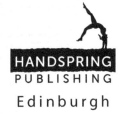

HANDSPRING
PUBLISHING
Edinburgh

HANDSPRING PUBLISHING LIMITED
The Old Manse, Fountainhall,
Pencaitland, East Lothian
EH34 5EY, Scotland
Tel: +44 1875 341 859
Website: www.handspringpublishing.com

First published 2017 in the United Kingdom by Handspring Publishing

First edition 1997, Churchill Livingstone
Second edition 2003, Churchill Livingstone
Third edition 2010, Churchill Livingstone

ISBN 978-1-909141-34-6

British Library Cataloguing in Publication Data
A catalogue record for this book is available from the British Library

Library of Congress Cataloguing in Publication Data
A catalog record for this book is available from the Library of Congress

Notice
Neither the Publisher nor the Authors assume any responsibility for any loss or injury and/or damage to persons or property arising out of or relating to any use of the material contained in this book. It is the responsibility of the treating practitioner, relying on independent expertise and knowledge of the patient, to determine the best treatment and method of application for the patient.

Commissioning Editor Mary Law
Copy-editor Stephanie Pickering
Designer Bruce Hogarth
Indexer Aptara
Typesetter DiTech Process Solutions
Printer Ashford Colour Press Ltd

The
Publisher's
policy is to use
paper manufactured
from sustainable forests

CONTENTS

	Contributors		vii
	Foreword		ix
	Preface		xi

Chapter 1 Objective: palpatory literacy   *Leon Chaitow*   1

Chapter 2 Palpation reliability and validity   *Michael Seffinger*   9

Special topic 1 Using appropriate pressure (and the myofascial pain index)   *Leon Chaitow*   27

Special topic 2 Structure and function: are they inseparable?   *Leon Chaitow*   31

Chapter 3 Fundamentals of palpation   *Leon Chaitow*   35

Special topic 3 Visual assessment, the dominant eye, and other issues   *Leon Chaitow*   55

Chapter 4 Palpating and assessing the skin   *Leon Chaitow*   59

Special topic 4 Source of pain: is it reflex or local?   *Leon Chaitow*   87

Special topic 5 The morphology of reflex and acupuncture points   *Leon Chaitow*   91

Special topic 6 Is it a muscle or a joint problem?   *Leon Chaitow*   93

Chapter 5 Palpating for changes in muscle structure   *Leon Chaitow*   97

Chapter 6 Fascial palpation   *Thomas W. Myers*   147

Chapter 7 Assessment of "abnormal mechanical tension" in the nervous system   *Leon Chaitow*   171

Special topic 7 Red, white and black reaction   *Leon Chaitow*   183

Special topic 8 Percussion palpation and treatment   *Leon Chaitow*   189

Special topic 9 Joint play/"end-feel"/ range of motion: what are they?   *Leon Chaitow*   197

Chapter 8 Palpation and assessment of joints (including spine and pelvis)   *Leon Chaitow*   203

Chapter 9 Accurately identifying musculoskeletal dysfunction   *Whitney Lowe*   235

Chapter 10 Evaluating movement   *Warrick McNeill and Sarah Mottram*   251

Special topic 10 Fibromyalgia palpation assessment   *Leon Chaitow*   261

Chapter 11 Palpating for functional "ease"   *Leon Chaitow*   265

Special topic 11 About hyperventilation   *Leon Chaitow*   283

Chapter 12	Visceral palpation and respiratory function assessment *Leon Chaitow*	289
Special topic 12	Synesthesia *Sasha Chaitow*	305
Chapter 13	Understanding and using intuitive faculties *Sasha Chaitow*	309
Special topic 13	Palpating the traditional Chinese pulses *Leon Chaitow*	317
Chapter 14	Subtle palpation *Leon Chaitow*	323
Chapter 15	Palpation and emotional states *Leon Chaitow*	357
	Appendix: Location of Chapman's neurolymphatic reflexes	373
	Index	377

CONTRIBUTORS

Sasha Chaitow PhD
Independent Researcher
Corfu, Greece

Whitney Lowe LMT
Director, Academy of Clinical Massage
Sisters, OR, USA

Warrick McNeill Grad Dip Phyty (NZ), MCSP
Director, Physioworks
Associate Editor, Journal of Bodywork and Movement
Therapies
London, UK

Sarah Mottram MSc MCSP
Director, Movement Performance Solutions
Bristol, UK

Thomas W. Myers LMT NCTMB CSI
Director, Anatomy Trains
Walpole, ME, USA

Michael A. Seffinger, DO
Professor
Department of Neuromusculoskeletal Medicine/Osteopathic
Manipulative Medicine (NMM/OMM)
College of Osteopathic Medicine of the Pacific
Western University of Health Sciences
Pomona, CA, USA

FOREWORD

The university at which I teach encourages students to frequently practice their palpation and assessment skills on fellow students and instructors. Some students have a natural ability to feel the structures they are palpating, while others are going through the motion of poking and prodding without understanding what their fingers should be experiencing. I am willing to let students practice these exercises on me because I was once at their level of inexperience. We all must start at the beginning of the path.

One of the exercises I was taught as a student in palpation class was to move my fingers over a sheet of paper until I could locate a single human hair hidden underneath the page by a fellow student. Over time, we would increase the number of pages to challenge each other and to continue improving our skills. We initially struggled to find the hair under one sheet of paper, but with practice we improved our sense of touch and could feel the minor shift in paper height even through many pages.

As such, palpation and assessment skills improve over time. As we learn to trust our abilities and instincts, we stop being concerned about our body mechanics during the assessment and start focusing on what we are feeling under our fingertips including the incredible variations in tissue height, density, temperature, and movement. We are continually learning the nuances of touch throughout our journey as manual medicine practitioners, fluidly moving between assessment and treatment of human structures and finding new variations with each patient we see.

Leon Chaitow has been my mentor and friend for many years. I have always been impressed by his ease at describing even the most complex issues in understandable terms. After dozens of publications on manual therapy, he has brought forward a revision of another incredible text. *Palpation and Assessment in Manual Therapy* brings our attention towards the most important aspect of everyday practice in manual medicine- the art, science, and intuition of palpation and assessment. This text poses many interesting questions about how and what we feel, bringing us back to the beginning of our education to rethink our own method of palpation. After many years in manual medicine, palpation and assessment become second nature

but include our own biases and expectations. Refocusing on the process and relearning different aspects of thought discussed in this text was educational, interesting, and exciting.

Leon Chaitow has many suggestions on how to focus on different aspects of palpation such as the external feel and temperature of the skin and moving from the superficial layers to the subcutaneous fat, fascia, vessels, and eventually muscle tissues and joint complexes, as well as the potential reasons for variability in the feel of these structures. Multiple exercises are included throughout the book that encourage refinement of the described techniques, which range from basic (such as the "hair through paper" exercise - see page 43) to advanced, making this text ideal for improving the skills of seasoned practitioners and students alike. Illustrated orthopedic tests, postural observation methods, and functional movement tests are all revisited, accompanied by commentary and discussion regarding variations that we may encounter in clinical practice.

The chapter on reliability and validity of palpation by contributing author Professor Michael (Mickey) Seffinger was particularly interesting, and includes research that describes the consistency of physical findings within practice. What he presents is that many manual medicine assessment techniques are neither accurate nor consistent; however, recommendations for improvement are offered along with quotes from experts such as Craig Liebenson and David Simons, providing suggestions as to how best to improve the reliability of our palpation assessments.

Contributions from other authors add a blend of different viewpoints to the text, including chapters on fascial palpation by Tom Myers, accurately identifying musculoskeletal dysfunction by Whitney Lowe, evaluating movement by Warrick McNeill and Sarah Mottram, and understanding and using intuitive faculties by Sasha Chaitow. Each chapter offers insight for contemplation by both new and experienced health care providers, supplementing and enhancing the chapters and discussions presented by the editor.

Of great interest to more advanced practitioners are chapters on visceral palpation, assessment of respiratory function, using intuition during palpation, and the effect of emotional states on palpatory findings. In practice, we all encounter patients who do not fully respond to treatment. Learning to reassess through different means may benefit our patients' overall outcomes. This text provides us with some novel thoughts to consider when that difficult patient once again comes for an appointment.

Congratulations to Leon Chaitow and the contributing authors on an intriguing book about manual therapies that encourages us to improve our palpation and assessment skills no matter how much experience we may have. Through this book, he is challenging us to continue to learn and to add even more pages over that strand of hair, to see what we feel.

Jerrilyn Cambron
Lombard, Illinois
December 2016

PREFACE

As Frymann (1963) noted: "Palpation cannot be learned by reading or listening; it can only be learned by palpation." Learning palpation should not be just about effort – it should be fun and it should be rewarding. Skillful palpation can be seen to represent "knowing in action" (Schön 1983), in which apparently spontaneous therapeutic skills emerge from a background of deep understanding and refined actions, acquired by diligent practice.

If manual treatment is to have an optimal therapeutic effect, it needs to relate to the requirements of the tissues, region, or person concerned. Haphazard or unstructured manual approaches are unlikely to achieve good results. The clinical decisions made as to what type, degree, and duration of treatment to offer will always depend on the training and belief system of the practitioner/therapist, responding to information gathered and interpreted, through history-taking, palpation, observation, and assessment.

Whether the therapeutic objective is to mobilize a joint, restore range of motion, release hypertonic, shortened soft-tissues, modify fibrosis, enhance circulation or drainage, or to tone weak or inhibited musculature, deactivate trigger points, or ease pain, or any of a range of other "bodywork" objectives, an adequate degree of appreciation of the nature and current level of dysfunction, as well as an ability to compare the current state with whatever is conceived of as "normal," before treatment commences, is desirable.

The ability of a practitioner seamlessly to switch from palpation/assessment to treatment, and back again, marks the truly skilled individual. Whether palpation and assessment are used to build a clinical picture from which treatment flows, or whether assessment/palpation and treatment are simultaneous, what is evaluated offers the basis for the intervention, a yardstick by means of which to measure progress, a documentable, ideally measurable, foundational (to the therapeutic endeavor) record of the current state of the target tissues.

It is true to say that much evaluation can now be performed using technology. Patients can be photographed, scanned, X-rayed, and in a multitude of other ways inves-

tigated as to the current state of their structures, functions, and dysfunctions. Biotechnology is advancing rapidly, and tools and equipment previously only available in hospital and major clinic settings are increasingly available to the individual practitioner and therapist, to assist in the clinical application of such methods.

• Does this make the ancient art of palpation redundant?
• Are assessments involving subjective judgment old-fashioned and inaccurate?

In recent years the value of palpation has been challenged, with research studies suggesting that reproducible results cannot always be demonstrated when the accuracy of palpation is tested. The reliability of palpation performed by individuals, as well as the degree of agreement between experts palpating the same patient, or tissues, is increasingly questioned. These issues have been diligently explored in Chapter 2.

The truth is that as with the acquisition of any skill there are a number of variables that can determine whether palpation is skilled, or not. These include:
• the quality of the teaching of the skill, particularly involving methods used in hands-on practice
• the degree of application and practice given to skill acquisition by the student of palpation – however experienced – involving the amount of time, number of repetitions, as well as the degree of focus and thought, applied to particular exercises, tasks, and methods
• the underlying depth of knowledge of anatomy, physiology and pathophysiology to which the findings can be applied, and from which interpretations and conclusions can be drawn.

This book contains a distillation of the methods and thoughts of hundreds of skilled individuals, from diverse therapeutic backgrounds. The commonality that emerges is that there is no equivalent in technology to replace what can be gleaned from truly skilful hands-on touch and assessment methods.

You are recommended to work through this book, chapter by chapter, exercise by exercise (more than once), recording your findings and refining your skills. This is as relevant to the student as to the person currently in active practice, for we should never cease striving for even better subtlety of palpation. I am immensely grateful to the gifted chapter authors for their insights and input that have helped to make the book less of a dry "how to" text, and more of an immersion in subtle skill refinement.

Whether palpating skin, muscle, fascia, neural structures or joints, the same message applies: repeat and repeat again, until what is observed, and what is perceived makes sense.

In the very first incarnation of this book, before it adopted its current title, the book was titled *Palpatory Literacy*, a phrase that emphasizes the ultimate goal of the reader (and the author and chapter contributors) that – like learning to read – this subtle art would become automatic, with the multiple sensory impulses reaching the brain being accurately interpreted.

Please enjoy the exploration of "what you feel."

Leon Chaitow ND, DO
Honorary Fellow, University of Westminster
Corfu, November 2016

References
Frymann V (1963) Palpation. Its study in the workshop. In: *Yearbook of the Academy of Applied Osteopathy*, pp 16–31. Carmel, California: Academy of Applied Osteopathy.
Schön D (1983) *The Reflective Practitioner*, London: Temple Smith.

Objective: palpatory literacy

Leon Chaitow

Therapists and practitioners who use their hands to treat soft tissues and joints need to be able, reliably and relatively swiftly, to feel, assess, and make a preliminary judgment as to the current status of those tissues:

- Does this seem to be normal?

- If abnormal, in what way?

- What assessments are needed to provide more information?

It should be obvious that in order to appreciate what is abnormal, it is necessary to be familiar with the way normal tissues and structures feel and behave. This requires appreciation of a wide range of physiological and pathological conditions and parameters, relating not only to the tissues being assessed, but also to other tissues associated with them, perhaps lying at greater depth or at a distance. The information a practitioner needs to gather is, therefore, likely to vary according to the therapeutic approach, possibly including:

- the range of motion

- the feel of joint play

- the relative weakness, shortness, or tightness in muscles

- the amount of induration, edema, or fibrosis in soft tissues

- possible distant postural, functional, or fascial influences, affecting the area being assessed

- identification of neurological influences, or reflex activity that might be influencing dysfunction

- a sense as to whether pathology – rather than dysfunction – is involved …

… and many other pieces of potentially useful information.

Karel Lewit (1999) described a major problem in learning to palpate: "Palpation is the basis of our diagnostic techniques [and yet] it is extremely difficult to describe exactly, in words, the information palpation provides." We will try, nevertheless, to do just this, with the help of numerous experts from a variety of disciplines, all the while keeping in mind the words of Viola Frymann (1963): "Palpation cannot be learned by reading or listening; it can only be learned by palpation."

Much of this book comprises descriptions of various forms of palpation, highlighting different ways in which information can be gathered, along with numerous examples of exercises that can help in the development of perceptive exploratory skills. Of course, what we make of the information we derive from palpation will depend upon how it fits into a larger clinical picture, which needs to be built up from case history taking and other forms of assessment. Such interpretation is essential in order for treatment to have any direction, since palpation is anything but an end in itself.

To be clear, the *interpretation* of the information deriving from palpation is not the major purpose of this text; rather, the purpose is *learning how to palpate and assess* – not how to offer interpretations. This focus on the process of learning how to palpate does not imply that interpretation of the gathered information is of only secondary importance, for it is not, but for this book to have ventured too far into the direction of interpretation and diagnosis would have expanded the text to an unmanageable size.

For example, in Chapter 3 ("Fundamentals of palpation"), which deals in part with the assessment of skin tone elasticity, there will be a focus on making an accurate assessment of local and general areas in which there is a relative loss of the skin's ability to stretch – possibly due to reflex activity. The section therefore deals with the art of palpation of these particular tissues in terms of their elasticity and adherence to underlying tissues. How elastic, how flexible, is the skin, and how well/symmetrically does it move over underlying structures? Various expert opinions will be provided as to what the finding of changes in local skin behavior *might* actually mean clinically, but it is not the aim of this book to offer a comprehensive survey of those topics, or to suggest definitive interpretations.

In other words, the individual therapist/practitioner needs to fit the acquired information into their own healthcare system, and to use it in accordance with whatever therapeutic methods are seen to be appropriate. The aim of the book is to help us identify what it is that is under our hands when they are in touch with the patient.

An analogy can be made between learning to make sense of information gathered from manual palpation and learning to make sense of some other form of information, for example, that relating to music. It is possible to learn how to read music, to understand its structure, the theory of harmony, tones, chords, and even something of the application of such knowledge to different forms of composition. However, this would not enable you to play an instrument. The instrument that therapists "play" is the human body, and the development of palpatory literacy allows us to begin the process of "reading" that body.

One of osteopathy's major figures, Frederick Mitchell Jr (1976), makes a different comparison when he equates palpatory literacy with visual literacy:

Visual literacy is developed in visual experiences, and the exercise of visual perceptions in making judgments. Visual judgments and perceptions may be qualitative, or quantitative, or both. Although the objectives in training the diagnostic senses do not include aesthetic considerations, aesthetic experiences probably are developmental in terms of visual literacy. In making aesthetic value judgments one must be able to discriminate between straight lines and crooked lines, perfect circles and distorted circles ... To evaluate the level of sensory literacy, one may (also) test for specific sensory skills in a testing situation.

Later chapters suggest ways in which this can be done.

Assumptions and paradoxes

The assumption is made that, if you are reading this book, you already have some knowledge of anatomy and physiology, and, ideally, of pathology. The way you will interpret the information gained by palpation depends on your underlying knowledge base. It is all too easy for practitioners (even those with wide experience) to feel what they "want" to feel, or what they expect to feel. A relative degree of objective detachment from the process of assessment is therefore helpful, and indeed necessary.

An open mind is also vital to the task of learning palpatory literacy. Those practitioners with the greatest degree of "rigidity" in terms of their training and the system of therapy they follow often have the hardest time allowing themselves to sense new feelings and become aware of new sensations. Those with the most open, most eclectic approaches (massage therapists are a prime example) usually find it easiest to "trust" their senses and feelings. The other side of the coin, however, is that many (though by no means all) such "open-minded" therapists also have the poorest knowledge of anatomy/physiology and pathology against which to relate their palpatory evaluations.

This paradox can only be resolved by highly trained professionals becoming more intuitive and open (see Chapter 13), trusting that they really are sensing very subtle sensations as they open themselves to developing the delicate skills necessary for many palpatory methods. At the same time, less "well-trained" professionals might need to accept the necessity of adding layers of knowledge to their existing intuitive and nurturing talents.

Unless a practitioner is able to "read" the mass of information that is present in all soft tissues, and is also able to relate this to the problems of the patient (as well as to a good deal of other diagnostic information), much potentially vital data may be missed.

No one in the osteopathic field has done more to stress the importance of sound palpatory skills than Viola Frymann, and we will be learning from a number of her observations as we progress through the text. She summed up the focusing of these skills, and the importance of making sense of them, when she said (Frymann 1963):

The first step in the process of palpation is detection, the second step is amplification, and the third step must therefore be interpretation. The interpretation of the observations made by palpation is the key which makes the study of the structure and function of tissues meaningful. Nevertheless it is like the first visit to a foreign country. Numerous strange and unfamiliar sights are to be seen, but without some knowledge of the language with which to ask questions, or a guide to interpret those observations in the life and history of the country, they have little meaning to us. The third step in our study then is to be able to translate palpatory observations into meaningful anatomic, physiologic or pathologic states.

Palpation objectives

Philip Greenman, in his superb analysis *Principles of Manual Medicine* (Greenman 1989), summarizes the five objectives of palpation. You, the practitioner/therapist, should be able to:

1. detect abnormal tissue texture

2. evaluate symmetry in the position of structures, both physically and visually

3. detect and assess variations in range and quality of movement *during* the range, as well as the quality of the end of the range of any movement

4. sense the position in space of yourself and the person being palpated

5. detect and evaluate change in the palpated findings, whether these are improving or worsening as time passes.

As we will see, others have suggested adding more subtle but apparently still palpable factors, such as energy variations, "tissue memory," and emotional influences, to these basic requirements of what can (and should) be palpated and assessed. The elements described by Greenman are, however, our major objectives in obtaining palpatory literacy.

Karel Lewit (1999), the brilliant Czech physician who has eclectically combined so much of osteopathic, chiropractic, physical therapy and orthopedic knowledge, makes the following statement of what our objective should be when palpating the patient:

Palpation of tissue structures seeks to determine the texture, resilience, warmth, humidity and the possibility of moving, stretching or compressing these structures. Concentrating on the tissues palpated, and pushing aside one layer after another, we distinguish skin, subcutaneous tissue, muscle and bone, we recognise the transition to the tendon, and finally the insertion. Palpating bone, we recognise tuberosities (and possible changes) and locate joints. Reflex changes due to pain affect all these tissues, and can be assessed by palpation; one of the most significant factors is increased tension.

Lewit's methods of ascertaining the presence of tense, tight tissues are examined in some detail in later chapters.

Regarding the learning process, Gerald Cooper (1977) says:

To begin to learn palpatory skill one must learn to practice to palpate bone or muscle or viscera. Gradually one learns to distinguish between a healthy muscle, a spastic muscle, and a flaccid one, and gradually one learns there is a difference in feel between a hard malignant tumor and a firm benign tumor. Palpation cannot be learned by reading or listening, it can only be learned by palpation.

This message is basic, and vital, and many experts repeat it. Read, understand and then practice, practice, and practice some more. It is the only way to become literate in palpation.

George Webster (1947) said:

We should feel with our brain as well as with our fingers, that is to say, into our touch should go our concentrated attention and all the correlated knowledge that we can bring to bear upon the case before us … The principle employed by Dr Still [founder of osteopathy] in so carefully educating his tactile sense … accounted for his success over such a wide field. He had a way of letting his fingers sink slowly into the tissues, feeling his way from the superficial to the deep structures, that gave him a comprehensive picture of local as well as general pathology.

On the learning of palpatory skills, Frederick Mitchell Jr (1976) states:

Although visual sensing of objects is done through an intervening medium (the atmosphere or other transparent material), students may be uncomfortable with the notion that palpation is also performed through an intervening medium. The necessity for projecting one's tactile senses to varying distances through an intervening medium, must seem mystical and esoteric to many beginning students. Yet even when one is palpating surface textures the information reaches one's nervous system through one's own intervening integument. Students are often troubled by the challenge of palpating an internal organ through overlying skin, subcutaneous fascia and fat, muscle, deep fascia, subserous fascia and peritoneum.

Becker, whose work is discussed in later chapters, suggested we palpate *through* our fingers, not *with* them.

Palpate by "feeling", not thinking

The exercises and advice in the text will hopefully overcome any concerns such as those expressed by Mitchell, for, along with the assertion of so many experts that palpation can only be learned by palpating, there is another common theme, which is that there needs to be a *trusting* of what is being felt, a suspension of critical judgment while the process of exploration is being carried out.

Later on, critical judgment becomes essential when interpreting what has been felt, but the process of "feeling" needs to be carried out with that faculty silenced. No one has better expressed this need than John Upledger (1987), the developer of craniosacral therapy, who stated:

> *Most of you have spent years studying the sciences and have learned to rely heavily upon your rational, reasoning mind. You probably have been convinced that the information which your hands can give you is unreliable. You may consider facts to be reliable only when they are printed on a computer sheet, projected on a screen or read from the indicator of an electrical device. In order to use your hands and to begin to develop them as reliable instruments for diagnosis and treatment, you must learn to trust them and the information they can give you.*

Learning to trust your hands is not an easy task. You must learn to shut off your conscious, critical mind while you palpate for subtle changes in the body you are examining. You must adopt an empirical attitude so that you may temporarily accept without question those perceptions which come into your brain from your hands. Although this attitude is unpalatable to most scientists it is recommended that you give it a trial. After you have developed your palpatory skill, you can criticize what you have felt with your hands. If you criticize before you learn to palpate, you will never learn to palpate, you will never learn to use your hands effectively as the highly sensitive diagnostic and therapeutic instruments which, in fact, they are.

"Accept what you sense as real" is Upledger's plea. This is a valid motto for the exploration of palpatory skills only if the palpation is accurately performed. As will be discussed in detail in the next chapter (and with periodic references in later chapters), the accuracy of palpatory findings is frequently questioned by researchers (Van Duersen et al. 1990; Panzer 1992; Vincent Smith & Gibbons 1999).

The ability of an individual practitioner to regularly and accurately locate and identify somatic landmarks and changes in function lies at the very heart of palpatory reliability. Upledger's injunction to "trust what you feel" is only valid if what you think you feel really is what you intended to feel, that the vertebra or rib being assessed is actually the one you meant to investigate!

W.G. Sutherland (1948), the primary osteopathic researcher into cranial motion, gave his uncompromising instruction as follows: "It is necessary to develop fingers with brain cells in their tips, fingers capable of feeling, thinking, seeing. Therefore first instruct the fingers how to feel, how to think, how to see, and then let them touch."

Palpation variations

As though the fears outlined by Mitchell were insufficient, and Upledger's and Sutherland's directions not difficult enough, there are also those therapists who make an assessment a short distance from the skin, although it should be clear that what they are "palpating" is rather different from the tissues that Mitchell's students were palpating.

This approach is far less indefensible than might be assumed, following the publication of the results of double blind studies into the use of "therapeutic touch" methods, in which no contact with the (physical) body is made at all. This will be discussed further in Chapter 14, where an array of methods aimed at increasing sensitivity to subtle energy patterns will be detailed.

Other forms of assessment involving very light skin contact, with the palpating hand(s)/digit(s) either stationary or moving in a variety of ways, will also be explored at length. Palpation of this sort often employs, as Lewit (1999) mentions, awareness of variations in skin tone, temperature, feel, and elasticity (which may reflect or be associated with altered electrical resistance) or other changes.

Some methods, such as the German system of *bindegewebsmassage* (connective tissue massage), employ a sequential examination of the relative adherence of different layers of tissue to each other, either at an interface (say, between muscle and connective tissue) or above it (skin over muscle,

muscle over bone and so on) (Bischof & Elmiger 1960). Lewit (1999) has also shown the relevance of identifying changes in skin adherence over reflexogenic areas that are active, such as trigger points, or as he terms these, "hyperalgesic skin zones."

Recent developments, as well as the reintroduction of older concepts, have led to methods of assessment of visceral structures in terms of both position and "motion," and some of the methods involved will be outlined, specifically those that involve evaluation of drag or tension on mesenteric attachments (Kuchera 1997). Craniosacral and "zerobalancing" methods (among others) involve the sensing of inherent rhythms, felt on the surface, to make assessments of relative physiological or pathological states or even, it is suggested, of "tissue memory" relating to trauma, either physical or emotional (Tozzi 2014). Variations on these methods will be examined and described in Chapter 13, together with exercises that can assist in developing appropriate degrees of sensitivity for their effective use.

Deeper palpation of the soft tissues, involving stretching, probing, compressing and the use of various movements and positions, is commonly employed to seek out information relating to local and reflex activity; these approaches are examined and explained, for example in Chapters 4 and 5. Such methods are frequently combined with the use of sequential assessment of the relative degree of tension (shortness), or strength, of associated muscles and such a sequence is described in detail in Chapter 5.

Examination of some of the ways in which joint status can be judged, from its "end-feel," when range of motion and motion palpation are used for this purpose, add a further dimension to the art of palpation and will be presented with appropriate exercises in Chapter 8.

And what of psychological implications? This latter element is something we should always be aware of, as there are few chronic states of dysfunction that are not overlaid (or often caused) by psychosomatic interactions. Indeed, research by German connective tissue massage therapists has clearly demonstrated specific, palpable, soft tissue changes that relate to particular emotional or psychological states (Chapter 15).

Osteopathy, chiropractic, physiotherapy, massage therapy, and a host of other systems associated with bodywork have all developed individualized diagnostic methods, some of which have become universally applied and valued

by other systems. In order not to upset professional sensitivities, credit will be given to the system that first developed particular palpatory methods, wherever this is known.

Poetry of palpation

Ida Rolf, the developer of structural integration, through the system known as Rolfing, gave an idea of just how exciting an experience palpation can be. She suggests (Rolf 1977) that the beginner in the art of palpation should feel their own thigh (as an example). Initially, she says, this will feel "undifferentiated," either overly dense or soft, lacking in tone, or as though large lumps were held together under the skin. These "extremes in the spectrum of spatial, material and chemical disorganization" make recognition of the ideally well-organized elements of the structures difficult. However, after appropriate normalization of such tissues the "feel" is quite different:

> You can feel the energy and tone flow into and through the myofascial unit ... dissolving the "glue" that, in holding the fascial envelopes together, has given the feeling of bunched and undifferentiated flesh.

As fascial tone improves, individual muscles glide over one another, and the flesh – no longer "too, too solid" – reminds the searching fingers of layers of silk that glide on one another with a suggestion of opulence.

Rolf's excitement is real. Palpation of the body should change with practice from being a purely mechanical act into a truly touching and moving experience, in all senses of those words.

Inspired by having studied with Rolf, Tom Myers (2001) has developed a model which demonstrates concrete fascial continuities, or networks. These anatomy "trains," or connective tissue lines or meridians, link all parts of the body in functional ways, and awareness of the connection patterns can change the way we see the musculoskeletal system and its problems. See Chapter 6 on fascial palpation for more on these concepts, described in Myers' own words.

Paul Van Allen (1964) pinpointed the need for concentrated application to the task of heightening one's perceptive (and therapeutic) skills:

> Let us lay down a few principles to guide us in the development of manual skills ... It is commonplace to accept the need for basic principles and for practice, in

developing manual skill to strike a golf ball, or a baseball, to roll a bowling ball, to strike a piano key or to draw a bow across strings, but we seldom, if ever any more, think of manual skills in osteopathic practice in this way. Is it possible that osteopathic manipulation began to lose its effectiveness and to fall into disrepute even among our own people, when students no longer practiced to see through how many pages of Gray's Anatomy they could feel a hair?

Note that this was written at a traumatic time for osteopathy in the United States, when 2000 Californian osteopaths had given up their DO status, and accepted MD status ("little md" was the derogatory comment of many at the time) in return for the turning of an osteopathic college into an allopathic medical school. A major resurgence of basic osteopathic teaching and skills has since reversed that catastrophe.

Describing what we feel

All therapists who use their hands may usefully ask themselves whether they spend enough time refining and heightening their degree of palpatory sensitivity. The answer in many cases may be "no," and hopefully this text will encourage a return to exercises such as the unusual application of Gray's Anatomy described above (a telephone directory was used for this purpose in the author's training, and is equally effective, but such directories are now fading into history as electronic versions take over).

Moving beyond his despair at the loss of interest in palpatory skills, Van Allen makes another useful contribution:

> We will understand better what we feel if we attempt to describe it. In describing what is experienced through palpation we try to classify the characteristics of tissue states, thus not only clarifying our own observations but broadening our collective experience by affording a better means of communication between us and discussing [osteopathic] theory and method. We are accustomed to describing crude differences in what we feel by touch, the roughness of the bark of a tree or of a tweed coat, the smoothness of a glass or silk. We must now develop a language of nuances and I shall suggest only a few words from many to apply to palpable tissue states in an effort to describe them accurately.

Van Allen then offers detailed descriptions of the meanings, as he sees them, of words such as "density," "turgidity," "compressibility," "tensile state" (or response to stretch), and "elasticity." His choice of words may not suit everyone but the idea is sound. We need to find a large variety of descriptive words for what we feel when we palpate, and the chapters covering various approaches to this most vital of procedures will hopefully inspire you to follow Van Allen's advice, to obtain a thesaurus and to look up as many words as possible in order to describe accurately the subtle variations in what is being palpated.

Viola Frymann reminds us that Dr Sutherland used the analogy of a bird alighting on a twig, and then taking hold of it, when he tried to teach his students how to palpate the cranium. Some of the exercises in this book are derived from Frymann's work, and in many of these she echoes Van Allen's idea that the student of palpation should also practice the art of describing what she is feeling, either verbally or in writing. Dr Frymann's words (Frymann 1963) may serve as a guide throughout this book:

> It is one thing to understand intellectually that physiological functions operate, and what may happen if they become disorganized. It is quite another thing, however, to be able to place the hands on a patient and analyze the nature and the extent of the disorganization and know what can be done to restore it to normal, unimpeded, rhythmic physiology. This then is the task before us; to know what has happened and is happening to the tissues under our hands, and then to know what can be done about it and be able to carry it through ... [however] ... palpation alone is virtually worthless without the rest of the patient evaluation. The value comes from the entire package – history, examination [including palpation], special tests, and response to treatment.

Interdisciplinary views

The comments at the start of this chapter regarding the need to become familiar with "normal" so that "abnormal" can be identified are echoed in a modern British osteopathic view offered by Stone (1999), who describes palpation as the "fifth dimension:"

Palpation allows us to interpret tissue function. Different histological make-up brings differing amounts of inherent pliability and elasticity; because of this a muscle feels completely different from a ligament, a bone and an organ, for example. Thus there is a "normal" feel to healthy tissues that is different for each tissue. This has to be learned through repeated exploration of "normal" and the practitioner builds his/her own vocabulary of what "normal" is. Once someone is trained to use palpation efficiently, then finer and finer differences between tissues can be felt. This is vital, as one must be able to differentiate when something has changed from being "normal" to being "too normal".

Touching on the palpatory qualities of tissues in relation to emotional states (see also Chapter 15), Stone continues:

Each practitioner must build up their own subjective description of what the tissue states mean to them clinically, whether this is to do with the degree of actual injury or some sort of emotional problem. Experience and careful reflection on the nature of the tissue reactions and responses to manipulations are an important part of maturing as a professional, and by their very nature are descriptive terms unique to the individual practitioner.

A challenging physiotherapy perspective is offered by Maitland (2001), one of the giants of that profession:

In the vertebral column, it is palpation that is the most important and the most difficult skill to learn. To achieve this skill it is necessary to be able to feel, by palpation, the difference in the spinal segments – normal to abnormal; old or new; hypomobile or hypermobile – and then be able to relate the response, site, depth and relevance to a patient's symptoms (structure, source and causes). This requires an honest, self-critical attitude, and also applies to the testing of functional movements and combined physiological test movements. It takes at least 10 years for any clinician (even one who has an inborn ability) to learn the relationship between her hands, the pain responses, and her mind.

Chiropractic examination depends a great deal on direct palpation, both static and active. Murphy (2000) describes that profession's modern perspective:

Palpation encompasses static palpation, such as for skin temperature and texture, masses, myofascial trigger points, or soft tissue changes; motion palpation for assessing joint function; and muscle length tests for assessing muscle function. So it is used in the detection of red flags for serious disease, the primary pain generator(s), and the key dysfunctions and dysfunctional changes. There is no substitute for good palpation skills in examining patients ... The two most important tools that are used in the process of examination are those of sight and touch (in addition to hearing) ... palpation in particular, is a skill that is invaluable in the assessment of locomotor system function.

American osteopathic medicine training places great emphasis on palpation skills. Kappler (1997) explains:

The art of palpation requires discipline, time, patience and practice. To be most effective and productive, palpatory findings must be correlated with a knowledge of functional anatomy, physiology and pathophysiology. It is much easier to identify frank pathological states, a tumor for example, than to describe signs, symptoms, and palpatory findings that lead to or identify pathological mechanisms ... Palpation with fingers and hands provides sensory information that the brain interprets as: temperature, texture, surface humidity, elasticity, turgor, tissue tension, thickness, shape, irritability, motion. To accomplish this task, it is necessary to teach the fingers to feel, think, see, and know. One feels through the palpating fingers on the patient; one sees the structures under the palpating fingers through a visual image based on knowledge of anatomy; one thinks what is normal and abnormal, and one knows with confidence acquired with practice that what is felt is real and accurate.

By heeding the words of the experts, quoted throughout this book, and by evaluating and reflecting on some of the insights to be found in the clinically relevant "Special topics" between chapters, as well as by assiduously practicing the exercises given in subsequent chapters, palpation skills can be refined to an extraordinary degree, bringing both satisfaction and benefit to practitioner and patient alike. The acquisition of greater skills will also reduce the frequency with which researchers find unreliability to be common. Issues of reliability are discussed in the next chapter.

Chapter 1

References

Bischof I and Elmiger G (1960) Connective tissue massage, in Licht S (ed) Massage, Manipulation and Traction. New Haven, CT: Elizabeth Licht.

Cooper G (1977) Clinical considerations of fascia in diagnosis and treatment. Newark, OH: Academy of Applied Osteopathy Yearbook.

Frymann V (1963) Palpation – its study in the workshop. Newark, OH: Academy of Applied Osteopathy Yearbook, pp 16–30.

Greenman P (1989) Principles of manual medicine. Baltimore: Williams and Wilkins.

Kappler R (1997) Palpatory skills, in Ward R (ed) Foundations for Osteopathic Medicine. Baltimore: Williams and Wilkins.

Kuchera W (1997) Lumbar and abdominal region, in Ward R (ed) Foundations for Osteopathic Medicine. Baltimore: Williams and Wilkins.

Lewit K (1999) Manipulation in rehabilitation of the motor system, 3rd edn. London: Butterworths.

Maitland G (2001) Maitland's vertebral manipulation, 6th edn. Oxford: Butterworth Heinemann.

Mitchell F Jr (1976) Training and measuring sensory literacy. Newark, OH: Yearbook of the American Academy of Osteopathy, pp 120–127.

Murphy D (2000) Conservative management of cervical spine syndromes. New York: McGraw-Hill.

Myers T (2001) Anatomy trains. Edinburgh: Churchill Livingstone.

Panzer DM (1992) The reliability of lumbar motion palpation. Journal of Manipulative and Physiological Therapeutics 15 (8): 518–524.

Rolf I (1977) Rolfing: The integration of human structures. New York: Harper and Row.

Stone C (1999) Science in the art of osteopathy. Cheltenham: Stanley Thornes.

Sutherland WG (1948) The cranial bowl. Mankato, MN: Free Press.

Tozzi P (2014) Does fascia hold memories? Journal of Bodywork and Movement Therapies 18 (2): 259–265.

Upledger J (1987) Craniosacral therapy. Seattle: Eastland Press.

Van Allen P (1964) Improving our skills. Carmel, CA: Academy of Applied Osteopathy Yearbook, pp 147–152.

Van Duersen L, Patijn J, Ockhuysen A and Vortman B (1990) The value of some clinical tests of the sacroiliac joint. Manual Medicine 5: 96–99.

Vincent Smith B and Gibbons P (1999) Inter-examiner and intra-examiner reliability of palpatory findings for the standing flexion test. Manual Therapy 4 (2): 87–93.

Webster G (1947) Feel of the tissues. Minneapolis, IN: Yearbook of the American Academy of Osteopathy, pp 32–35.

Michael Seffinger

Manual practitioners rely on palpation to determine where to manipulate and what techniques to use, and to assess the patient's response. Although palpatory tests can be described and taught, there is no standard method of palpation required or used by all manual practitioners. Despite the fact that palpatory diagnostic procedures are variable between manual practitioners, in general the goal is similar, that is, to identify the reasons for dysfunction and suffering that are amenable to manual treatment. Diagnostic palpation is used to identify abnormal structures and functions; more specifically, it aims to:

- detect asymmetry of, or locate specific anatomical landmarks
- identify altered range or resistance to passive joint or tissue motion
- assess non-bony ("soft") tissues for altered tone and tension levels, resistance or compliance to manual pressure and shearing forces, warmth or coolness, swelling or inflammation, fibrous or scar tissue
- find points or areas of tenderness.

There are many palpatory tests that can be used to detect the above findings on physical examination. However, which tests are best to use in clinical practice? Moreover, which of the above findings are possible to palpate with precision and accuracy? In theory, the more precise (reliable) and accurate (valid) a palpation procedure is, the more certain will be the clinical diagnosis, leading to the most appropriate and effective treatment.

This chapter will define the terms "reliability" and "validity," describe how the reliability and validity of palpatory tests are determined, and summarize the results of reliability and validity studies, including recent scientific literature reviews (Seffinger et al. 2004; van Trijffel et al. 2005; Stochkendahl et al. 2006; Hollerwöger 2006; May et al. 2006; Hancock et al. 2007; Stuber 2007; Rubenstein and van Tulder 2008; Haneline et al. 2008; Laslett 2008; Murphy et al. 2008; Haneline & Young 2009; Stovall & Kumar 2010; Triano et al. 2013; Póvoa et al. 2015). Finally, experts from various professions provide insightful responses to questions related to the results of palpation reliability and validity studies.

What is meant by reliability?

Reliability measures the concordance, consistency, or repeatability of outcomes. Using archery as an example, if an archer hits the target around the periphery, though not the bull's eye at the center, again and again with each successive arrow, then he is considered to be reliable in hitting the target in general, even though he is not hitting the intended area in the center. Hitting the bull's eye would mean the archer is accurate. Hitting the target in general again and again means the archer is reliable. Thus, reliability is not synonymous with accuracy.

In relation to palpation, reliability means that a clinician can report the same feeling assessed by his or her hand repeatedly with consistency. For example, when a clinician states "this muscle is firm every time I press on it," he or she is reliably stating that the muscle feels firm. The muscle itself may or may not be firm, as there may be a hard cyst under it that gives the impression that the muscle itself is firm. Nevertheless, the examiner is considered reliable, even if not accurate. *Intra-examiner reliability* refers to this ability to agree with one's own previous manual assessment. *Inter-examiner reliability* means two or more examiners agree on each other's manual assessment.

The reliability of a palpatory test is its capacity to provide the same information on repeated application. This depends primarily on three factors:

1. stability of the palpatory findings
2. variability inherent in the method of palpation
3. skill of the examiner.

Precision is the measure of the variability in a test, and is often used synonymously with reliability. A tight cluster of arrows around an area within the target means the archer was precise, even though they did not hit the bull's eye. A palpatory test is precise if it repeatedly measures the same thing with little variation. If a palpation test is precise and accurate, then it is both reliable and has validity.

Why is reliability important in palpatory diagnosis?

Reliability is most important when there is no gold standard test that can tell of the existence of a phenomenon. Since there are no gold standard tests for most palpatory procedures used to determine where and what to manipulate, the most reproducible, reliable procedure is considered the gold standard. If two or more examiners can agree that a palpatory finding is present, there is more confidence that the finding actually exists. In this sense, reliability of a palpatory procedure is used synonymously with "accuracy" or "validity." Unless a more accurate method of evaluation is used, such as an ultrasound (US) imaging machine for assessing soft tissue integrity and fluid content, the most reliable palpatory test is the most accurate test available. This is why the most reliable palpatory tests are sought after, to improve the chance that the examiner will make an accurate diagnosis, which should lead to the correct treatment that will relieve suffering and assist in the patient's recovery.

How is palpation reliability determined?

Reliability of a palpatory procedure is determined by comparing the reproducibility and concordance of diagnostic findings from the same examiner and from different examiners palpating the same subject or group of subjects. Variables that affect the reliability of a test are listed in Table 2.1. Palpation reliability studies use a variety of combinations of these variables to assess their effect on the reliability of palpatory procedures.

Researchers most commonly use the kappa (κ) statistic to account for the possibility of chance agreement. Kappa values range from -1 to +1, with 0 indicating that the examiner(s) results are no better than chance alone and thus the procedure is not reliable. A negative value indicates that the diagnostic procedure tested is less reliable than chance alone. Acceptable values for the determination of a reliable test vary among researchers. Kappa values recommended by Fleiss (1981) are listed in Table 2.2.

Table 2.1

Independent variables in palpatory reliability studies
Amount of subcutaneous fat in the patient that may affect palpation accuracy of locating anatomical landmarks
Anatomical variants in patients (need to be screened for prior to the study)
Education level of the examiners
Examiner consensus on the palpatory procedures to be used and the criteria for a positive result
Examiner level of familiarity (experience) with the tests to be used (pre-study training)
Gender of the patients or examiners
Presence or lack of symptoms in the patients
Stability of the phenomenon being palpated over time and in response to being palpated
The palpatory experience (skill) level of the examiners

Table 2.2

Levels of agreement: interpretation of the kappa value (Fleiss 1981)	
Kappa value (κ)	Interpretation
κ <0.4	Poor
κ 0.4–0.75	Good or moderate
κ >0.75	Excellent or substantial

Since examiners alter their methods of palpation over time, and learn shortcuts from the experience they gain, they need to be re-calibrated, just like an instrument used in laboratory experiments. Thus, examiners need to meet often during a study and reassess their procedures, re-train and regain agreement on their results of the palpatory tests being used to determine where to manipulate (Degenhardt et al. 2005, 2010). Additionally, it has been emphasized that anatomical variations, especially between males and females, need to be considered more carefully when identifying landmarks for palpatory reliability tests (Snider et al. 2008).

How reliable are manual diagnostic procedures?

Systematic literature reviews assess the quality of the research designs and reporting methods utilized in palpation reliability studies, in essence analyzing the reproducibility of the studies themselves. The overall results of these systematic reviews on the reliability of spinal palpatory procedures are as follows:

- *Anatomical landmark identification* and assessment of symmetry are not reliable; however, adjusting the criteria for agreement by enlarging the area of the target improves reliability. Assessing regional variations of the landmarks, as in assessment for scoliosis, kyphosis, for example, have moderate to substantial reliability.

- *Active regional* range of *motion* is more reliable than passive *segmental* range of motion. Cervical, thoracic and lumbar *intersegmental spinal passive* motion palpatory tests have good reliability in some studies, but low reliability in others.

- *Soft tissue* tests assessing for *tissue texture abnormalities*, altered compliance or the presence of muscle tension are in general not reliable other than the skin-rolling technique to determine subcutaneous tissue tension.

- Soft tissue or osseous *pain provocation* tests are most reliable. Pain provocation is in reality a test of the reliability of the patient to state the degree of pain felt when a tender spot is palpated by an examiner; it is not truly a palpatory sensation that the examiner has to interpret.

- *Intra*-examiner reliability is better than *inter*-examiner reliability. Overall, an examiner's field of expertise, experience level, consensus on procedures used, training just prior to the study or use of symptomatic subjects does not necessarily improve reliability.

Additional studies have found the following:

- Identification of lumbar spine spinous processes using multiple bony landmarks is more accurate than using one landmark (Snider et al. 2011).

- Clinicians seem to be more precise in identifying hypomobile spinal vertebral segments than hypermobile ones. Passive posterior–anterior assessment of the *least mobile lumbar spinal joint* in prone patients with low back pain has good inter-examiner reliability ($\kappa = 0.71$); however, reliability is poor ($\kappa = 0.29$) in identifying the *most mobile segment* (Landel et al. 2008).

- Having a standard point of reference improves reliability as is seen in the study of chiropractic students evaluating the intersegmental motion of the cervical spine of three subjects, two of whom each had a congenitally fused vertebra at C2–3 and the other at C5–6. Identification of the segment of greatest hypomobility had very good reliability overall ($\kappa = 0.65$), with substantial ($\kappa = 0.76$) and moderate ($\kappa = 0.46$) agreement for hypomobility at C2–3 and C5–6 respectively (Humphreys et al. 2004).

- Combining motion tests with pain provocation increases reliability as demonstrated by kappa values of at least 0.4 when testing thoracic and lumbar intervertebral joint mobility with pain response and end range pain in lumbar flexion and extension in adolescent patients (Aartun et al. 2014). This has been corroborated in the adult cervical spine as well (Maigne et al. 2009).

- Triano et al. (2013) reviewed a series of studies that demonstrated that motion palpation is more reliable between clinicians when performed on patients who have pain in the region being assessed; joints and muscles in the painful region tend to be more easily recognizable as stiff and hypomobile as well as painful upon motion. A case in point is the study by Manning et al. (2012), which showed that in patients with neck pain, examiners demonstrated acceptable reliability (kappa at least 0.4) of palpation tests for hypomobility, range of motion end-feel, and pain provocation.

- Additionally, reliability increases for spinal segmental motion tests when the examiner's confidence level in the findings is factored into the equation; the more confident the clinicians feel about their diagnosis, the more reliable the test becomes (Cooperstein et al. 2013). Some researchers argue that the kappa value alone cannot determine the reliability of a test as the prevalence of the characteristic being studied, the nature of the sample population, the bias of the examiners and the threshold of how much reliability is "good enough" to make a clinical diagnosis are variables that need to be considered in the interpretation of the data (May et al. 2006). Cooperstein (2012) demonstrated that the selection of appropriate statistical tests and analysis is key to the accuracy of reliability study results and their interpretation.

- The reliability of palpatory procedures for other body regions and joints besides the spine has also been assessed.

Sacroiliac joint

- Palpatory tests for sacroiliac (SI) joint mobility are in general not reliable (Robinson et al. 2007).

- Using a cluster of pain provocation tests improves reliability (Laslett et al. 2005; Van der Wurff et al. 2006; Robinson et al. 2007).

- Combining motion tests with pain provocation tests increases reliability even more (Arab et al. 2009).

- Using the most reliable test among a series of tests increases reliability (Tong et al. 2006).

Hip

- FABER test, log roll test and assessment of greater trochanteric tenderness have acceptable reliability for patients with musculoskeletal hip pain (kappa values greater than 0.4) (Martin & Sekiya 2008).

Leg length

- Leg length symmetry assessment at the medial malleoli has been shown to have acceptable reliability (kappa at least 0.4) (Woodfield et al. 2011; Holt et al. 2009).

Shoulder

- Range of motion and strength testing of the upper limb are reliable.

- Assessing shoulder motion restriction has good to excellent reliability, especially when pain is present, for example, scapulothoracic motion in patients with shoulder pain (Baertschi et al. 2013).

- Palpatory tests for generalized joint hypermobility (GJH) and benign joint hypermobility syndrome (BJHS) are reliable (Juul-Kristensen et al. 2007).

- In patients with shoulder impingement syndrome, the painful arc, empty can and external rotation resistance tests have moderate to substantial reliability (kappa ranges from 0.45 to 0.67) and the Neer and Hawkins–Kennedy tests have fair reliability (kappa ranges from 0.39 to 0.40) (Michener et al. 2009).

Hand

- Palpation for swelling and pain on resisted movement have poor reliability, but there is moderate to good reliability for joint bony contour or size changes and tenderness (Myers et al. 2011).

- Finger hypermobility as per the Beighton Joint Mobility Index has moderate (kappa at least 0.4) reliability (Aartun et al. 2014).

Knee

- Tests for knee joint instability are not reliable (Malanga et al. 2003).

Myofascial trigger points

- Myofascial trigger points are more reliable in certain muscles, for example, trapezius, gluteus medius, and quadratus lumborum (Myburgh et al. 2008); the reliability is acceptable (kappa at least 0.4) for pain provocation and tenderness, but not for taut band, jump sign, or tissue texture abnormalities (Lucas et al. 2009).

Primary respiratory mechanism

- Reliable palpation of the cranium and/or sacrum for inherent rhythmic motion called the primary respiratory mechanism has not been demonstrated (Sommerfeld et al. 2004).

- Palpation of cranial strain patterns, the cranial rhythmic impulse rate, and cranial quadrants for restricted motion has moderate to substantial (kappa ranges from 0.52 to 0.82) intra-examiner reliability (Halma et al. 2008).

The art of diagnostic palpation

Each practitioner develops his or her own method of obtaining information by palpation that fits his or her own skill level and ability to interpret the sensations. There is a high degree of art in palpation, as the interpretation of the sensation is dependent on the experience, knowledge, and skill of the examiner. A clinician is going to be less reliable in performing and interpreting a palpatory test if he or she does not practice. But some clinicians have a compassionate and caring bedside manner about them that gains patients' confidence and trust, even if they use unreliable methods. Other clinicians have an extremely sensitive sense of touch that very few other examiners can match.

Many of the palpatory exercises and procedures in this book have not yet been evaluated for reliability. However, they are skills recommended by expert practitioners in determining dysfunction in the patient that, in their experience, can be improved by applying manual treatment procedures. The exercises in this book will prove to be very useful in developing skills that can be evaluated by very sensitive machines and found to be accurate. This leads us to the next section on the validity or accuracy of diagnostic palpatory tests.

What is meant by validity?

Validity measures the extent to which a palpatory test actually does what it is supposed to do. It is the degree to which the results of measurement correspond to the true state of the phenomenon being measured (Feinstein 1987). It is synonymous with accuracy and veracity. The archer who hits the bull's eye is considered to be accurate in shooting an arrow. The archer may not hit it repeatedly. If his arrow misses the bull's eye, yet is closer to it than another archer's arrow, he is considered to be more accurate than the other archer. This is the same with a palpatory test. If it measures its intended target, it is considered accurate. If it does this irregularly, but more often than another palpatory test, it is considered more accurate than the other test. For example, the accuracy of palpation to determine the firmness of a muscle depends on whether the muscle is indeed firm when the examiner feels it to be so. If a standard measuring device is used to identify the nature of the muscle in question, and it is found to indeed be firm, then the palpatory procedure used to assess the muscle, that is, pressing upon

it, is considered valid. A valid palpatory test is determined by its ability to detect what a reference, or gold standard, measuring device can detect. Just as the bow and arrow is only as accurate in hitting the bull's eye as the archer using it, a palpatory test is only as accurate as the examiner using it. Sometimes one examiner is more accurate than another because of training or experience.

Validity does not imply reliability or reproducibility. If a palpatory procedure accurately assesses a true phenomenon, but only some of the time, then it is not reliable. If you can palpate a supine patient's ischial tuberosity using only your forefinger 60% of the time, but 100% of the time when you use your palm, then using the palm is a more accurate method for the intended target. So, a valid test is most useful when it is reproducible or reliable. Conversely, a reliable method is most useful when it is also accurate or valid.

Clinicians, educators, and researchers also consider a palpatory test valid if the examiner using it interprets it with accuracy. A series of palpatory tests used by an examiner is considered valid if the examiner comes up with an accurate assessment, since the assessment cannot be made by one palpatory test alone. There is some debate about whether it is the examiner that is accurate or whether it is the palpatory procedures used that are accurate. This is why inter-examiner palpatory diagnosis validity studies are necessary to discern between the two possibilities.

There are various types of validity research studies. There are qualitative studies which rely on an examiner's opinion or interpretation alone. Then there are quantitative studies in which the examiner's findings are compared to a reference standard, usually an instrument measuring the same or a related phenomenon. Although the concept of validity differs in qualitative and quantitative research, this chapter focuses on the concepts used in quantitative research.

The reference standard

Definition: A *reference standard* (also called the *gold standard*) is a measure proven through research to have a high sensitivity and specificity for a phenomenon or condition that it purports to measure, or is one that is accepted by consensus of experts in the field as the best available for determining the presence or absence of a particular phenomenon.

Caveat: When there is no perfect reference standard, as in the case of measurement of a patient's sense of pain upon palpation, then *pragmatic criteria* can be used as a reference standard (Knottnerus 2002). The visual analog pain scale has been used as a pragmatic reference standard for palpatory pain provocation tests for several decades (Price et al. 1983).

Selecting an appropriate reference standard for validity studies is not as simple as one would predict. For example, Jende and Peterson (1997) studied cervical spinal motion palpation; they used an X-ray as the reference standard and assumed (took it at face value) that motion, or lack thereof, was related to bony position. However, palpation of cervical joint motion to identify restriction is not always related to bony position as measured by an X-ray; asymmetric muscle tension that restricts motion may not alter static bony position on X-ray. Another common example is when an instructor uses a palpatory procedure to show a student how to tell in which direction a vertebra is thought to be rotated. The student takes it on face value, or face validity, that the palpatory test actually can help to discern the vertebra's position or motion characteristics. In this case, the instructor is the reference standard. However, the instructor may or may not be a reliable or an accurate palpator. In spite of the common perception or belief that motion tests are valid and reliable for assessment of presence or absence of restricted vertebral motion, there is no evidence to support this concept. A case in point is the inability of results from lumbar spine passive accessory motion testing designating segmental levels of joint motion restriction to match findings from dynamic magnetic resonance imaging (MRI) (Landel et al. 2008).

There are three steps to palpation recognition: (1) detection by the hand, (2) transmission by the peripheral nerves to the central nervous system and brain, and (3) interpretation of the sensations by the brain. Thus, researchers counter-argue, the hand is only the interface between the brain and the object being palpated. What they say needs validation is the interpretation made by the brain of every palpatory sensation. Training the brain's interpretation using biofeedback and instrumentation is one method educators are beginning to employ in teaching palpation. Once a reference or gold standard is established for a palpatory test, students can be trained to meet the accuracy level of that reference standard.

The reason it is important to understand the different types of validity studies is that when researchers profess that a palpatory procedure is valid or accurate, one must determine what is actually being tested and proved valid: the palpatory procedure itself, the interpretation of what the examiner feels, or the identification of where to manipulate. Validating one aspect of palpation does not translate into making the other aspects valid. Conversely, invalidating one aspect of a palpatory test does not invalidate the other aspects. Clinically, it is important to be able to validate all three stages of palpation: what is felt at the fingers, how it is interpreted, and what is diagnosed using that interpretation.

Why is validity important in palpatory diagnosis?

Six blind men palpating different parts of an elephant may feel six different sensations and interpret their findings differently: as an animal that is like a fan (ear), a tree (leg), a wall (body), a rope (tail), a spear (tusk) or a snake (trunk). Each may be reliable in describing again and again what he is sensing, but the interpretation is not accurate. They are each palpating only one aspect of the entire entity. Their palpatory skills lack validity or accuracy since they have no gold standard method of evaluating what they feel. It can be argued that if they palpated the entire animal in a series of tests, then they would have more inter-examiner reliability, but they would still not be accurate. Vision adds that gold standard. Likewise, palpators use visualization of the symmetry of anatomical landmarks to validate what they feel with their hands. However, some of the problems that manual practitioners attempt to fix with manipulation techniques cannot easily be seen with the eyes as they are subtle tissue texture changes, motion restrictions and resistance to provocative motion or pressures applied by the examiner's hands. If the sensations felt by the palpating hand could be validated by an accurate instrument, then the palpator would have more confidence in the interpretation of his or her findings. Intra-examiner and inter-examiner reliability would likewise improve. Does such an instrument exist?

There are no instruments that can evaluate every aspect of the dysfunction that palpators assess. When there is no instrument to act as the reference or gold standard, it is the most experienced or most reliable palpator who becomes the reference standard. One would think that the more accurate the palpatory test, the more reliable it is likely to be. Although a bow and arrow offer an archer an accurate means of hitting a bull's eye a few times out of 10, this would not necessarily be accurate or reliable in another's hands. Similarly, an expert palpator may use valid palpatory tests with precision and reliably, but another palpator may only occasionally be accurate or reliable. So, both validity and reliability are necessary. Study, practice, experience and conscientious skill development are cornerstones of the palpatory literacy foundation. This book will serve the clinician well by providing a clear explanation of a compendium of palpatory assessment skills and development exercises from masters around the world.

How is validity of palpatory procedures determined?

Validity of a palpatory test is determined by measuring how well it performs against a reference or "gold" standard. This chapter will focus on the validity of palpatory tests as assessed by sensitivity and specificity in accordance with recommendations from systematic reviews (Najm et al. 2003).

Sensitivity and specificity are merely mathematical expressions of the ability of a palpatory test to detect the presence and absence of a true phenomenon. For example, a clinician attempts to detect if a cervical vertebra is rotated to the right by palpation, and an X-ray is used as a reference or gold standard measurement. If the clinician correctly detects the rotated vertebra by palpation alone 90% of the time, and also correctly detects a normal vertebra 90% of the time, then the palpatory test is considered to be sensitive in that it detects the true state of the structure, also called a true positive, with very few false negatives, that is, rotated vertebrae that the examiner missed. The palpatory test is also very specific, in that it also enables the clinician to detect the absence of the condition, in this case a non-rotated vertebra. This is because he detected the true negatives and very few false positives, that is, vertebrae that he thought were rotated but which were not. Both sensitivity

and specificity are needed to determine the content validity of a palpatory diagnostic test.

Since no test has perfect sensitivity and specificity, combinations of tests are used to increase the likelihood of making the most accurate diagnosis. Although it would be ideal if each palpatory test was at least 90% sensitive and specific, it is most important for the most sensitive and specific tests, or combination of tests that together are most sensitive and/or specific, be used for clinical decision making.

The ability of a palpatory procedure to correctly detect both the presence and absence of a finding is called its overall *accuracy*. If a person has low back pain and on palpatory examination, the clinician detects tissue texture changes, restricted lumbar joint motion and tenderness of the spinous processes, there is evidence to diagnose somatic dysfunction. Some patients have evidence of somatic dysfunction although they do not complain of low back pain. The palpation used may be considered accurate in detecting somatic dysfunction. But if the patient's complaint of low back pain is used as a reference standard, then the tests would be considered as inaccurate (at selecting which patients are complaining of pain). So, when hearing or reading about the alleged inaccuracies of palpation, ask what reference standard it is being compared to. The use of different reference standards within a population being studied, and the accuracy of the alternative reference standards used when there is no gold standard available, increases the risk of bias in the study (Naaktgeboren et al. 2013).

How valid are manual diagnostic procedures?

Most palpation validity studies are of the construct, criteria, or predictive validity types. There are very few content validity palpation studies. Their results can be grouped into the categories of the type of palpatory test or the region of the body assessed for dysfunction that indicates need for manual therapy.

Anatomical landmark assessment

Palpatory identification of anatomical landmarks and assessment of symmetry of bilateral landmarks has varied degrees of accuracy:

- Pinpoint assessment of midline landmarks, such as locating spinous processes using X-ray as the reference standard has not been shown to be accurate (Robinson et al. 2009).

- Palpatory tests for cervical spine landmarks have poor to moderate accuracy ranging from 51% to 87.8% using a variety of tests and radiographic reference standards (Póvoa et al. 2015).

- Experienced clinicians were more accurate than students in bilateral anterior iliac spine landmark assessments for symmetry using a pelvic anatomical model as the reference standard when the amount of asymmetry exceeded 5 mm. Using the evaluator's "dominant eye" in the midline to assess bilateral symmetry of landmarks did not improve accuracy. Evaluations were even more accurate when the asymmetry was 10 mm (Lee et al. 2015).

- Shaw et al. (2012) demonstrated accuracy of digital pressure palpation to determine tissue depth and interpretation of asymmetry of lumbar vertebral transverse processes both before and after spinal manipulation in healthy subjects using ultrasonography as the reference standard. Further studies using this reference standard are warranted.

Palpatory tests for spinal motion

Palpatory tests for range and quality of motion of small joints, such as the spinal zygapophyseal or facet joints, are difficult to assess for accuracy due to lack of a gold standard. A plastic spinal model with fixed joints has been employed with some success. These studies demonstrated that intervertebral motion tests are inaccurate palpation methods of assessment for hypomobile or fixed joints (Najm et al. 2003). However, passive spinal motion tests on humans have some validity:

- Humphreys et al. (2004) assessed the ability of chiropractic students to identify the most hypomobile cervical joint in patients with congenital fusion of a single cervical joint as the reference standard using an intersegmental lateral side bending palpatory test with the patient in the seated position. Sensitivity was low, but specificity of the procedure was high. When the students identified a hypomobile spinal segment, it was

indeed the fused vertebra (few false positives); but they also missed the fused vertebra much of the time (many false negatives).

- Fritz et al. (2005) assessed passive lumbar motion tests in combination with other non-palpatory tests to predict lumbar hypermobility compared to an X-ray reference standard. They found that the two most predictive factors of hypermobility were increased lumbar flexion range of motion and a lack of hypomobility during lumbar intervertebral palpatory motion testing. The presence of both findings increased the probability of instability from 50% to 93%.

- Abbott et al. (2005) assessed the validity of lumbar spine passive accessory intervertebral motion tests (PAIVMs) and passive physiological intervertebral motion tests (PPIVMs) by physical therapists trained in manual therapy using X-rays as the reference standard. PAIVMs and PPIVMs tests are highly specific, but not sensitive for the detection of translational lumbar segmental instability.

Pain provocation

- Pain provocation is one of the most accurate methods of identifying *where* a patient hurts, although it may not be able to identify *why*. Although palpation can certainly elicit pain, contrary to popular belief, using a visual analog scale or a patient's subjective report of pain as reference standards, palpation is not consistently a highly accurate method of determining the *cause or location of joint pain* (Najm et al. 2003). However, digital pain provocation has higher accuracy at detecting painful joints than motion testing (Najm et al. 2003). If a person is tender to palpation, it is likely that there is indeed something wrong at that location (specificity is high). However, if a patient is not tender, it does not mean that there is nothing wrong at that location (sensitivity is low). Pain at the end range of passive motion tests, such as Kemp's test (also known as the quadrant test or extension-rotation test), which is used by clinicians to identify vertebral facet joint pain often indicative of "facet syndrome" in the cervical, thoracic, or lumbar spine, has not demonstrated accuracy using facet block injections as the reference standard (Stuber et al. 2014).

Palpation tests to identify viscerosomatic reflexes indicative of visceral disease

There are no well-designed content validity studies that have demonstrated accuracy of palpation tests evaluating paraspinal soft tissue tension, tenderness, or costal and/or vertebral motion restriction for evidence of distinct viscerosomatic reflex pathology indicative of organic disease. However, Kumarathurai et al. (2008) assessed the relationship between chest wall muscle tenderness and myocardial perfusion imaging in patients with stable or suspected angina. They found that presence of tender chest wall muscles upon digital palpation was associated with a normal myocardial perfusion study. A follow-up to this study demonstrated that *reproducible* chest wall tenderness (CWT) in emergency room patients complaining of chest pain helps to rule out acute coronary syndrome (ACS), whereas *non-reproducible* chest wall tenderness helps to rule it in (Gräni et al. 2015):

- Non-reproducible CWT had a high sensitivity of 92.9% (95% CI 66.1% to 98.8%) for ACS and the presence of *reproducible CWT ruled out* ACS (p = 0.003) with a high negative predictive value (98.1%, 95% CI 89.9% to 99.7%).

- Conversely, *non-reproducible CWT ruled in* ACS with low specificity (48.6%, 95% CI 38.8% to 58.5%) and low positive predictive value (19.1%, 95% CI 10.6% to 30.5%).

Validity of diagnostic palpation in various body regions

Shoulder

Whereas single tests have not been very accurate (Hegedus et al. 2012), the best combination of tests for making the diagnosis of impingement syndrome of any degree is (Park et al. 2005):

- a positive Hawkins–Kennedy impingement sign

- a positive painful arc sign

- weakness in external rotation with the arm at the side.

Michener et al. (2009) found that if three out of five tests for impingement (Neer, Hawkins–Kennedy, painful arc, empty can, and external rotation) were positive, accuracy

was sufficient, but if fewer than three of five tests were positive, they were not sufficiently accurate to make the diagnosis, and, in fact, serve to rule it out.

To diagnose a full-thickness rotator cuff tear, the best combination of tests, when all three are positive, is (Park et al. 2005):

- the painful arc

- the drop-arm sign

- weakness in external rotation.

For a glenoid labrum tear (Walsworth et al. 2008):

- The combination of popping or catching with a positive crank or anterior slide result or a positive anterior slide result with a positive active compression or crank test result suggests the presence of a labral tear.

- The combined absence of popping or catching and a negative anterior slide or crank result suggests the absence of a labral tear.

Palpatory tests for tendonitis or tendon rupture in patients with rheumatoid arthritis are not accurate (Kim et al. 2007).

Knee

Orthopedic palpatory assessments of knee joint stability or ligament laxity that have high predictive validity are (Hing et al. 2009):

- the Lachman test for anterior cruciate ligament tear

- the posterior drawer test for posterior cruciate ligament tear.

For diagnosing meniscal tears (Hing et al. 2009):

- The McMurray test is the most accurate test when positive. It is not sensitive, however, so it has a lot of false negatives; thus, a negative test may miss an actual meniscal tear. It should therefore be combined with other tests, such as joint line tenderness, and a good history.

Pelvis: sacroiliac joint

Single palpatory tests for the sacroiliac (SI) joint for pain are not accurate at identifying it as the source of low back pain; however, a series of pain provocation tests increases their validity when combined (Van der Wurff et al. 2006; Stuber 2007).

- Pelvic distraction, thigh thrust, compression, and sacral thrust tests, in combination, are accurate in detecting the SI joint as a source of pain (Laslett et al. 2005; Laslett 2008). It is only necessary to use two of four of these tests to have the best predictive power of determining that the SI joint was the patient's pain source. When all tests do not provoke pain, the SI joint can be ruled out as a source of the pain.

- Hancock et al. (2007) performed a systematic review of validity studies that evaluated various tests used to identify the source of low back pain, including SI joint pain palpatory provocation tests. Combinations of SI joint provocation tests had a moderate degree of validity.

- Patrick's F-Ab-ER-E (flexion, abduction, external rotation; extension) test, and other SI joint pain provocation tests, such as the transverse anterior distraction compression test (gapping test), and/or transverse posterior distraction test (Gaenslen's test) are not accurate using double fluoroscopy-guided joint anesthetic blocks as the reference ("gold") standard (Eskander et al. 2015).

- Researchers have questioned the validity of using joint block injections as a standard reference for assessing the accuracy of palpatory or provocative manual SI joint tests to determine if it is the source of a patient's low back or leg pain, when it is not in itself a valid procedure for eliminating SI joint inflammation or pathology as a source of low back or leg pain (Berthelot et al. 2006; Hansen et al. 2007). Also, many studies support using provocative maneuvers as being accurate at identifying the SI joint as a source of pain, but just as many refute their accuracy; thus, evidence is limited at this time, requiring further rigorously designed studies.

- In a study examining palpatory diagnostic procedures of the SI joint in patients with lumbar-pelvic pain, researchers found that the results of a validated (sensitive and/or specific) pain provocation test, or cluster of tests, do not correlate with those obtained from a validated motion test, or cluster of motion tests, in identifying the SI joint as the cause of the patient's problem (Soleimanifar et al. 2016). Although combining pain provocation and motion tests increases interexaminer

reliability in locating manipulable dysfunctions of the SI joint, both these types of tests are not necessarily going to be positive, as they measure different pathologies; the SI joint may not be the cause of both the lumbar-pelvic pain and the motion dysfunction. It is probable that in many cases, the lumbar-pelvic pain is referred to the SI joint from the lumbar spine, for example. It is commonly taught and found in practice that joint motion dysfunction and joint pain go hand in hand, but this is not what was found in this study. It is not yet known whether this is peculiar to the SI joint or applicable to other joints as well.

Lumbar spine

- Manual assessment of spinal stiffness using posterior to central anterior palm pressure to determine indication for providing spinal manipulation for vertebral joint hypomobility is neither sensitive nor specific using mechanized indentation as a standard reference (Koppenhaver et al. 2014).

- Most palpation tests have low accuracy by themselves; however, accuracy is increased with patient verbal reports of pain during palpation (Phillips & Twomey 1996). Forced lumbosacral extension and percussion of lumbar spinous processes assessing for pain were inaccurate alone, but combinations of both observational and palpatory tests which included at least one painful movement (active or passive) are accurate at determining pain in the lumbar region for patients complaining of low back pain (Leboeuf-Yde & Kyvik 2000).

Cervical spine

- The cervical flexion-rotation test is very accurate (91%) in assessing motion restriction at C1–2 related to cervicogenic headache (Ogince et al. 2007).

- In a landmark study, Jull et al. (1988) compared manual diagnosis in predicting which joints were causing neck pain in 20 consecutive symptomatic patients to the criterion standard of local anesthetic blocks. Manual examination that assessed joint motion end-feel, quality of motion and pain upon passive motion testing is 100% sensitive and 100% specific at identifying both symptomatic and asymptomatic joints *when all patients are in pain.*

However, a larger (128 patients) follow-up study with *both symptomatic and asymptomatic patients*, using more rigorous statistical analysis, indicated cervical spine palpation to detect cervical joint pain as the cause of the neck pain was not accurate (King et al. 2007). Carragee et al. (2007) point out that the anesthetic block of pain as a reference standard for spinal joint pain is unproven and flawed. Additionally, what King et al. also fail to acknowledge is that although manual therapy is often directed at reducing or eliminating pain, it is also used to restore proper motion and function. Although pain may linger, clinical trials have shown that once proper motion and function is restored, pain usually subsides or resolves (Hurwitz et al. 2008).

Kinematic analysis has shown promise in evaluating motion characteristics of the cervical spine as a reference standard for passive and active motion assessment in patients with neck pain (Rutledge et al. 2013). Using kinematic analysis instrumentation, Vorro et al. (2013) found that blinded clinicians assessing cervical spine passive motion in patients with neck pain used decreased angular velocities when compared to angular velocities measures during cervical spine passive motion assessment of asymptomatic patients. This may explain why accuracy is improved when there is pain in the region being assessed. The clinician likely senses increased resistance, or altered quality of motion, in the surrounding soft tissues and joints and thus moves slower during the passive assessment process.

Cranial motion palpation

Although content validity studies are lacking, it is of interest to note the results of a construct validity study that showed that it is possible to palpate motion in the range of several tens of micrometers, which is within the range reported for calvarial motion in response to intracranial pressure fluctuations (10–50 micrometers) (Kasparian et al. 2015).

Since palpation is not consistently reliable or accurate, experts in the field need to provide guidance and perspectives to understand how this information affects clinical practice, clinical decision making, and patient care. The next section addresses this need.

Can the reliability and validity of diagnostic palpatory tests be improved?

Nyborg and Smith (2013) propose that attention to the inherent strengths and weaknesses of the sensory organs within the palpating hand should lead to the design of more precise and accurate diagnostic tests. They recommend the following:

- Use fingertips instead of palm pressure to assess passive intervertebral motion.

- Do not over-analyze first impressions of the findings.

- Use light touch rather than heavy pressure to assess motion.

- Focus on the initial motion felt rather than the end range of motion.

- Conform the palpating fingertips or hand to the structures being palpated.

- Keep hands and fingers active and practice palpation and other psychomotor activities.

- Combine visualization and visual imagery with palpation to enhance sensory discrimination.

- Pay attention to the test and its intended finding.

- Test movement slowly.

The palpation reliability debate: the experts' opinions

In the October 2001 issue of the *Journal of Bodywork and Movement Therapies* (JBMT), the editorial raised questions as to the value, validity, and accuracy of palpation methods in assessing musculoskeletal dysfunction (Chaitow 2001). Many research publications cast doubt on inter- and intra-rater reliability and accuracy in the performance of manual forms of assessment.

In order to elicit the perspectives of experts from various professions regarding the research literature on the reliability and validity of palpatory diagnostic procedures, JBMT invited a number of eminent clinicians and researchers to answer a series of questions which had been compiled in consultation with various experts. Professions represented in the responses include medicine

(David Simons and Karel Lewit), osteopathy (Peter Gibbons and Philip Tehan), chiropractic (Craig Liebenson and Don Murphy), physiotherapy (Joanne Bullock-Saxton and Dianne Lee) and massage therapy (Shannon Goosen). The following is a summary of their responses, edited from the original published version to spotlight their opinions and recommendations that are still pertinent. In their published replies, they cited recent relevant literature to support their points of view. These literature citations have been removed from the summary below. The responses they provided, however, remain intact as they are indeed timeless and are as applicable today as they were at the turn of the century; they are still excellent guideposts for future manual practitioners, educators and researchers.

Questions and answers

Question 1. Does the poor inter-observer reliability of palpation methods make you question the validity and usefulness of an examination based upon this skill? If not, why not?

Answer "The question about palpation's reliability should not be turned against palpation, but should be turned towards asking how to develop reliable, responsive, and valid instruments. The difficulty of establishing motion palpation's reliability may, in fact, point to the conclusion that our ability to measure the parameters involved in motion palpation is insufficient … While we strive to establish proof as our goal for creating a "best practice" scenario, we are a long way from being able to reasonably justify throwing away such a safe, low cost, although admittedly difficult to measure, technique as palpation of joint, muscle or soft tissue motion and stiffness … In fact, simply because palpation is too complex to measure with a gold standard instrument like seeing with photography, or hearing with tape recorders, this does not make palpation useless. Palpation is much more than just pressure (algometry), it involves proprioception, motion, and tension. The fact that it cannot be copied is no reason to abandon it. Manipulative techniques are best performed after first sensing with the hands such things as resistance and tension. One's level of technique depends on the capacity to feel (i.e., the palpatory skill), as well as to interpret what is felt. In fact, it could be argued that without the ability to palpate, good manipulative technique is unimaginable.

It is precisely the wealth of information, i.e., its sophistication including feedback with the patient, which makes it less reliable, or more precisely less reproducible. Clinically, palpation is a highly valued method because it tells the experienced examiner where the patient feels pain. Areas of increased tension, especially myofascial trigger points, are signposts for the clinician. If palpation were to be abandoned what is to fill its void? The field of manual medicine has a long way to go scientifically, but abandoning palpation for a "more sophisticated" analysis would be a memorable error … We should learn about palpation's limitations and focus on incorporating sturdier assessment tools. However, manual medicine practitioners should not abandon palpation of joints, muscles, and soft tissues any more than an internist should abandon palpating the abdomen or a cardiologist abandon auscultating the chest. The direction of combining several techniques to accurately classify and, therefore, accurately treat patients seems to show great promise at this point."

Craig Liebenson DC and Karel Lewit MD

Answer "I would not want to be without them in the clinic … I believe that we have not been able to show inter nor intra tester reliability when motion (either active or passive) of these joints is assessed because we have not paid attention to the dynamic and changing nature of the individual being tested. To investigate, determine and then compare findings such as articular range of motion implies that the tester "knows" what the range of motion for that joint should be. In addition, we have assumed that the range of motion will be constant from moment to moment for that individual … Unless trials are repeated and motions averaged, reliability is impossible, not because the tester can't feel what's happening but because the subject keeps changing from moment to moment."

Diane Lee MCPA

Answer "If used appropriately, applying the most effective means and the most clinically appropriate criteria, palpation methods can be an excellent tool in patient examination. It must be noted, however, that the patient examination has many aspects, starting with history taking, through neurologic and general physical examination, to pain provocation and functional examination. It is from the entire clinical exam that we draw conclusions as to diagnosis, and thus management strategy, not from any one assessment tool."

Donald R. Murphy DC, DACAN

Answer "There are many components of the clinical examination leading to a final diagnosis. Poor inter-observer reliability of palpatory findings should not be considered as necessarily devaluing the use of palpation as a diagnostic tool. Different practitioners respond in different ways to different palpatory cues, formulating their own manipulative prescription based upon individual experience. We believe that reliability of palpatory diagnosis could be improved by:

1. standardization of palpatory assessment procedures

2. utilization of multiple tests

3. increased focus upon linking palpation with pain provocation.

... Research to date has largely focused upon the reliability of palpation in diagnosis but has not adequately explored the relationship between palpatory skills and the delivery and monitoring of manipulative techniques. Even where diagnosis is not predicated upon the use of palpatory cues, palpation is still critical to the safe and effective application of "hands on" techniques. While there is obviously a need to continue research and improve our abilities within the area of palpatory diagnosis, we believe the debate should also address another area where the skills of palpation make a significant impact. This is in the delivery of "hands on" technique in a pain free, safe, and effective manner. Proficiency in the delivery of manipulative technique takes training, practice, and development of palpatory and psychomotor skills. We would contend that highly refined palpatory skills are essential for the development of the psychomotor skills necessary to perform manual therapy techniques."

Peter Gibbons MB, BS, DO, DM-SMed and Philip Tehan DipPhysio, DO, MPA

Question 2. How do you think palpation and clinical assessment should be taught/studied so that its validity and clinical potential can be best demonstrated?

Answer "In order to really be proficient in palpation one needs hundreds of hours of training and feedback.

Structural evaluation also takes hundreds of hours to learn. Therapists need more training in the context of what they are evaluating and palpating. This needs to be done with a multidisciplinary training team, where they are asked the difficult questions of 'How do you know that?' and 'Are you sure that you are where you think you are, and can you prove it?' If no one asks these questions, it may be easy to assume knowledge which is in fact absent."

Shannon Goossen BA, LMT, CMTPTMA

Answer "In my experience of teaching physical therapists, the most effective way to teach palpation of MTrPs is one-on-one training. Have the student first study (and learn) that muscle's attachments, structure, and function, then understand what they are looking for in their examination, and finally realize the pathophysiological basis for the MTrP's clinical characteristics. At that point, I have the student examine one of my muscles (the SCM for pincer palpation and the third finger extensor for flat palpation for starters). First, I check the muscle myself to make sure I know what is there and then see what they can find. If they are having trouble finding it, it is easy for me to see why based on what I see them doing and what their palpation of that muscle feels like compared to what it felt like when I palpated myself. This process can be applied to most of the muscles in the body. Another approach that is less demanding of teaching time is to have the students work in teams of three and have them take turns being paired examiners of the subject. Each examiner examines the muscle with the other examiner blinded and fills out a worksheet listing individual examination findings and what MTrPs were found. After the second examiner fills out a similar worksheet, they then compare results and, with the help of an instructor, see how they could have examined the muscle so they would have agreed as to their findings. The person who served as subject then similarly examines one of the previous examiners."

David G. Simons MD

Answer "I think the teaching methods for translatoric and angular motion analysis in the spine and pelvis are fine. What we need to consider is how we are interpreting the findings from these assessments. Just because a joint has decreased amplitude of motion does not mean that the joint is stiff or hypomobile. Excessive activation of the deep stabilizers for that joint will increase compression and restrict the available range. We need to apply a clinical reasoning process from a number of different tests to reach a mobility diagnosis of hypomobility, hypermobility, or instability. This cannot be reached from one test alone and yet too often we are being asked (in research) to make statements regarding range of motion based on one test. To demonstrate validity for the test procedures I believe we need to really look at the inclusion criteria of the subjects and include subjects on the basis of a biomechanical assessment regardless of location and behavior of pain. Pain has no relevance on motion. Exquisitely painful joints can have full range of motion whereas non-painful joints can be totally blocked in all directions."

Diane Lee MCPA

Answer "First, I think that students should be taught to palpate for both joint restriction and pain provocation when palpating joints, as this is the only method that has been shown to be reliable, and should be taught tissue texture changes during joint and myofascial palpation of other tissues. When I was in school (some time ago!), there was no systematic method applied to teaching students the art of palpation. One was just told to palpate as many patients as possible, and eventually one would "get the hang of it." It would be much more effective to teach the art of palpation, and to develop the sensitivity to detect differences in texture, movement, and muscle activity, in a stepwise fashion, starting with simple tasks, and gradually progressing to more difficult tasks. There is some recent evidence that suggests that starting with non-biologic materials may be an effective starting point for students to be able to detect levels of stiffness in isolation from the other nuances of biological tissue."

Donald R. Murphy DC, DACAN

Question 3. Should we depend less on palpation and assessment methods in clinical settings, since their reliability seems to be so poor?

Answer "I believe that palpation forms one component of a large range of potential assessment procedures to assess components of the muscular, articular, and neural systems. Following a thorough subjective examination, decisions are made by the clinician regarding the appropriate musculoskeletal structures to assess. Responses to various assessments provide the necessary information to assist clinicians in generating a hypothesis about the nature of the problem, and the most likely dysfunctional structure to manage. During the examination of the patient, a suite of positive tests will be identified, and the nature of the responses recorded, to provide baseline data prior to application of an intervention. Once a decision is made about diagnosis and the form of management, treatment may commence, followed by re-evaluation of the positive tests in order to ascertain the influence of treatment. Such review of management confirms the clinician's assumptions based on the suite of tests and ultimately improves the efficacy of patient management."

Joanne Bullock-Saxton PhD, MApp Phty St (Manips), BPhty (Hons)

Answer "No. We should learn how to improve our palpation skills and concentrate on a better understanding of what it is that we are palpating."

David G. Simons MD

Acknowledgment: Shana Feinberg for assistance with updating the references for this chapter.

References

Aartun E, Degerfalk A, Kentsdotter L and Hestbaek L (2014) Screening of the spine in adolescents: Inter- and intra-rater reliability and measurement error of commonly used clinical tests. BioMed Central Musculoskeletal Disorders 15: 37.

Abbott JH, McCane B, Herbison P et al. (2005) Lumbar segmental instability: A criterion-related validity study of manual therapy assessment. BioMed Central Musculoskeletal Disorders 6: 56.

Arab AM, Abdollahi I, Joghataei MT et al. (2009) Inter- and intra-examiner reliability of single and composites of selected motion palpation and pain provocation tests for sacroiliac joint. Manual Therapy 14 (2): 213–221.

Baertschi E, Swanenburg J, Brunner F and Kool J (2013) Interrater reliability of clinical tests to evaluate scapulothoracic motion. BioMed Central Musculoskeletal Disorders 14 (1): 1–15.

Berthelot J, Labat J, Le Goff B, Gouin F and Maugars Y (2006) Provocative sacroiliac joint maneuvers and sacroiliac joint block are unreliable for diagnosing sacroiliac joint pain. Joint Bone Spine 73 (1): 17–23.

Carragee EJ, Haldeman S and Hurwitz E (2007) The pyrite standard: The Midas touch in the diagnosis of axial pain syndromes. Spine Journal 7 (1): 27–31.

Chaitow L (2001) Palpatory accuracy: Time to reflect. Journal of Bodywork and Movement Therapies October 5 (4): 223–226.

Cooperstein R (2012) Interexaminer reliability of the Johnston and Friedman percussion scan of the thoracic spine: Secondary data analysis using modified methods. Journal of Chiropractic Medicine 11 (3): 154–159.

Cooperstein R, Young M and Haneline M (2013) Interexaminer reliability of cervical motion palpation using continuous measures and rater confidence levels. Journal of the Canadian Chiropractic Association 57 (2): 156–164.

Degenhardt BF, Snider KT, Snider EJ et al. (2005) Interobserver reliability of osteopathic palpatory diagnostic tests of the lumbar spine: Improvements from consensus training. Journal of the American Osteopathic Association 105 (10): 465–473.

Degenhardt B, Johnson J, Snider K and Snider E (2010) Maintenance and improvement of interobserver reliability of osteopathic palpatory tests over a 4-month period. Journal of the American Osteopathic Association 110 (10): 579–586.

Eskander JP, Ripoll JG and Calixto F (2015) Value of examination under fluoroscopy for the assessment of sacroiliac joint dysfunction. Pain Physician 18: E781–E786.

Feinstein A (1987) Clinemetrics. New Haven, CT: Yale University Press.

Fleiss J (1981) Statistical methods for rates and proportions, 2nd edn. New York: John Wiley.

Fritz JM, Piva SR and Childs JD (2005) Accuracy of the clinical examination to predict radiographic instability of the lumbar spine. European Spine Journal 14: 743–750.

Gräni C, Senn O, Bischof M et al. (2015) Diagnostic performance of reproducible chest wall tenderness to rule out acute coronary syndrome in acute chest pain: A prospective diagnostic study. British Medical Journal Open 5 (1): e007442 (accessed online October 21, 2015).

Halma KD, Degenhardt BF, Snider KT et al. (2008) Intraobserver reliability of cranial strain patterns as evaluated by osteopathic physicians: A pilot study. Journal of the American Osteopathic Association 108 (9): 493–502.

Hancock MJ, Maher CG, Latimer J et al. (2007) Systematic review of tests to identify the disc SIJ or facet joint as the source of low back pain. European Spine Journal 16: 1539–1550.

Haneline MT and Young M (2009) A review of intraexaminer and interexaminer reliability of static spinal palpation: A literature synthesis. Journal of Manipulative and Physiological Therapeutics 32 (5): 379–386.

Haneline MT, Cooperstein R, Young M and Birkeland K (2008) Spinal motion palpation: A comparison of studies that assessed intersegmental end feel vs excursion. Journal of Manipulative and Physiological Therapeutics 31 (8): 616–626.

Hansen HC, McKenzie-Brown AM, Cohen SP et al. (2007) Sacroiliac joint interventions: A systematic review. Pain Physician 10: 165–184.

Hegedus EJ, Goode AF, Michener L et al. (2012) Which physical examination tests provide clinicians with the most value when examining the shoulder? Update of a systematic review with meta-analysis of individual tests. British Journal of Sports Medicine 46 (14): 964–978.

Hing W, White S, Reid D and Marshall R (2009) Validity of the McMurray's test and modified versions of the test: A systematic literature review. Journal of Manual and Manipulative Therapy 17 (1): 22–35.

Hollerwöger D (2006) Methodological quality and outcomes of studies addressing manual cervical spine examinations: A review. Manual Therapy 11: 93–98.

Holt KR, Russell DG, Hoffman NJ et al. (2009) Interexaminer reliability of a leg length analysis procedure among novice and experienced practitioners. Journal of Manipulative and Physiological Therapeutics 32 (3): 216–222.

Humphreys BK, Delahaye M and Peterson CK (2004) An investigation into the validity of cervical spine motion palpation using subjects with congenital block vertebrae as a "gold standard." BioMed Central Musculoskeletal Disorders 5: 19.

Hurwitz EL, Carragee EJ, van der Velde G et al. (2008) Treatment of neck pain: Noninvasive interventions. Results of the Bone and Joint Decade 2000–2010 Task Force on Neck Pain and its Associated Disorders. Spine 33 (45): S123–S152.

Jende A and Peterson CK (1997) Validity of static palpation as an indicator of atlas transverse process asymmetry. European Journal of Chiropractic 45: 35–42.

Jull G, Bogduk N and Marsland A (1988) The accuracy of manual diagnosis for cervical zygapophysial joint pain syndromes. Medical Journal of Australia 148: 233–236.

Juul-Kristensen B, Røgind H, Jensen DV et al. (2007) Inter-examiner reproducibility of tests and criteria for generalized joint hypermobility and benign joint hypermobility syndrome. Rheumatology (Oxford) 46 (12): 1835–1841.

Kasparian H, Signoret G and Kasparian J (2015) Quantification of motion palpation. Journal of the American Osteopathic Association 115(10): 604–610.

Kim HA, Kim SH and Seo YI (2007) Ultrasonographic findings of the shoulder in patients with rheumatoid arthritis and comparison with physical examination. Journal of Korean Medical Science 22: 660–666.

King W, Lau P, Lees R et al. (2007) The validity of manual examination in assessing patients with neck pain. Spine Journal 7: 22–26.

Knottnerus JA, van Weel C and Muris JW (2002) Evidence base of clinical diagnosis: Evaluation of diagnostic procedures. British Medical Journal 324: 477–480.

Koppenhaver S, Hebert J, Kawchuk G, Childs J et al. (2014) Criterion validity of manual assessment of spinal stiffness. Manual Therapy 19 (6): 589–594.

Kumarathurai P, Farooq M, Christensen H et al. (2008) Muscular tenderness in the anterior chest wall in patients with stable angina pectoris is associated with normal myocardial perfusion. Journal of Manipulative and Physiological Therapeutics 31 (5): 344–347.

Landel R, Kulig K, Fredericson M et al. (2008) Intertester reliability and validity of motion assessments during lumbar spine accessory motion testing. Physical Therapy 88 (1): 43–49.

Laslett M (2008) Evidence-based diagnosis and treatment of the painful sacroiliac joint. Journal of Manual and Manipulative Therapy 16 (3): 142–152.

Laslett M, Aprill CN, McDonald B et al. (2005) Diagnosis of sacroiliac joint pain: Validity of individual provocation tests and composites of tests. Manual Therapy 10: 207–218.

Leboeuf-Yde C and Kyvik KO (2000) Is it possible to differentiate people with or without low-back pain on the basis of tests of lumbopelvic dysfunction? Journal of Manipulative Physiological Therapeutics 23: 160–167.

Lee AS, Pyle CW and Redding D (2015) Accuracy of anterior superior iliac spine symmetry assessment by routine structural examination. Journal of the American Osteopathic Association 115 (8): 482–489.

Lucas N, Macaskill P, Irwig L, Moran R and Bogduk N (2009) Reliability of physical examination for diagnosis of myofascial trigger points: A systematic review of the literature. Clinical Journal of Pain 25 (1): 80–89.

Maigne JY, Chantelot F and Chatellier G (2009) Inter-examiner agreement of clinical examination of the neck in manual medicine. Annals of Physical Rehabilitation Medicine 52 (1): 41–48.

Malanga GA, Andrus S, Nadler SF et al. (2003) Physical examination of the knee: A review of the original test description and scientific validity of common orthopedic tests. Archives of Physical Medicine and Rehabilitation 85: 592–603.

Manning DM, Dedrick GS, Sizer PS and Brismée JM (2012) Reliability of a seated three-dimensional passive intervertebral motion test for mobility end-feel and pain provocation in patients with cervicalgia. Journal of Manual and Manipulative Therapy 20 (3): 135–141.

Martin RL and Sekiya JK (2008) The interrater reliability of 4 clinical tests used to assess individuals with musculoskeletal hip pain. Journal of Orthopedic Sports Physical Therapy 38 (2): 71–77.

May S, Littlewood C and Bishop A (2006) Reliability of procedures used in the physical examination of non-specific low back pain: A systematic review. Australian Journal of Physiotherapeutics 52: 91–102.

Michener LA, Walsworth MK, Doukas WC and Murphy KP (2009) Reliability and diagnostic accuracy of 5 physical examination tests and combination of tests for subacromial impingement. Archives of Physical Medicine and Rehabilitation 90 (11): 1898–1903.

Murphy DR, Hurwitz EL and Nelson CF (2008) A diagnosis-based clinical decision rule for spinal pain, part 2: Review of the literature. Chiropractic and Osteopathy 16: 7.

Myburgh C, Larsen AH and Hartvigsen J (2008) A systematic critical review of manual palpation for identifying myofascial trigger points: Evidence and clinical significance. Archives of Physical Medicine and Rehabilitation 89 (6): 1169–1176.

Myers HL, Thomas E, Hay EM and Dziedzic KS (2011) Hand assessment in older adults with musculoskeletal hand problems: A reliability study. BioMed Central Musculoskeletal Disorders 12: 3.

Naaktgeboren CA, de Groot JAH, van Smeden M et al. (2013) Evaluating diagnostic accuracy in the face of multiple reference standards. Annals of Internal Medicine 159: 195–202.

Najm WI, Seffinger MA, Mishra SI et al. (2003) Content validity of manual spinal palpatory exams: A systematic review. BioMed Central Complementary and Alternative Medicine 3: 1.

Nyborg RE and Smith AR (2013) The science of spinal motion palpation: A review and update with implications for assessment and intervention. Journal of Manual and Manipulative Therapy 21 (3): 160–167.

Ogince M, Hall T, Robinson K and Blackmore AM (2007) The diagnostic validity of the cervical flexion–rotation test in C1/2-related cervicogenic headache. Manual Therapy 12: 256–262.

Park HB, Yokota A, Gill HS et al. (2005) Diagnostic accuracy of clinical tests for the different degrees of subacromial impingement syndrome. Journal of Bone and Joint Surgery in America 87: 1446–1455.

Phillips DR and Twomey LT (1996) A comparison of manual diagnosis with a diagnosis established by a uni-level lumbar spinal block procedure. Manual Therapy 1: 82–87.

Póvoa L, Ferreira A and Silva J (2015) Validation of palpatory methods for evaluating anatomical bone landmarks of the cervical spine: A systematic review. Journal of Manipulative and Physiological Therapeutics 38 (4): 302–310.

Price DD, McGrath PA, Rafii A et al. (1983) The validation of visual analogue scales as ratio scale measures for chronic and experimental pain. Pain 17: 45–56.

Robinson HS, Brox JI, Robinson R et al. (2007) The reliability of selected motion and pain provocation tests for the sacroiliac joint. Manual Therapy 12 (1): 72–79.

Robinson R, Robinson HS, Bjork G and Kvale A (2009) Reliability and validity of a palpation technique for identifying the spinous processes of C7 and L5. Manual Therapy 14 (4): 409–414.

Rubinstein SM, van Tulder M (2008) A best-evidence review of diagnostic procedures for neck and low-back pain. Best Practices and Research in Clinical Rheumatology, 22(3): 471–482.

Rutledge B, Bush TR, Vorro J et al. (2013) Differences in human cervical spine kinematics for active and passive motions of symptomatic and asymptomatic subject groups. Journal of Applied Biomechanics 29 (5): 543–553 [Epub 2012 Nov 21].

Seffinger MA, Najm WI, Mishra SI et al. (2004) Reliability of spinal palpation for diagnosis of back and neck pain: A systematic review of the literature. Spine 29: E413–E425.

Shaw KA, Dougherty JJ, Treffer KD and Glaros AG (2012) Establishing the content validity of palpatory examination for the assessment of the lumbar spine using ultrasonography: A pilot study. Journal of the American Osteopathic Association 112 (12): 775–782.

Snider KT, Kribs JW, Snider EJ et al. (2008) Reliability of Tuffier's line as an anatomic landmark. Spine 33 (6): E161–E165.

Snider KT, Snider EJ, Degenhardt BF et al. (2011) Palpatory accuracy of lumbar spinous processes using multiple bony landmarks. Journal of Manipulative Physiological Therapeutics 34 (5): 306–313. doi:10.1016/j.jmpt.2011.04.006 (accessed September 29, 2016).

Soleimanifar M, Karimi N and Arab AM (2016) Association between composites of selected motion palpation and pain provocation tests for sacroiliac joint disorders. Journal of Bodywork and Movement Therapies, epub June 16. Available online at http://dx.doi.org/10.1016/j.jbmt.2016.06.003 (accessed September 29, 2016).

Sommerfeld P, Kaider A and Klein P (2004) Inter- and intraexaminer reliability in palpation of the "primary respiratory mechanism" within the "cranial concept." Manual Therapy 9: 22–29.

Stochkendahl MJ, Christensen HW, Hartvigsen J et al. (2006) Manual examination of the spine: A systematic critical literature review of reproducibility. Journal of Manipulative Physiological Therapeutics 29 (6): 475–485.

Stovall BA and Kumar S (2010) Anatomical landmark asymmetry assessment in the lumbar spine and pelvis: A review of reliability. Physical Medicine and Rehabilitation 2 (1): 48–56.

Stuber KJ (2007) Specificity sensitivity and predictive values of clinical tests of the sacroiliac joint: A systematic review of the literature. Journal of the Canadian Chiropractic Association 51 (1): 30–41.

Stuber K, Lerede C, Kristmanson K, Sajko S and Bruno P (2014) The diagnostic accuracy of the Kemp's test: A systematic review. Journal of the Canadian Chiropractic Association 58 (3): 258–267.

Chapter 2

Tong HC, Heyman OG, Lado DA and Isser MM (2006) Interexaminer reliability of three methods of combining test results to determine side of sacral restriction sacral base position and innominate bone position. Journal of the American Osteopathic Association 106 (8): 464–468.

Triano JJ, Budgell B, Bagnulo A et al. (2013) Review of methods used by chiropractors to determine the site for applying manipulation. Chiropractic and Manual Therapies 21: 36.

Van der Wurff P, Buijs EJ and Groen GJ (2006) A multitest regimen of pain provocation tests as an aid to reduce unnecessary minimally invasive sacroiliac joint procedures. Archives of Physical Medicine and Rehabilitation 87: 10–14.

Van Trijffel E, Anderegg Q, Bossuyt PM et al. (2005) Inter-examiner reliability of passive assessment of intervertebral motion in the cervical and lumbar spine: A systematic review. Manual Therapy 10: 256–269.

Vorro J, Bush TR, Rutledge B and Li M (2013) Kinematic measures during a clinical diagnostic technique for human neck disorder: inter- and intraexaminer comparisons. Biomedical Research International. doi: 10.1155/2013/950719. Epub 2013 Feb 16 (accessed September 29, 2016).

Walsworth MK, Doukas WC, Murphy KP et al. (2008) Reliability and diagnostic accuracy of history and physical examination for diagnosing glenoid labral tears. American Journal of Sports Medicine 36 (1): 162–168.

Woodfield HC, Gerstman BB and Olaisen HR (2011) Interexaminer reliability of supine leg checks for discriminating leg-length inequality. Journal of Manipulative Physiological Therapeutics 34 (4): 239–246.

Special topic 1

Using appropriate pressure (and the myofascial pain index)

Leon Chaitow

When palpating lightly, advice varies as to how to learn to achieve appropriate levels of contact pressure. Upledger and Vredevoogd (1983) speak of 5 grams of pressure, which is very light indeed. Many experts advise discovering how hard you can press on your own (closed) eyeball before discomfort starts, as a means of learning just how lightly to press. Other advice includes keeping an eye on the degree of blanching of the nailbed, to ensure uniformity of pressure (Wolfe et al. 1990).

In truth, the art of palpation, and of using applied pressure, requires sensitivity, involving awareness of when tissue tension/resistance is being "met" and when overcome. This is particularly important in the evaluation mode of neuromuscular technique (see Chapter 5).

When we palpate more deeply or apply digital pressure to a tender point in order to ascertain its status ("Does it hurt?", "Does it refer?", etc.), it is important to have some way of knowing that the pressure being applied is uniform. For example, when assessing people with the symptoms of fibromyalgia, the criteria for a diagnosis depend upon 11 of 18 designated sites testing as positive (i.e., hurting severely) on application of 4 kg of pressure (Wolfe et al. 1990). If it takes more than 4 kg of pressure to produce pain, the point does not count in the tally. (See Special topic 10 for details of the areas palpated in fibromyalgia assessment.)

The question then is, how does a person learn to apply 4 kg of pressure, and no more? It has been shown that, using a simple technology (such as bathroom scales), physical therapy students can be taught to accurately produce specific degrees of pressure on request. Students have been tested

applying posteroanterior pressure force to lumbar tissues. After training, using bathroom scales to evaluate pressure levels, the students showed significantly reduced error both immediately after training, as well as a month later (Keating et al. 1993).

The term *pressure threshold* is used to describe the *least* amount of pressure required to produce a report of pain and/or referred symptoms when a trigger point is compressed (Hong et al. 1996). Myburgh et al. (2008) showed that there is moderately good evidence for the reproducibility of trigger point palpation of the trapezius when evaluating for local tenderness, and of the gluteus medius and quadratus lumborum when seeking evidence of referred pain from trigger points. It is obviously useful to know how much pressure is required to produce pain and/or referred symptoms and whether this degree of pressure is different before and after treatment, or at a subsequent clinical encounter (see pain index discussion below).

Use an algometer?

Without a measuring device such as an algometer there would be no accurate means of achieving or measuring a standardized degree of pressure application. An algometer is a hand-held, spring-loaded, rubber-tipped pressure-measuring device that offers a means of achieving standardized pressure application. Using an algometer, sufficient pressure to produce pain is applied to palpated or preselected points, at a precise 90° angle to the skin. The measurement is taken when pain is reported.

Baldry (referring to research by Fischer) discusses algometer use (he calls it a "pressure threshold meter") and suggests it should be employed to measure the degree of pressure required to produce symptoms "before and after deactivation of a trigger point, for when this is successful, the pressure threshold over the trigger point increases by about 4 kg" (Baldry 1993; Fischer 1988). (Special topic Fig. 1.1.)

Valuable as it is in research, and in training pressure sensitivity, use of an algometer is not really practical in everyday clinical work. It is, however, an important tool in research, as an objective measurement of a change in the degree of pressure required to produce symptoms. It also helps a practitioner to train themselves to apply a standardized degree of pressure when treating, and to "know" how hard they are pressing.

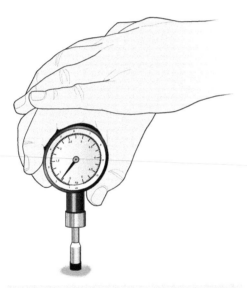

Figure ST 1.1
Pressure algometer

Myofascial pain index (MPI)

One use of an algometer is to identify a "myofascial pain index" (MPI). This is an objective base that is calculated from the patient's subjective pain reports when pressure is applied to test points. The calculation of the MPI determines the average degree of pressure required to evoke pain in a trigger or tender point.

Using an algometer, pressure is applied to each of the points being tested (which could be the 18 fibromyalgia test points – see Special topic 10) or, more logically, a selection of active trigger points identified by standard palpation. Pressure is applied using the algometer at a precise 90° angle to the skin, sufficient to produce pain, with the pressure measurement being taken when this is reported. The values are recorded and then averaged, producing a number, which is the MPI. This allows comparison at a later stage to see whether the trigger point requires greater pressure to produce pain, indicating that it is less active, or the same or less pressure, indicating that it has not changed or is more sensitive.

Pick's palpation guidelines

Pick (1999) has given extremely useful suggestions regarding the levels of pressure that he recommends in cranial assessment and treatment (see Special topic Fig. 1.2). These guidelines are equally useful in general palpation.

Pick describes:

- Surface level: first contact, molding to the contours of the structure, *no actual pressure*.

- Working level: "The working level … is the level at which most manipulative procedures begin. Within this level the practitioner can feel pliable counter-resistance to the applied force. The contact feels noninvasive … and is usually well within the comfort zone of the subjects. Here the practitioner will find maximum control over the intracranial structures."

- Rejection levels: Pick suggests these levels are reached when tissue resistance and/or discomfort/pain are noted. Rejection will occur at different degrees of pressure, in different areas, and in different circumstances, and is not recommended in the therapeutic setting.

So, how much pressure should be used? Ideally, not enough to hurt, and yet enough to be effective.

1. when working with the skin: surface level

2. when palpating for trigger points: working level

3. when testing for pain responses, and when treating trigger points: rejection level.

When you are applying pressure at the rejection level there is a feeling of the tissues pushing you away, and you have to overcome the resistance to achieve a sustained compression.

Special topic Exercise 1.1 *Variable pressure*

- Perform the application of digital pressure to each level described above – surface, rejection and working – using either a finger or a thumb on a variety of tissue areas: on the gluteal region, on a lightly muscled area of the forearm, on the cranium, close to the spine, and on the anterior neck muscles, as examples.

- Try to locate areas to practice on that are hypertonic and/or flaccid, so that you learn to apply appropriate pressure to a range of tissue types and tones.

- If no palpation partner is available practice this on yourself.

- Touch the tissues, and then *slowly* apply pressure (sink into the tissues) until you feel a sense of "rejection" – as though the tissues are pressing back against your digit or are resisting further pressure.

- Then try to identify a point somewhere between these two levels – between superficial and deep.

- When you do so you will be touching tissues, and the pressure you are applying will match the tone of those tissues.

- This will be very similar to what is being achieved during NMT evaluation (see Chapter 5), only in this instance the pressure is static rather than on the move.

- Practice this approach until you can rapidly identify the "working level" of different tissues in all parts of the body.

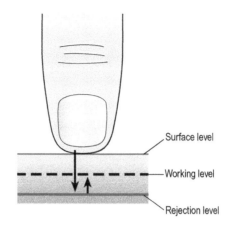

Figure ST 1.2
The concept of a "working level." Surface level involves touch without any pressure at all. Rejection is where pressure meets a sense of the tissues "pushing back" defensively. By reducing pressure slightly from the rejection level, the contact arrives at the working level, where perception of tissue change should be keenest, as well as there being an ability to distinguish normal from abnormal tissue (hypertonic, fibrotic, edematous, etc.) (after Dr Marc Pick DC 1999).

References

Baldry P (1993) Acupuncture trigger points and musculo-skeletal pain. Edinburgh: Churchill Livingstone.

Fischer A (1988) Documentation of muscle pain and soft tissue pathology, in Kraus H (ed) Diagnosis and treatment of muscle pain. Chicago, IL: Quintessence, pp 55–65.

Hong C-Z, Chen Y-N, Twehouse D and Hong D (1996) Pressure threshold for referred pain by compression on trigger point and adjacent area. Journal of Musculoskeletal Pain 4 (3): 61–79.

Keating J, Matuyas T and Bach T (1993) The effect of training on physical therapist's ability to apply specified forces of palpation. Physical Therapy 73 (1): 38–46.

Myburgh C, Larsen AH and Hartvigsen J (2008) A systematic, critical review of manual palpation for identifying myofascial trigger points: Evidence and clinical significance. Archives of Physical Medicine and Rehabilitation 89 (6): 1169–1176.

Pick M (1999) Cranial sutures. Seattle: Eastland Press, pp xx–xxi.

Upledger J and Vredevoogd J (1983) Craniosacral therapy. Seattle: Eastland Press.

Wolfe F, Smythe H, Yunus M et al. (1990) The American College of Rheumatology 1990 criteria for the classification of fibromyalgia: Report of the Multicenter Criteria Committee. Arthritis and Rheumatism 33: 160–172.

Special topic 2

Structure and function: are they inseparable?

Leon Chaitow

One of the oldest maxims in osteopathic medicine highlights the interdependence of structure and function: structure determines (or strongly influences) function and vice versa. Anything that causes a change in structure will cause function to modify, and any functional change will result in structural change (for example, fibrosis of muscle, alteration in length of any soft tissue, change in joint surface smoothness).

There is no way that a shortened or fibrosed muscle can function normally; there will always be a degree of adaptation, a modification from normal patterns of use, some degree of compensation, malcoordination, or imbalance in the way it works.

Similarly, all changes in the way any part of the body is used (breathing function is a good example), or the way the whole body is used (posture, for example), which varies from the way it was designed to work, will produce alterations in structure. If posture is poor or habitual use is incorrect (sitting cross-legged and writing with the head tilted to one side are common examples) structural changes will develop in response to, or in order to support and cement, these functional changes.

Examples are given in Chapter 12 of the biomechanical changes that emerge when respiratory function modifies chronically, emphasizing that there is a function–structure–function continuum.

On a cellular level as well

When a force is applied to tissues, the mechanical load is transferred to individual cell surfaces, and from these to linked cytoskeletal elements that form the framework of the cell. These may either distort or break (Wang & Stamenovic 2000).

Mechanotransduction describes processes in which cells and tissues respond to alterations in their architectural features, with consequent changes in their shape being mirrored by modification of biological function. As the structural form of cells alter in response to applied load – for example involving forces such as torsion, tension, shear, compression, stretch, bending and friction – processes are triggered involving chemical signaling that profoundly influence cellular behavior and development, including gene expression (Hicks et al. 2012).

Kumka and Bonar (2012) explain that mechanotransduction occurs "as cells convert a diversity of mechanical stimuli, transmitted throughout the extracellular matrix, into chemical activity to regulate morphology and function of tissues."

Ingber (2000) explains further:

> *The functional state of the cell appears to "self-organize" as a result of the architecture and dynamics of its underlying regulatory network. In this context, tensegrity-based changes in cytoskeletal structure may influence cell phenotype, switching on the basis of their ability simultaneously to alter the biochemical activities of multiple cytoskeleton-associated signaling components throughout the cell.*

Ingber's research into bone density loss in astronauts (on behalf of NASA) demonstrated that the collapse of the cytoskeleton's tensegrity struts in zero gravity causes cells to warp, and this is one reason for the cells' inability to process calcium and other nutrients normally, leading to the loss of bone density (Ingber 1999). Here we see a picture of complex structural adaptations and modification, determining the efficiency of metabolic function and gene expression, at the cellular level.

And on a larger scale as well

We can summarize factors that produce functional and subsequently structural change as involving overuse, misuse, abuse and disuse, which in turn can be reduced to one word: stress. Conversely, when we palpate structure and identify alterations from the expected norm, we should be able to confirm related functional changes.

For example, if we palpate shortened or fibrosed soft tissues, it should be possible to register that the area does not function normally (e.g., when a shortened hamstring is palpable the leg will be restricted during a straight-leg raising test, as well as when normal functional demands are made of that muscle).

It is worth considering, however, that just because something is other than the way it "should" be, this does not mean that it needs to be modified by treatment or rehabilitation exercises. Take, for example, the same short hamstring muscle mentioned above. There may be times when this is actually serving a useful purpose; for instance, if there is a dysfunctional and unstable sacroiliac joint a tight hamstring that places additional load on the sacrotuberous ligament might be acting as a stabilizing influence (see Chapter 8). In such a situation stretching the tight hamstring group might make these muscles more "normal" but could produce instability in the sacroiliac joint (Vleeming et al. 1997).

Similar consideration should be given to the presence of active trigger points, which may be serving some stabilizing function because they produce heightened tone in the muscles in which they exist, as well as in the muscles to which they refer (Chaitow & DeLany 2000).

When we observe functional change we should readily be able to identify structural alterations as well. Thus, when posture or breathing function is not as it should be, we should target the tissues that are most likely to carry evidence of associated structural change, as well, of course, as those structures (and behaviors) that may be influencing these stresses.

On a more local scale, when skin elasticity (a function that depends on normal structure) is reduced, we know that underlying reflex change (function) is involved (see Chapter 4).

Palpation and observation are as inseparable as structure and function and this should be kept in mind both during our exploration of palpatory methods that experience both structure and function, and also as we observe the physical manifestation of these two concepts – what the body looks and feels like, and what its functions look and feel like.

When we palpate we are feeling structure, the physical manifestation of functional tissues and units, and we are also sensing the changes that take place as a result of the functioning of the body or part. When we observe we are seeing these same things.

Ida Rolf (1977) suggests that we have an ever-enquiring mind focused on what we are feeling and that we should ask ourselves:

What is structure? What does it look like? What am I looking for when I look for structure, and how do I recognise it? Structure in general, structure in human bodies in particular – what is its function? What is its mechanism? To what extent can it be modified in humans? If you modify the physical structure of a body, what have you modified, and what can you hope to influence?

So, how accurate are our observations and palpations?

References

Chaitow L and DeLany J (2000) Clinical applications of neuromuscular techniques, vol 1 (Upper body). Edinburgh: Churchill Livingstone.

Hicks M, Cao TV, Campbell DH and Standley PR (2012) Mechanical strain applied to human fibroblasts differentially regulates skeletal myoblast differentiation. Journal of Applied Physiology 113 (3): 465–472.

Ingber D (1999) How cells (might) sense microgravity. FASEB Journal S1: 3–15

Ingber D (2000) Cancer as a disease of epithelial–mesenchymal interactions and extracellular matrix regulation. Differentiation 70: 547–560.

Kumka M and Bonar J (2012) Fascia: A morphological description and classification system based on a literature review. Journal of the Canadian Chiropractic Association 56 (3): 179–191.

Rolf I (1977) Rolfing: The integration of human structures. New York: Harper and Row.

Vleeming A, Mooney V, Dorman T, Snijders C and Stoeckart R (eds) (1997) Movement, stability and low back pain. Edinburgh: Churchill Livingstone.

Wang N and Stamenovic D (2000) Contribution of intermediate filaments to cell stiffness, stiffening, and growth. American Journal of Physiology. Cell Physiology 279 (1): C188–C194.

Viola Frymann (1963) has summarized the potential that palpation offers the healing professions:

The human hand is equipped with instruments to perceive changes in temperature, surface texture, surface humidity, to penetrate and detect successively deeper tissue textures, turgescence, elasticity and irritability. The human hand, furthermore, is designed to detect minute motion, motion which can only be detected by the most sensitive electronic pick-up devices available. This carries the art of palpation beyond the various modalities of touch into the realm of proprioception, of changes in position and tension within our own muscular system.

These words define the instruments we use, and the tasks we perform, when we palpate.

Different parts of the human hand are more, or less, able to discriminate variations in tissue features, such as relative tension, texture, degree of moisture, temperature and so on. This highlights the fact that your overall palpatory sensitivity depends on a combination of different perceptive (and proprioceptive) qualities and abilities. These include the ability to:

- register temperature variations
- differentiate subtle differences in a spectrum of tissue tone, ranging from very flaccid and soft to degrees of hypertonicity and spasm
- register the existence and size of extremely small entities, such as are found in fibrotic tissue or areas of induration
- sensitively distinguish between a variety of tissue textures and types, ranging from muscle to fascia and bone.

Irvin Korr (1970) helps us to understand just why the hand is so delicately able to perform its many tasks:

Where do we find the greatest number of muscle spindles? Exactly where they logically belong. If the muscle spindle has to do with finely-tuned muscle activity, with measuring gains in extremely small lengths of muscle fibers, one would expect that for more complex movement patterns, as in the muscles of the hand, we would have a very large number of muscle spindles. And this is exactly what we find. The num-ber of spindles per gram of muscle is only 1 in the latissimus dorsi; in the hand the number is close to 26. Functionally this is of great significance.

Physiology of touch

Palpatory perception depends largely on variations in the number and type (see summary in Box 3.1) of sensory neural receptors located in the skin and tissues, since this determines discriminatory capabilities.

Box 3.1 Receptors and perception	
Mechanoreceptors	
Light touch	Meissner's corpuscle
	Merkel's disc
	Hair-root plexus
Deep pressure	Pacinian corpuscle
Crude touch	Thought to be Krause's end-bulb
	Thought to be Ruffini's ending
Proprioception	
Muscle length, tendon and limb	Muscle spindle position
	Golgi tendon organ
	Joint/kinesthetic receptors
Nociceptors	
Pain	Free nerve endings
Thermoreceptors	
Warmth	Thought to be free nerve endings
Cold	Thought to be free nerve endings
Internal temperature	Hypothalamic thermostat

- Light touch is generally accepted to be achieved via mechanoreceptors (such as Meissner's corpuscle and Merkel's disc, as well as hair-root plexi) lying in the skin, muscles, joints, and organs. They respond to mechanical deformation resulting from pressure, stretch, or hair movement. It is in the skin that the greatest number of these receptors are found.

- Cruder touch perception is thought to relate to Krause's end-bulb, Ruffini's ending, and Pacinian corpuscles.

- Sensations of heat and cold are detected by thermoreceptors that are considered to be the free nerve endings in the skin.

- If cold is intense, detection is by nociceptors – specialized pain detectors – that are also free nerve endings.

Different parts of the hand have varying sensitivities

Kappler (1997) notes that although for some people, the palmar surface of the hand – including the finger pads, not tips – are best for fine assessment of texture, and the presence of pulsations, induration, edema, and moisture, as well as for the mobility of organs (see Chapter 12). The palmar surface of the fingers and the ulnar surface of the hand are also the most effective palpation contacts for discrimination of subtle motions; however, temperature variations are usually more keenly noted by the dorsum of the hand, particularly the dorsum of the second, third, and fourth fingers.

Sensory neurons link the skin of your palpating hand with the spinal cord or brainstem. These serve an area of skin called a receptive field, of which there are many on the surface of the hand, some of which overlap. The degree of tactile sensitivity of any area is in direct proportion to the number of sensory units present, as well as to the degree of overlap of receptive fields.

Two-point discrimination test

Small receptive fields with many sensory units obviously have the highest degree of discriminatory sensitivity. You can test this as follows:

- Two sharp points are touched to the skin of the area being tested.

- The distance between these points is varied, until the shortest distance is reached at which it is still possible to discern that two points, and not one point, are being touched (Fig. 3.1).

- Measurement of the minimum separable distance between two tactile points of stimulus proves that the greatest degree of spatial discrimination exists on the surface of the tongue, the lips, and the fingertips (1–3 μm).

- In contrast, the backs of the hands, the back, and the legs all have a poor degree of sensitivity to spatial discrimination (50–100 μm).

Not only is there a difference of perception relating to spatial accuracy, but also one relating to intensity of sensation. For example, an indentation of 6 micrometers can be registered on the finger pads, while an indentation of 24 micrometers is required before the sensors in the palm of the hand reach their threshold, and perceive the stimulus.

Kappler (1997) notes that movements with an amplitude as small as a tenth of a millimeter (i.e., a ten-thousandth of a meter, a micrometer) can be sensed by skilled palpation touch, and that the most sensitive parts of the hand surface where this can register are likely to be the pads (not the tips) of the thumb and first two fingers (where more nerve endings are found than anywhere else in the hands).

The sensitivity threshold on the backs of the hands (despite poor spatial discrimination sensitivity here – see above), trunk, and legs is some 10–20 times higher than the fingertips, which, along with the tongue, are the most sensitive palpatory units available to us.

Contrasting views

It is not likely that any clinical value can relate to the tongue's sensitivity, and therefore our focus needs to be on the remarkable discriminatory features of the fingertips and finger pads so that we can enhance palpatory literacy (Uddin et al. 2014). This is a popular idea; however, some prominent dissenters (Upledger & Vredevoogd 1983; Kuchera & Kuchera 1994) suggest that proprioceptive capabilities can be improved by using a whole-hand contact (see later in this chapter).

Variations

Variations in sensitivity highlight the marked degree of differences in discriminatory abilities between individuals. This may be because of anatomical differences, such as the number of receptors per square centimeter, something that

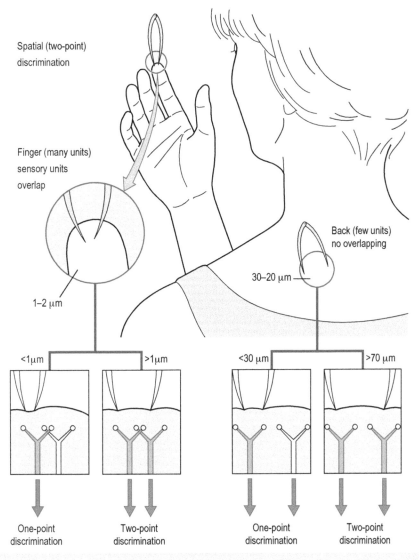

Spatial (two-point) discrimination

Finger (many units) sensory units overlap

Back (few units) no overlapping

30–20 μm

1–2 μm

<1μm   >1μm   <30 μm   >70 μm

One-point discrimination   Two-point discrimination   One-point discrimination   Two-point discrimination

Figure 3.1

Tactile discrimination. *Spatial discrimination*: in the two-point test, the spatial discriminative ability of the skin is determined by measuring the minimum separable distance between two tactile point stimuli. The back of the hands, the back and legs rate low (50–100 μm) in this ability. The fingertips, lips and tongue rate high (1–3 μm). *Intensity discrimination*: sensitive areas are also better able to discriminate differences in the intensity of tactile stimuli. Therefore, an indentation of 6 μm on the fingertip is sufficient to extract a sensation. This threshold is four times higher in the palm.

would clearly modify the degree of perception possible. In any comparative study of human (or animal) anatomy, there are clear and marked variations in size, number, and position of almost all structures, including neural receptors.

Physiological differences also abound, so not everyone will have the same degree of sensitivity when they palpate. Some will find it easy to perceive delicate pulsating rhythms, whereas others may have to work long and hard to do so.

Receptor adaptation

Anatomical differences are not the only factors involved in variations in palpatory sensitivity; we have to try to overcome, by constant effort, a physiological response that "switches off" (or decreases) the rate of firing of receptors when stimuli are maintained. This relates to what are called "*rapidly firing receptors,*" that tend to lose their sensitivity on any sustained contact. Those receptors responsible for fine touch and pressure adapt rapidly. Under normal conditions this is thought to have value in preventing constant awareness of whatever is touching the body (clothing, for example), but it is a nuisance for anyone involved in palpation assessment.

By contrast, mechanoreceptors, serving joint and muscle, are *slow* adapters, as are pain receptors. Some experts, such as Upledger and Vredevoogd (1983), suggest that use of the proprioceptive receptors should be incorporated into our palpatory endeavors. Their slow adaptation certainly supports this suggestion with the alteration in sensitivity resulting from rapid adaptation to light touch. The exercises later in this chapter will assist in this.

Filtering information

Although fine-touch receptor adaptation may reduce sensitivity, at times too much information is being received, and some filtering of information is required in order to make sense of what is being touched.

Kappler (1997) summarizes this as follows.

A more significant component [of palpation skills] is to be able to focus on the mass of information being perceived, paying close attention to those qualities associated with tissue texture abnormality, and bypassing many of the other palpatory clues not relevant at the time. This is a process of developing mental filters ... The brain cannot process everything at once. By concentrating only on the portion you want, it becomes easy and fast to detect areas of significant tissue texture abnormality.

Kappler et al. (1971) tested this concept, and found that when they compared student examiners with experienced practitioner examiners, although the students recorded *more* palpation findings, the practitioners recorded *more significant* findings. The experienced practitioners were

filtering out the unimportant, and focusing on what was meaningful, rather than being "overwhelmed with the mass of palpatory data."

Clearly how we interpret what we feel matters, and exercises later in this chapter will focus on learning discrimination.

Where do we palpate?

According to many experts (see below), it is the pads of the fingers or thumbs that have the greatest discriminatory ability to measure variations in whatever is being felt.

- The skin surface itself, with its range of variations from hot or warm, to cool or cold; thick or thin; dry, oily, or moist; puffy or firm; smooth or rough and so on, is usually best assessed with the pads of the fingers or the palm.

- The dorsum of the hand appears to be best for measuring the skin surface for temperature and moistness variations. However, this remains unproven.

- Assessment of the distance of structures from the surface, their depth, as well as their relative size, is usually best achieved by the fingertips/pads, and to some extent the palms of the hands. The palms and fingertips are also thought to be the most useful contacts for perception of variations in the status of osseous structures, through skin, fat, fascia, and muscle (Upledger & Vredevoogd 1983).

- Kuchera and Kuchera (1994) suggest that the coordinated involvement of the palmar surfaces of the hands and the fingers is the best approach for evaluating the shapes and contours of tissues and objects.

- The whole hand, including the fingers (possibly also the forearms and wrists), makes an accurate measuring instrument – with the hands being molded to the surface, 'listening' for subtle physiological motions, such as primary respiratory motion, in cranial osteopathic terminology, or visceral motion when organ position and function are being assessed. It is claimed that subtle variations in amplitude and direction of such movement, as well as the frequency of cycles of activity, can be assessed in this way – with practice (Upledger & Vredevoogd 1983).

Palpation of movement

If palpation is going to move beyond a simple assessment of the obvious characteristics of the tissues themselves, the hands need to register movement, pulsations, and minor tremors and rhythms, along with variations in all or any of these, during palpation. The palmar finger surfaces seem to be the most efficient for picking up very fine vibration. Walton (1971) summarized this as follows:

Most authorities agree ... that the pads of the fingers are the most sensitive portions of the hands available to diagnosis; that part of the pad just distal to the last interphalangeal articulation is the most sensitive. Also – the thumb and first two fingers are the best to use.

Sutton (1977) differentiates the loci of sensitivity in the hands:

The pads of the fingers are most sensitive for fine tactile discrimination and require light touch. The dorsal surfaces of the hands are most sensitive to temperature changes, while the palmar surfaces of the metacarpo-phalangeal joints are more sensitive to vibratory changes. The center of the palm is sensitive to gross shape recognition.

These ideas will be expanded on, with exercises for enhancement of palpatory skills as we progress.

Ford (1989) reminds us that we commonly "project" our sense of touch, giving the example of writing with a pencil. We feel the texture of the page on which we are writing, not at our skin surface or in our fingertips, but at the end of the pencil, thus demonstrating how our proprioceptive awareness can be projected. Ford suggests you experiment by:

Changing the pressure with which you grasp the pencil – you'll quickly discover that you can't write. The pressure exerted to hold the pencil needs to be constant so you can extend your perception to [the] pencil tip and thereby control the complex task of writing. A good craftsperson knows this instinctively. The woodworker's sense of touch extends to the teeth of the saw, a machinist's to the end of a wrench, a surgeon's to the edge of a scalpel, an artist's to the tip of a brush.

In days gone by, when a physician had to diagnose by touch: "A good practitioner did not feel a tumor at his fingertips but he projected his vibratory and pressure sensations into the patient." So we regularly project our sense of touch beyond our physical being and, in palpation, says Ford: "We merely make the ordinarily unconscious process available to our conscious mind. In so doing we cross the delicate boundary between self and other, to explore, to learn and ultimately to help."

Mitchell et al. (1979), in their classic text on muscle energy techniques, explain what they believe palpation to be aiming at: "Palpation is the art of feeling tissues with your hands in such a manner that changes in tension and position within these tissues can be readily noticed, diagnosed and treated." This is the very simplest aim of palpation, for the method and the instrument (finger pads? whole hand?), it seems, can vary, and the objectives can become ever more refined.

Mitchell (1976), writing alone this time, examined the subject of the training and measurement of sensory literacy (he coupled visual and palpatory literacy in the term "sensory literacy") in a wider sense:

The necessity for projecting one's tactile senses to varying distances through an intervening medium must seem mystical and esoteric to many beginning students. The projection of the palpatory sense through varying thicknesses of tissue is actually a refinement of the sense of tension and hardness. This sense is capable of even further refinement, through perceptual eidetic imagery, to be able to recognize, characterize, and quantify potential energies in living tissues. Thus some osteopaths are able to read in the tissues the exact history of past trauma.

Achieving the ideal of skilled palpation requires mastery of a number of subtle abilities. For example, Kappler (1997) suggests we need to be able to estimate:

- the weight of objects
- the amount of pressure needed to move them
- the resistance being exerted against any pressure we may be applying.

These skills are necessary to discriminate accurately the variations in motion of tissues, whether we are moving them, or whether the movement is generated from the tissues themselves (muscular movement, for example), or whether movement derives from some inherent motion (pulsation, etc.).

Localizing dysfunction: practical value of skilled palpation

As we progress through the chapters that aim to build palpation skills, we should arrive at a point where specific dysfunctional tissues can be localized for therapeutic attention. In osteopathic medicine the locality of a dysfunctional musculoskeletal area is noted as having a number of common characteristics, summarized by the acronym ARTT (sometimes rearranged as TART). These characteristics are further evaluated and defined in later sections of the book as they apply to skin, muscle, joints, etc.

Gibbons and Tehan (2001) explain the basis of osteopathic ARTT palpation, when assessing for somatic dysfunction (their particular focus is on spinal and joint dysfunction), as follows:

A relates to asymmetry

DiGiovanna (1991) links the criteria of asymmetry to a positional focus, stating that the "position of the vertebra or other bone is asymmetrical." Greenman (1996) broadens the concept of asymmetry by including functional, in addition to structural, asymmetry.

R relates to range of motion

Alteration in range of motion can apply to a single joint, several joints, or a region of the musculoskeletal system. The abnormality may be either restricted or increased mobility and includes assessment of quality of movement and "end-feel."

T relates to tissue texture changes

The identification of tissue texture change is important in the diagnosis of somatic dysfunction. Palpable changes may be noted in superficial, intermediate, and deep tissues. It is important for clinicians to be able to distinguish normal from abnormal.

T relates to tissue tenderness

Undue tissue tenderness may be evident. Pain provocation and reproduction of familiar symptoms are often used to localize somatic dysfunction.

How valid is the ARTT model?

Fryer et al. (2004) have confirmed that sites in the thoracic paravertebral muscles, identified by deep palpation as displaying "abnormal tissue texture," also showed greater tenderness than adjacent tissues, thus confirming the T and T elements of ARTT.

In a follow-up study, Fryer et al. (2005) examined the possibility that tissue texture irregularity of paravertebral sites might be due to greater cross-sectional thickness of the paraspinal muscle bulk. Diagnostic ultrasound showed that this was not the case.

A further study (Fryer et al. 2006) examined the electromyographic (EMG) activity of deep paraspinal muscles, lying below paravertebral thoracic muscles, with "altered texture," that were also more tender than surrounding ones. This demonstrated increased EMG activity in these dysfunctional muscles, that is, they were hypertonic.

Blending the elements

Denslow (1964) makes it clear that while each of the various ARTT elements can be palpated for and assessed separately, students should start the process of assessing for dysfunction by thinking of these as separate activities. Over time, he suggests, "these elements will be blended into a single procedure … to secure, more or less simultaneously, information concerning tenderness, tissue tone, motion and alignment." Denslow also notes that the changes being assessed have been given a number of titles by different researchers and clinicians, including "faulty mechanics" (Goldthwait 1937), "trigger zones" [or points] (Travell 1951), "segmental neuralgia," and hyperalgesic zones (Lewit 1992). Additionally these changes may be described as "subluxations" and "facet syndrome" in chiropractic, as well as "osteopathic lesions" and "somatic dysfunctions" in osteopathic medicine.

If an area "feels" different from usual, and/or appears different, symmetrically speaking (one side from the other), and/or displays a restriction in normal range of motion, and/or is tender to the touch, dysfunction and distress are present. The nature of the dysfunction is not revealed, merely its presence. These elements, together with the history and presenting symptoms, can then usefully be related to the degree of acuteness or chronicity, so that tentative conclusions can be reached as to the nature of the problem, and what therapeutic interventions are most appropriate.

Exercises are presented in various chapters, but particularly Chapters 5 and 8, in which ARTT characteristics are evaluated.

Specific objectives

Walton (1971), discussing physical examination as it relates to superficial and then deep palpation, points to specific objectives that should be looked for:

There are five types of change to be noted by superficial palpation in both acute and chronic lesions: skin changes, temperature changes, superficial muscle tensions, tenderness, and oedema.

And for deeper palpation:

The operator increases the pressure on his palpating fingers sufficiently to make a contact with the tissues deep in the skin ... six types of change may be noted: mobility, tenderness, oedema, deep muscle tension, fibrosis and interosseous changes. All but fibrosis can be perceived in both acute and chronic lesions.

In order to achieve the basic objective of being able to assess and judge such changes, education of the hands and development of heightened proprioceptive sensibility in the detection and amplification of subtle messages are required (see Exercises 3.12–3.14 in particular). This should then be followed by appropriate interpretation of the information.

- *Detection* is a matter of being aware of the possible findings and practicing the techniques required to expose these possibilities.

- *Amplification* requires localized concentration on a specific task and the ability to block out extraneous information.

- *Interpretation* is the ability to relate the information received via detection and amplification.

As indicated in Chapter 1, it is the detection and amplification aspects of palpation with which we are largely concerned, since what you subsequently do with any information thus gathered (i.e., how you interpret it) will largely depend upon your training and belief system.

Philip Greenman (1989) has defined the three stages of palpation as being *reception, transmission, and interpretation*, and he offers a useful caution, that care be taken over the hands ("these sensitive diagnostic instruments") as we develop coordinated, symmetrical skills, linked with our visual sense.

Avoidance of injury abuse is essential, hands should be clean, and nails an appropriate length. During the palpation the operator should be relaxed and comfortable to avoid extraneous interference with the transmission of the palpatory impulse. In order accurately to assess and interpret the palpatory findings it is essential that the physician concentrate on the act of palpation, the tissue being palpated, and the response of the palpating fingers and hands. All extraneous sensory stimuli should be reduced as much as possible. **Probably the most common mistake in palpation is the lack of concentration by the examiner.** [My emphasis]

Moving beyond the physical assessments towards the palpation of subtle circulatory and energy rhythms and patterns, as described in craniosacral therapy, "zero balancing," and the work of various osteopathic researchers, requires that palpation skills be further refined (see Chapter 15).

Where then should we begin in the process of developing and/or enhancing our proprioceptive and palpatory skills? Exercises that can help in this task have been formulated by many experts, and a good starting point would be to practice the following examples until you are comfortable with your ability to obtain the information demanded, without undue difficulty. These exercises are based on the advice and work of numerous individuals who have described specific methods for the acquisition of high levels of palpatory literacy. They are meant to be introduced more or less in the sequence in which they are presented in the book, in order to gradually refine sensitivity.

Important comparative descriptors

Before starting these exercises (which are not only useful for beginners but are excellent for refreshing the skills of the more experienced therapist), it is useful to prepare a number of comparative descriptive terms for that which will be palpated. Thus, we should have a number of what Greenman (1989) calls "paired descriptors." These can include:

- superficial/deep
- compressible/rigid
- warm/cold
- moist or damp/dry
- painful/pain-free
- local or circumscribed/diffuse or widespread
- relaxed/tense
- hypertonic/hypotonic
- normal/abnormal

   and so on … .

It is also useful to begin, when appropriate, to think in terms of whether any abnormality is acute, subacute, or chronic (Box 3.2).

In making such an assessment you might wish to couple this with information from the patient in order to confirm the accuracy or otherwise of the finding. Thus, if tissue feels chronically altered, and the patient confirms that the area has been troublesome for longer than 4 weeks, an accurate "reading" was made. (Obviously, in many instances, acute exacerbation of a chronic area of dysfunction may be what is being palpated, a confusing but useful palpatory exercise.)

The degree of change should also be noted, using a subjective scale for conditions that seem to be mild, moderate or severe. A simple numerical code can be used to identify where on this scale the palpated tissues lie.

Box 3.2 Acute, subacute, and chronic

In general terms:

1. acute conditions relate to the past few weeks
2. subacute to between 2 and 4 weeks
3. chronic to longer than 4 weeks

Palpation exercises

Viola Frymann (1963) summarized some very simple starting points for developing sufficient sensitivity to commence efficient palpation of the living body. When we come to palpating tissue, she advises that we palpate direct, not through clothing, and that we remain as relaxed as possible during the whole process. This is important, as unnecessary tensions interfere with perception.

It is also vital that we use only sufficient weight in our contact with the region being palpated, and that this contact should be slowly applied to allow time for "attunement" to the tissue being assessed. The gauging of tissue resistance is attained by the application of your own muscle sense, your work sense. It is not merely a contact sense, but involves sensations deriving from work being done by the muscles. The objective of the following series of simple exercises is to begin to refine these palpation skills.

Some of Frymann's exercises help to increase the sensitivity required for very light palpation, needed for noting elasticity, turgor, moisture, sebaceous activity, relative warmth or coldness of tissues, and so on. It is strongly suggested that all of the exercises in the book be practiced many times, and that even experienced individuals, with well-evolved skills in this field, go back to some of the apparently simple exercises from time to time. It is a process that can be regarded as a voyage of discovery. A sense of profound satisfaction awaits you when you realize just how much you can learn to read tissues with your sense of touch.

Exercise 3.1 *Coin Palpation*

Time suggested **several minutes at a time with each hand**

- Have an assortment of different denomination coins, in a container.
- Remove one coin at a time, with your eyes closed.
- Carefully feel each side of the coin and decide, by virtue of its size and weight, what value it represents.
- Carefully palpate and identify which is heads, and which is tails.
- Do the same with a number of different size/value coins.
- Repeat at regular intervals until you can identify and name the coins.

Exercise 3.2 *Coin Through Paper Palpation*

Time suggested **2–4 minutes with each hand**

- Place a coin under a telephone directory, or other thick, soft-covered book.
- Try to find the coin by careful palpation of the upper surface.
- If this is too difficult at first, do it initially with a magazine, gradually increasing the thickness of the barrier between your fingers and the coin, until the telephone directory itself presents no problem.
- Incorporate variations in which you use different parts of the hand to palpate for the coin.

Exercise 3.3 *Hair Through Paper Palpation*

Time suggested **2–4 minutes with each hand**

- Place a human hair under a page of a telephone directory, and palpate for it through the page, eyes closed.
- Once this becomes relatively easy, place the hair under two pages, and then three, doing the same thing, feeling slowly and carefully for the slight variations of the surface overlaying the hair.
- Now how long does it take you to feel the hair?
- Repeat until it is easy and quick.
- Incorporate variations in which you use different parts of the hand to palpate for the hair.

Exercise 3.4 *Inanimate Object Discrimination*

Time suggested **3–5 minutes with each hand**

- Sit at a table (blindfolded) and try to distinguish variations between objects on the table, made out of different materials: wood, plastic, metal, bone and clay, for example.
- Describe what you feel – shape, temperature, surface texture, resilience, flexibility, etc.
- Do materials of organic and non-organic origin have a different feel?
- Describe any differences you noted.

Chapter 3

Exercise 3.5 *Wood Density Palpation*

Time suggested 5 minutes with each hand

Van Allen (1964) developed a training method for enhancing perception of what he termed tissue "density." He obtained several blocks of wood, measuring 2 × 4 × 18 inches (5 × 10 × 46 cm), of very soft wood (pine), and of progressively harder woods (cherry, walnut, maple). He states:

Sliding one's fingers over these blocks revealed the differences in density and was a good exercise in developing tactile sensitivity. In some of these blocks I bored inch [1.9 cm] holes from the underside, half the length, to within a quarter of an inch [0.6 cm] of the upper surface, and poured the holes full of lead, peaning it solidly with a ball-pean hammer. The blocks appeared uniform as they lay face up, with the leaded ends, some one way and some another. It was not too hard for most observers to tell which end was which as they slid their fingers over them. Osteopathic physicians varied widely in their ability to do this, some detecting the differences in one sweep of the fingers, others requiring many trials.

Those who did better in the "test" were the practitioners known for their palpatory skills.

Reproducing Van Allen's blocks, lead and all, may be somewhat difficult, but obtaining blocks of wood of uniform size but of differing density should not be difficult; schools teaching manual therapy should have a variety of these for their students to palpate and assess.

Exercise 3.6 *Black Bag/Box Palpation*

Time suggested 5 minutes with each hand

Mitchell (1976) suggested different ways of performing a basic palpation exercise. He urged paired students to palpate a number of objects (unseen by the student to be tested) which were inside a box (or bag) with an opening through which the palpating student could reach to palpate.

Mitchell suggested that such a "black box" could be used as the first stage of learning to assess temperature, texture, thickness, humidity, tension or hardness, shape (stereognosis), position, proprioception, size, motion proprioception, and so on.

Method: The hand palpates a hidden object (made of plastic, bone, metal, wood, ceramic, glass, etc.) and the student indicates what the object is, as well as what material it is made of, before bringing it out of the bag/box.

Exercise 3.7 *Layer Palpation Using Inanimate Materials*

Time suggested 5–10 minutes with each hand

- An elaboration on the use of a "black box" would be to enhance discriminatory faculties by including a variety of materials made of rubber, plastic, wood, metal, and so on of *varying thicknesses* in the "box." Both the material and its relative thickness should be estimated on palpation, and the results discussed.

- The materials in the box could also contain another variation, in which a rough textured material, say sandpaper of different degrees of roughness, could be covered by varying thicknesses of foam. Multiple variations could be created for the tuning of palpatory skills: "Layers of materials of varying tension and hardness could be superimposed. For example, somatic soft tissues overlaying bone could be simulated with stratified layers of foam padding, sheet rubber, and vinyl fabric" (Mitchell 1976).

In this way, a training device, with variable tensions, could be constructed, simulating muscular spasm, fibrotic changes, edema and bony structures, felt through varying thicknesses of soft tissue: "It would be reasonable to expect that training with such devices would increase a student's confidence in his/her ability to tell the difference between spastic muscle and bone, or between hypertrophied muscle and contracted muscle."

Exercise 3.8 *Palpation of Bone, Real and Plastic*

Time suggested **5–7 minutes using both hands**

Frymann (1963) suggested that the next objective should be to move from tools, to begin to increase the student's ability to study anatomy, using the hand instead of the eye. Her suggested exercise was as follows:

- Sit, with eyes closed, or wearing a blindfold, while palpating one of the cranial bones, or any other bone, real or plastic if you are unfamiliar with cranial structures.

- Articular structures should be felt for, and described in some detail (ideally with someone else handing the bone to you and with findings being spoken into a tape recorder for self-assessment later, when the object/bone can be studied with eyes open).

- The bone should be named, sided, and its particular features discussed.

- If you are new to cranial structures this is an excellent educational method for becoming familiar with their unique qualities.

While palpating this bone you should be asking:

- What is the nature of this object, is it plastic or bone?

- Can you discern attachment sites on the bone?

Then describe the difference in feel and character between plastic and real bone.

- Bone, although no longer living, has a slight compressive resilience that plastic never has; nor can plastic achieve the detail of sutural digitation that bone contains.

- Careful fingering of the unseen object would establish its shape and if anatomy is well enough understood, it could then be named and sided.

- The whole process of palpating is enhanced, suggests Frymann, if the arms are supported, so that the hands and fingers are unaffected by the weight of the arms.

Discussion regarding Exercises 3.1–3.8

Regular repetition, on a daily basis for a few minutes at a time, of the sort of exercises outlined above will bring a rapid increase in sensitivity and this is desirable as a prerequisite to palpating living tissue. Such exercises should continue even when you have moved on to palpating the living body. What should emerge with repetition of these exercises is a discriminatory facility, in which the *qualities* and *characteristics* of different materials, whether organic or inorganic, including their slightly raised surface elevations and depressions, and their temperatures when compared with each other, are all readily noted.

After building up sensitivity in palpation using inanimate objects it is time to move towards palpation of living tissues. The ability to know what normal tissue feels like is a most useful palpatory exercise, since anything that feels other than normal is bound to offer evidence of dysfunction. This suggests that it is useful to perform palpation exercises with a wide range of people who are relatively young and "normal," as well as individuals who are older, or who have suffered injury or stress in the tissues you intend palpating. It is my personal experience that the most "normal" muscles available for palpation are those belonging to preschool children, and even this group is often already dysfunctional in terms of muscular hypertonicity.

Exercise 3.9 *Living Bone Palpation*

Time suggested **5–7 minutes with each hand**

Whichever bone is used in the previous exercise (cranial or otherwise), this should be followed by a blindfolded palpation of the same bone in a live subject, with its contours, sutures (if cranial), resilience, and observed (not initiated) motion being felt for and described.

The person being palpated could be either lying down or seated.

When comparison is made with the live bone in this way, similarities and differences should gradually become apparent. The differences between the dead and live bone should be described and defined, ideally into a tape recorder.

Obviously, the living bone would not be palpated directly but through superficial tissue. This requires that the palpation become discriminating. Frymann (1963) talks of the "automatic selection device of our consciousness," filtering out information offered by soft tissues that overlie the bone that is being assessed.

If the bone chosen has superficial musculature the palpation should start lightly, just above and then on the skin itself, with gradual increasing pressure, to eventually have contact with the contours of the bone in question.

By applying attention to what is being palpated (for several minutes in the early stages), subtle awareness of motion *inherent in the live bone's existence* might also become apparent.

If this is a cranial bone, there are three rhythms that may be sensed – pulsation, respiration, and a slower rhythmic motion – and it is often possible to learn to focus gradually on one or other of these at will, filtering out the others.

We will come to exercises that will improve such discrimination later in the book.

Notes

Before attempting the next few exercises (Exercises 3.10–3.14 inclusive) you may find it useful to skip ahead to Chapter 13 (by Sasha Chaitow), particularly Exercises 13.1, Part 2, and Exercise 13.2; both of these focus on intuitive faculties and the topic of encouraging "superior knowing" – seeing with the "mind's eye."

Exercise 3.10 *Palpating for Inherent Motion*

Time suggested **not less than 5 minutes**

In order to begin to study and analyze more subtle movements, Frymann (1963) suggests that the student of palpation should feel for a rhythmic motion, by placing one hand on a spinal segment from which stems the neurological supply to an area that is simultaneously being palpated by the other hand. Examples include the upper thoracic

spine and the heart region, or the midthoracic spine and the liver.

By patiently focusing for some minutes, eyes closed, on what is being felt, she states, "a fluid wave will eventually be established between the two hands."

● Can you feel this, or something like it?

● If so, try to put what you are feeling into words.

Exercise 3.11 *Simultaneous Palpation of Normal and Abnormal Tissues*

Time suggested **not less than 5 minutes**

Mitchell (1976) suggests that palpation be simultaneously performed on normal tissues and those of individuals affected by pathology such as limb paralysis, inflammation, spasm or extreme hypertonicity, or some internal pathological or pathophysiological process.

Such a simultaneous palpation exercise might mean literally having a hand on the normal and the abnormal tissues at the same time, or palpating them sequentially, moving from one to the other and back again, seeking words to describe the differences you feel.

Simultaneous palpation of normal and diseased or distressed tissues offers an educational opportunity that all practitioners and students involved in bodywork should aim to experience.

Describe the different "feel" of normal and abnormal tissue, or simply of hypertonicity and hypotonicity, for example, after palpating for several minutes.

Exercise 3.12 *Frymann's Forearm Palpation for Inherent Motion*

Time suggested **10 minutes**

Frymann (1963) simplifies the initial palpation of living tissue, compared with non-living (sparing us the task of finding a warmed-up corpse).

● In order to become familiar with an unhurried contact with living tissue, Frymann suggests that the student of palpation should sit at a table, opposite a partner, one of whose arms rests on the table, flexor surface upwards. That arm should be totally relaxed.

- The student lays a hand onto that forearm with attention focused on what the palmar surface of the fingers are feeling; the other hand is resting on the firm table surface. This is to provide a *contrast reference* as the living tissue is palpated, to help to distinguish a region in motion from an area not in motion.

- Both elbows of the person who is palpating should rest on the table so that no stress builds up in the arm or shoulders.

- With eyes closed, unhurried focus and concentration should then be projected into what the fingers and palm are feeling, attuning to the arm surface being touched.

- Gradually, focus should be brought to the deeper tissues, under the skin as well (without any particular increase in contact pressure from the palpating hand) and finally, to the underlying bone.

- When the feel of the structure being touched and what lies below (skin, muscle, bone, etc.) has been sensed, the function of the tissues should be considered.

- Feel for pulsations and rhythms, periodically varying the pressure of your contact hand.

- Pay no attention to the structure of skin, or muscle, or bone. Wait patiently until you become aware of motion.

- Observe and describe that motion, its nature, its direction, its rhythm and amplitude, its consistency or its variation.

- Perform the same exercise on different parts of the body, and on different people, of varying body types, ages, genders.

This entire palpation exercise should take not less than 5 minutes, and ideally 10, and should be repeated with the other hand to ensure that palpation skills are not one-sided.

Remember that the objective of this exercise is to acclimatize you to evaluating inherent motion (minute pulsations, rhythms) once you have noted the structural aspect of what you are palpating.

Exercise 3.13 *Bimanual Inherent Motion Palpation 1*

Time suggested **5–10 minutes**

When you have palpated an arm (or thigh, or indeed any other part of the body) to the point where you are clearly picking up sensations of motion and rhythmic pulsation with one hand, place your other hand on the opposite side *of the same limb.*

- Is this hand picking up the same motions?

- Are the sensations similar, with the same rhythm previously noted, and is there the same degree of amplitude to the motion as the first sensation?

- In health, they will be the same. When there is a difference it may represent some form of dysfunction.

- Perform the same exercise on different parts of the body and on different people, of varying body types, ages, genders.

Exercise 3.14 *Bimanual Inherent Motion Palpation 2*

Time suggested **not less than 7 minutes**

Frymann (1963) suggests that on another occasion (or at the same session) you palpate one limb with one hand (say, upper arm) and another limb (say, thigh, for example) with the other and that you "rest in stillness until you perceive the respective motions within."

- Ask yourself whether any subtle rhythms you are feeling are synchronous and moving in the same direction.

- Are they consistent or do they appear to periodically undergo cyclical changes?

- You may actually sense, Frymann suggests, that the sensation being felt seems to pull in one direction more than another, with little or no tendency to return to a balanced neutral position.

- This, she suggests, may represent a pattern established as a result of trauma. Careful questioning may confirm the nature and direction of a previously experienced blow or injury.

- Perform the same exercise on different parts of the body and on different people, of varying body types, ages, genders.

Exercise 3.15 *Radial Pulse Assessment*

Time suggested 5–7 minutes with each hand

Upledger (Upledger & Vredevoogd 1983) suggests that palpation and assessment of more obvious pulsating rhythms should be practiced, for example involving the cardiovascular pulses. He describes the first stages of this learning process thus:

With the subject lying comfortably supine, palpate the radial pulses. Feel the obvious peak of the pulsation. Tune in also to the rise and fall of the pressure gradient.

- How long is diastole?
- What is the quality of the rise of pulse pressure after diastole? Is it sharp, gradual, smooth?
- How broad is the pressure peak?
- Is the pressure descent rapid, gradual, smooth or stepped?

Memorize the feel of the subject's pulse so that you can reproduce it in your mind after you have broken actual physical contact with the subject's body. You can often sing a song after you have heard it a few times; similarly, you should be able to mentally reproduce your palpatory perception of the pulse after you have broken contact.

Upledger then suggests you do the same thing with the carotid pulse, and subsequently palpate both radial and carotid pulses at the same time, and compare them.

Notes

See also Special topic 13, on traditional Chinese pulse palpation.

Fryman's views on pulse taking

There are some very important lessons to be learned when performing simple pulse taking. Frymann (1963) analyzed some of the almost instinctive strategies we adopt if we do this well, and which all should consider as they perform Exercise 3.15.

1. If the patient has a relatively normal systolic pressure (120 mmHg) light digital pressure on the pulse will obliterate it.

2. If the applied pressure is very light, only a very faint sensation will be palpated, if anything at all.

3. If, however, a light initial pressure is gradually increased, a variety of pulsation sensations will be noted, until the pulse is obliterated when the digital pressure overcomes the blood pressure.

Frymann notes that this is how blood pressure was assessed before the introduction of the sphygmomanometer.

Students of palpation should experiment with variation of the degree of pressure, noting the subtle differences that are perceived. In doing this we are learning to control the degree of applied digital pressure so that we meet the demands of particular tissues, in order to gain optimal access to the locked-in information. Issues regarding application of pressure are discussed in Special topic 1.

Frymann (1963) states:

The examiner must supply the equal and opposite force to that of the tissue to be studied, [for example] the pressure in the eyeball can be estimated by attaining a balance of pressure between the examining finger and the intraocular pressure. The maturity of an abscess can be estimated similarly. Action and reaction must be equal.

This is an important lesson in learning palpation and is echoed in later chapters when neuromuscular evaluation (NMT) methods are discussed and practiced, for example in Chapter 5.

Exercise 3.16 *Discrimination of Information Palpation*

Time suggested 3–5 minutes

- Lay both hands on the upper thorax of a supine individual and palpate cardiovascular activity.

- Focusing on the various characteristics of the perceived pulsations, alter your focus to the breathing pattern and its multiple motions.

- Practice switching attention from the sensations associated with breathing to cardiovascular activity and back again, until you are comfortable with the idea of screening out "background" information from that which you want to examine.

- To highlight the subtle cardiovascular motions, have the person being palpated hold the breath for a few seconds at a time.

Accurate evaluation of many functional and pathological states depends upon the ability to filter out that information which you require from the many other motions and sensations which are being picked up by the palpating hands. This is an exercise to revisit many times.

Greenman's palpation exercises

Philip Greenman (1989, 1996) has described some excellent exercises for both beginners and the more experienced, to increase their palpation skills. These have been summarized as follows.

Exercise 3.17 *Forearm Layer Palpation (A: skin)*

Time suggested **7 minutes**

Sit with a partner, facing each other across a narrow table (Fig. 3.2). You are going to examine each other's left forearms with your right hands, so rest your left forearm on the table, palm downwards, and place your right (palpating) hand and fingers on your partner's left forearm, as he/she rests a hand and fingers on your forearm, just below the elbow.

The initial evaluation, without movement, calls for you to focus on what is being felt, noting the contours of your palpating partner's arm under the (very) light touch of your hand.

Project your thoughts to the sensors in your palpating hand, focusing first on the attributes of the skin in touch with your contact hand, which should initially be still.

- How warm/cool, dry/moist, thick/thin, rough/smooth is the palpated skin?

- You and your partner should now turn the forearm over, so that the same questions can be answered regarding the volar surface.

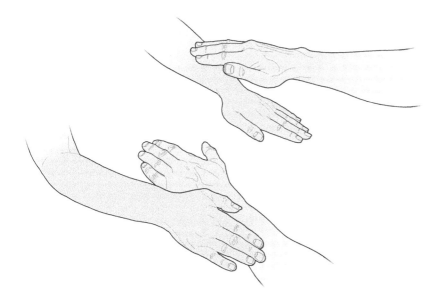

Figure 3.2
Forearm palpation exercise.

Compare what was palpated on the dorsal surface with what was palpated on the volar surface. Evaluate and put words to the differences noted in skin texture, temperature, thickness and so on.

Now, using the lightest ("feather-like") touch of one finger pad, run this along the skin of the forearm.

- Are there any areas which feel less smooth, which have an apparent roughness or moist feel, where your finger pad "drags"?

- Now, using a light pincer contact, lift a fold of skin and assess its elasticity and the speed with which it returns to normal when you release it. Do this on both surfaces of the forearm and compare these, as well as over areas of skin where "drag" was noted when you were lightly stroking with a finger pad. Record your findings.

Notes

The importance and meaning of variations in skin texture will be discussed fully in the next chapter.

Exercise 3.18 *Forearm Layer Palpation (B: skin on subcutaneous fascia)*

Time suggested **5 minutes**

- In the same position, make small hand motions while a firm contact is being maintained with the skin, moving this in relation to its underlying tissues.

- Move your hand both longitudinally and horizontally, in relation to the forearm, and evaluate what is being palpated as you move the skin on the subcutaneous fascial tissues.

- Try to assess its thickness and elasticity, its "tightness or looseness."

- Do the surface tissues move, glide, slide, more freely in some directions compared with others?

- Compare the findings from the dorsal and volar surfaces of your partner's forearm and also compare variations in areas where skin texture, "drag," etc. were different in the earlier palpation.

- Write down or record your findings.

Exercise 3.19 *Forearm Layer Palpation (C: blood vessels)*

Time suggested **5 minutes**

- With this same contact, palpate the subcutaneous fascial layer for the arteries and veins that lie in it.

- Use an anatomical atlas if you are rusty regarding this aspect of anatomy.

- In particular, find and palpate the radial artery.

- Identify (i.e., name) and describe as many of the blood vessels you can feel as possible, from wrist to elbow.

- Assess the difference in size, texture and quality of perceived internal motion of fluids as you compare veins and arteries.

- Have your palpation partner clench a fist and note what happens to the blood vessels over the course of a minute or so.

Exercise 3.20 *Forearm Layer Palpation (D: deeper fascia)*

Time suggested **5 minutes**

- In the same position, concentrate attention on the deeper fascia that surrounds, invests, and separates muscle, by increasing your hand pressure *slightly*.

- Use slow horizontal movements of the hands/fingers in order to try to identify thickened areas of fascia that act as envelopes that compartmentalize and separate muscle bundles.

- It is in the subcutaneous, and deeper, fascial layers that much somatic dysfunction is to be found, ranging from trigger points to stress bands, relating to overuse, misuse, or abuse.

- Look in particular for a sense of hardness, or thickening, that suggests dysfunction.

- Palpate as much of the fascia between the elbow and wrist as possible, and note your findings.

Exercise 3.21 *Forearm Layer Palpation (E: muscle fibers)*

Time suggested 5–7 minutes

- With the same position and contact, feel through the fascia to locate muscle bundles and fibers.

- Note their relative degrees of pliability or hardness and see whether you can feel their directions of action.

- You and your partner should now slowly open and close the left fist in order to tense and relax the muscles being palpated.

- Sense the variations in tone in the muscle fibers as this happens, particularly the difference between tissues with increased tone and relaxed tissue.

- Next you and your palpating partner should both hold your left fists closed, quite strongly, as you each palpate the hypertonic state of the forearm muscles, a useful preparation for what will be palpated in most patients, where overuse, misuse, or abuse has been operating.

- Describe the textures and variations in tone that you have noted during this exercise.

Exercise 3.22 *Forearm Layer Palpation (F: musculotendinous interface)*

Time suggested 5–7 minutes

The arm being palpated should now be relaxed.

Move your palpating fingers down the forearm toward the wrist and identify the interface between muscle and tendon (musculotendinous junction).

Continue to palpate the tendon itself, onwards towards its point of attachment, where the tendon is bound to the wrist by an overlying structure, the transverse carpal ligament.

Palpate this and see whether you can identify the various directions of fiber angle.

- Which way does the tendon run?

- Which way does the ligamentous structure run?

- Describe in writing or on tape the characteristics and "feel" of what you have palpated.

Review an anatomy/physiology text to help evaluate the accuracy of what you thought you were feeling.

Exercise 3.23 *Forearm Layer Palpation (G: active elbow joint)*

Time suggested 7 minutes

Move back up to the elbow and with your middle finger resting in the hollow on the dorsal side of the elbow and your thumb on the ventral surface of the elbow, palpate the radial head. Feel its shape and texture.

- How hard is it?

- Does it move on slight pressure?

- What do you feel if you move your finger and thumb slightly higher on the elbow, over the joint space itself?

You should not be able to feel the joint capsule, unless there exists gross pathology of the joint. Your contact is just above the joint.

Have your partner slowly, actively, pronate and supinate the arm and note what you feel between your finger and thumb.

- How does the end of range of motion vary with the action of pronation and supination?

- Is it symmetrical?

- Describe the end-feel (see Special topic 9 on "End-feel").

- Which end of range seems firmer/tighter (which has the harder end-feel) – supination or pronation?

Record your findings.

Exercise 3.24 *Forearm Layer Palpation (H: passive elbow joint)*

Time suggested 5 minutes

Now use your left hand to hold the hand and wrist of the arm you are palpating with your right hand. Introduce passive supination and pronation as you palpate the joint.

Assess the total range of motion as you slowly perform these movements.

You are receiving two sets of proprioceptive information at this stage, from the palpating hand and from the one which is introducing motion.

Describe the range and the end-feel, in both supination and pronation when these are passively introduced, as well as comparing active (as in the previous exercise) with passive findings.

- Does supination or pronation have the harder or softer end-feel, and which seems to have the greatest range of motion?

- Are you aware of the build-up of tension in the tissues ("bind") as you approach the end of the range of movement?

- Are you equally aware of the sense of tissue freedom ("ease") as you move away from that barrier?

Try to become aware of "ease" and "bind" as you move the joint in varying directions.

- Can you find a point of balance somewhere between the ends of range of motion in pronation and supination where tissues feel at their most free?

- If so, you have found what is called the physiological neutral point, or point of balance, which is a key feature of functional osteopathic treatment.

We will be returning to this concept and will perform more exercises involving the neutral point in later chapters.

Discussion regarding exercises 3.9–3.24

The exercises covered in this segment have focused on enhancing perception of subtle motions, inherent movements and pulsations, that might derive from a variety of sources.

Kappler (1997) has noted that:

Inherent motion is activity unconsciously generated within the body such as respiratory motion or peristalsis … [and] is postulated to occur in several ways, biochemically at the cellular or sub-cellular level; as part of multiple electrical patterns; as a combination of a number of circulatory and electrical patterns; as some periodic pattern not yet understood.

The term "entrainment" is sometimes used to describe the way in which multiple pulsations and rhythms in the body combine to form a harmonic palpable sensation (Oschman 2001). Physicists use entrainment to describe a situation in which two rhythms that have nearly the same frequency become coupled to each other. Technically, entrainment means the mutual phase locking of two or more oscillators. There are suggestions that evidence exists of therapeutic influences from this phenomenon; for example, in a setting such as craniosacral therapy, the multiple rhythms and pulsations of the therapist might influence the more dysfunctional rhythms of the patient to return to a more normal state (Chaitow 1999; Oschman 2001).

The palpation exercises in the early part of this chapter are designed to encourage awareness of subtle motions, largely outside the conscious influence of the person being assessed. In these as well as in the later exercises, especially those involving the musculoskeletal structures of the forearm, Greenman cautions that the most common errors might involve:

- a lack of concentration

- the use of excessive pressure

- too much movement.

In other words, when performing these palpations, touch lightly and slowly, and above all focus on what you are feeling, if you want to learn to palpate effectively.

Palpation skill status

The exercises in this chapter will help you to gain (or enhance) an ability to differentiate (and describe) the shape, size, texture, flexibility and temperature of varying thicknesses and combinations of a variety of inorganic materials; to become able to discriminate between organic and inorganic, living and dead materials and tissues, as well as living tissues in varying states of health, and the first stages of assessment of body pulsations and rhythms, with the facility to screen one from another, at will, being a key stage in developing palpatory literacy.

It may also be possible for you now to sense the residual forces associated with "tissue memory," a concept which will be examined more closely in later chapters.

These exercises can all be varied and altered to meet particular needs. They represent the ideas of some of the leading experts, and provide a starting point in the adventure in exploration of inner space that follows.

References

Chaitow L (1999) Cranial manipulation: Theory and practice. Edinburgh: Churchill Livingstone.

Denslow J (1964) Palpation of the musculoskeletal system. Journal of the American Osteopathic Association 63 (7): 23–31.

DiGiovanna E (1991) Somatic dysfunction, in DiGiovanna E and Schiowitz S (eds) An Osteopathic Approach to Diagnosis and Treatment. Philadelphia: JB Lippincott, pp 6–12.

Ford C (1989) Where healing waters meet. New York: Station Hill Press.

Fryer G, Morris T and Gibbons P (2004) The relationship between palpation of thoracic paraspinal tissues and pressure sensitivity measured by a digital algometer. International Journal of Osteopathic Medicine 7 (2): 64–69.

Fryer G, Morris T and Gibbons P (2005) The relationship between palpation of thoracic tissues and deep paraspinal muscle thickness. International Journal of Osteopathic Medicine 8 (1): 22–28.

Fryer G, Morris T, Gibbons P et al. (2006) The activity of thoracic paraspinal muscles identified as abnormal with palpation. Journal of Manipulative and Physiological Therapeutics 29 (6): 437–447

Frymann V (1963) Palpation – its study in the workshop. Newark: Yearbook of the American Academy of Osteopathy, pp 16–30.

Gibbons P and Tehan P (2001) Spinal manipulation: Indications, risks and benefits. Edinburgh: Churchill Livingstone.

Goldthwait J (1937) Body mechanics, 2nd edn. Philadelphia: JB Lippincott.

Greenman P (1989) Principles of manual medicine. Baltimore: Williams and Wilkins.

Greenman P (1996) Principles of manual medicine, 2nd edn. Baltimore: Williams and Wilkins.

Kappler R (1997) Palpatory skills, in Ward R (ed) Foundations for Osteopathic Medicine. Baltimore: Williams and Wilkins.

Kappler R, Larson N and Kelso A (1971) A comparison of osteopathic findings on hospitalized patients obtained by trained student examiners and experienced physicians. Journal of the American Osteopathic Association 70 (10): 1091–1092.

Korr I (1970) Physiological basis of osteopathic medicine. New York: Postgraduate Institute of Osteopathic Medicine and Surgery.

Kuchera W and Kuchera M (1994) Osteopathic principles and practice, 2nd edn. Columbus, OH: Greyden Press.

Lewit K (1992) Manipulative therapy in rehabilitation of the locomotor system, 3rd edn. London: Butterworths.

Mitchell F (1976) Training and measuring sensory literacy. Newark, OH: Yearbook of the American Academy of Osteopathy, pp 120–127.

Mitchell F, Moran P and Pruzzo N (1979) An evaluation of osteopathic muscle energy procedure. Valley Park, MI: Pruzzo.

Oschman J (2001) Energy medicine. Edinburgh: Churchill Livingstone.

Sutton S (1977) An osteopathic method of history taking and physical examination. Journal of the American Osteopathic Association 77 (7): 845–858.

Travell J (1951) Pain mechanisms in connective tissues, in Regan C (ed) Transactions of 2nd Conference on Connective Tissues. New York: Josiah Macy Foundation, pp 86–125.

Uddin Z, MacDermid JC and Hyungjoo HH (2014) Test–retest reliability and validity of normative cut-offs of the two devices measuring touch threshold: Weinstein Enhanced Sensory Test and Pressure-Specified Sensory Device. Hand Therapy 19 (1): 3–10.

Upledger J and Vredevoogd W (1983) Craniosacral therapy. Seattle: Eastland Press.

Van Allen P (1964) Improving our skills. Newark, OH: Academy of Applied Osteopathy Yearbook, pp 147–152.

Walton W (1971) Palpatory diagnosis of the osteopathic lesion. Journal of the American Osteopathic Association 71: 117–131.

Special topic 3

Visual assessment, the dominant eye, and other issues
Leon Chaitow

Many experts advise that, before starting to palpate, you should identify your dominant eye. Almost all of us have one eye that dominates, and the reasoning is that during the application of assessment procedures you should position yourself, in relation to the patient or body part, so that the dominant eye has the clearest possible view of what is being observed.

Clearly this is of little importance when palpating with the eyes closed (a common recommendation to reduce distractions and enhance palpation sensitivity). There will, however, be many instances when visual impressions need to be combined with palpation, for example, in use of the "red reaction" (see, for example, the assessment of ASIS levels as described in Chapter 8).

Assessing the dominant eye

- Hold both arms in front of you and with the hands, create a "triangular" space through which, with both eyes open, you can observe some object across the room (Special topic Fig. 3.1.).

- Close one eye. If the object is still in the triangle, you now have your dominant eye open.

- If, however, the image shifts out of the triangle when only one eye is open, open the closed eye and close the open eye, and the image should shift back into clear view, inside the triangle.

- The eye that sees the same view as was seen when both eyes were open is the one to use in close observation of the body.

- If the patient is on an examination table, you should approach from the side that allows your dominant eye to be closest to the center of the couch.

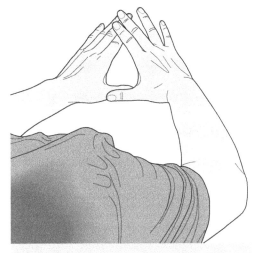

Figure ST 3.1
Creating a triangle through which to look.

Using peripheral vision

- In some instances, when symmetrical motion is being observed, such as when bilateral rib function is being assessed, it is a mistake to closely observe one side and then the other.

- You should instead rely on the sensitive discrimination that peripheral vision offers.

- Focus on a point between your two moving fingers, which rest on the ribs, and allow your peripheral vision to judge variations in range of motion, as the patient breathes.

The use of the dominant eye will be referred to in various exercises when it is appropriate.

By the way, if you are right-handed with a dominant left eye, or left-handed with a dominant right eye, both of which are unusual combinations, you would probably make an excellent batsman in cricket or hitter in baseball!

Body position and the eyes

Vladimir Janda (1988) points to the existence of oculopelvic and pelviocular reflexes which indicate that any change in pelvic orientation alters the position of the eyes, and vice versa. He also discusses the fact that eye position modifies muscle tone, particularly the suboccipital muscles (for example, look upwards and extensors tighten, look down and flexors tone to prepare for activity, etc.).

The implications of modified eye position, due to altered pelvic and head positions, therefore add yet another set of factors to be considered as we try to ensure that observational and palpatory efficiency are optimal (Komendatov 1945).

"Sensory literacy"

Frederick Mitchell Jr (Mitchell 1976), writing on the topic of training and measurement of sensory literacy, discussed the various "parts" of vision. As Mitchell puts it, can you judge, visually, the following:

- Does the patient have good or poor posture, and if poor, how poor?
- Is a laceration 2.5 cm or 3 cm in length?
- Are the iliac crests equal in height?
- Is the patient's head tilted, and by how many degrees?
- Is one knee larger than the other?
- Is dermatosis violaceous or merely pink?

In order to make such judgments, Mitchell lists the need to be able to:

1. identify and discriminate color hues and saturations
2. quantify "rectilinear length measurements, angular measurements, curvilinear and arcuate shapes, and their radius of curvature"
3. sense horizontal and vertical frames of reference, in which to make quantitative judgments
4. appreciate motion, absolute motion, or subjective awareness of motion, in relation to himself, or relative motion of one thing to another thing
5. demonstrate depth perception and the ability to estimate length and proportion.

All sighted individuals have these skills, but the degree of keenness is variable, and Mitchell suggests ways of measuring and of enhancing "visual literacy" by means of training devices which, for example, simulate an extremity's range of motion or leg length differences in a supine patient or levels of iliac crest height in a standing patient.

When such tools are utilized in classroom settings, the student remains unaware of the true angle or length or height until having made an estimation. There then needs to be an immediate feedback of information because, as Mitchell explains:

Success builds confidence. Failure destroys confidence. It is not unlikely that self-confidence may be an essential ingredient of reliability in accuracy of visual judgment. As accuracy and reliability in making visual judgments increases the student learns to avoid parallax errors and to deal with the possibilities of optical illusion.

Eye dominance appears to be a significant element in the accuracy of visual judgment and becoming aware of backgrounds.

Lighting is also a part of the training process and is important in eliminating optical illusions as a source of error.

Visual assessment in a physical examination

Dinnar et al. (1982) provide the following summary of the questions you might ask yourself during the visual component – observation – of a physical examination, in which screening occurs from three viewpoints: posterior, lateral, and anterior.

You might assess your ability to make these observations now, before you start to work your way through the many exercises in this book, and perhaps some time later when you have applied the exercises and hopefully enhanced those skills.

Special topic exercise 3.1 *Postural Screening*

Time suggested: 15 minutes

This visual screening is designed to give an initial impression – it is not diagnostic.

The patient is standing.

1. Posterior view

- Are shoulders and scapulae asymmetrical (unequal)?
- Is there a lateral curvature of the midspinal line?
- Is the head held to one side?
- Is the pelvic position asymmetrical (are crests level)?
- Is there obvious flatness or fullness of the paravertebral muscle mass?
- Are the feet placed symmetrically or not?
- Are the positions of the knees symmetrical?
- Is the body rotated as a whole?
- Are the Achilles tendons deviated or symmetrical?
- Are the positions of the malleoli symmetrical in relation to the heels?
- Are arm positions symmetrical?
- Are the fat folds (creases) at the waist symmetrical?
- Is there any obvious morphological asymmetry of the posterior skin surface such as scars, bruises?

2. Lateral view

- Are the knees relaxed or locked in extension?
- Are the normal spinal curves exaggerated or reversed?

- Is the body displaced relative to the center of gravity; for example, is the head position balanced?
- Is there any obvious morphological asymmetry of the lateral skin surface such as scars, bruises?

3. Anterior view

- Are the shoulder levels symmetrical at the mid-sternal line?
- Is the head tilted to one side?
- Does the normal horizontal clavicular line deviate?
- Is the pelvic position asymmetrical (are crests level)?
- Are the patellae deviated laterally or medially?
- Is there any obvious morphological asymmetry of the anterior skin surface such as scars, bruises?

References

Dinnar U, Beal M, Goodridge J et al. (1982) An osteopathic method of history taking and physical examination. Journal of the American Osteopathic Association 81 (5): 314–321.

Janda V (1988), in Grant R (ed) Physical therapy in the cervical and thoracic spine. New York: Churchill Livingstone.

Komendatov G (1945) Proprioceptivnije reflexi glaza i golovy u krolikov. Fiziologiceskij Zurnal 31: 62.

Mitchell F (1976) Training and measurement of sensory literacy. Journal of the American Osteopathic Association 75 (6): 874–884.

When you palpate the skin, you are in touch with the boundary that separates the individual from the outside world. This offers a rich potential source of information. Contact with someone else's skin can break emotional and resistance barriers. This process can be seen as both a unique privilege and an opportunity, which can be used to great advantage by those bodyworkers who focus on both the mind and the physical condition of their patients. The body surface seems to reflect the state of the mind intimately, altering its electrical as well as its palpable physical properties.

Deane Juhan (1987) has set the scene for our understanding of the skin's importance:

The skin is no more separated from the brain than the surface of a lake is separated from its depths; the two are different locations in a continuous medium. "Peripheral" and "central" are merely spatial distinctions, distinctions which do more harm than good if they lure us into forgetting that the brain is a single functional unit, from cortex to fingertips and toes. **To touch the surface is to stir the depths.** [My emphasis]

Learning to read changes on this surface is not easy, but contact with it provides a chance for exploration of much that is obvious, and much that is deeply hidden. We will examine various concepts that relate to the mind–body link in Chapter 15. However, at this stage we need to look more closely at some of the physical characteristics of the skin.

As mentioned in the previous chapters, the changes that should easily be read by the palpator include the relative degree of:

- warmth/coolness
- dryness/dampness
- smoothness/roughness
- elasticity/rigidity

… as well as the relative degree of thickness of the skin, in the region.

Much research and clinical experience suggests that altered skin physiology of this sort is often an end-result of dysfunction, involving the sympathetic nervous system, especially as it relates to the musculoskeletal system (Gutstein 1944; Korr 1977; Lewit 1999) (see Box 4.1).

Aspects of skin physiology

In order to understand some of the dynamics involved in skin function and dysfunction, as well as some of the potential pitfalls possible in skin palpation, a brief examination of some aspects of the physiology of skin is necessary.

Credit for much of the material in this section should go to Adams and colleagues (1982), a group of American researchers. Their review is a brilliant examination of some of the many interacting elements that make the skin such a critical area in palpation.

Box 4.1   Skin as a monitor of reflexive behavior

Brugger (1962) has described pseudoradicular syndromes that are distinct from root syndromes, and that derive from a "nociceptive somatomotoric blocking effect", in tissues such as joint capsules, tendon origins, and other local (to joint) tissues. These painful reflex effects are noted in muscles and their tendinous junctions, as well as the skin. Dvorak and Dvorak (1984) include in this category of referred pain and symptoms the phenomena of viscerosomatic and somatovisceral influences, in which, for example, organ dysfunction is said to produce tendomyotic changes (Korr 1975).

The reflex changes that can be observed or palpated include various patterns of vasomotor abnormality such as coldness, pallor, redness, cyanosis, etc.

Gutstein (1944) maintained that normalization of skin secretions, and therefore of hair and skin texture and appearance, can be achieved by the removal of active trigger points in the cervical and interscapular areas. The conditions of hyper-, hypo-, and anhidrosis may accompany vasomotor and sebaceous dysfunction. Gutstein observed that abolition of excessive

---

Box 4.1 *continued*

perspiration as well as anhidrosis followed appropriate treatment.

Korr (1970, 1976, 1977) noted in his research that readings of resistance to electricity in the paraspinal skin of an individual showed that there were often marked differences, with one side showing normal electrical resistance and the other showing reduced resistance (an area of segmental facilitation). When "stress" (e.g., compression or needling) was applied elsewhere in the body and the two areas of the spine were monitored, it was the area of facilitation that showed a marked rise in electrical (neurological) activity (Fig. 4.1).

Beal (1985) has described this phenomenon as resulting from afferent stimuli, arising from dysfunction of a visceral nature.

- The reflex is initiated by afferent impulses arising from visceral receptors being transmitted to the dorsal horn of the spinal cord, where they synapse with interconnecting neurons.

- The stimuli are then conveyed to sympathetic and motor efferents, resulting in changes in the somatic tissues, such as skeletal muscle, skin, and blood vessels.

- Abnormal stimulation of the visceral efferent neurons can result in hyperesthesia of the skin and associated vasomotor, pilomotor, and sudomotor changes.

- The first signs of such viscerosomatic reflexive influences are vasomotor (increased skin temperature) and sudomotor (increased moisture of the skin) reactions, skin textural changes (e.g., thickening), increased subcutaneous fluid and increased contraction of muscle.

Beal (1983) suggests that palpation should pay attention to the various soft tissue layers, particularly the skin, looking for changes *in texture, temperature and moisture.*

Lewit (1992) also emphasizes the value of light skin palpation in identifying areas of facilitation (sensitization). He notes that these signs tend to disappear if the visceral causes improve; however, when such changes become chronic:

- trophic alterations are noted, with increased thickening of the skin and subcutaneous tissue, and localized muscular contraction

- deeper musculature may become hard, tense, and hypersensitive

- there may be deep splinting contractions, involving two or more segments of the spine, with associated restriction of spinal motion

- the costotransverse articulations may be significantly involved in such changes.

Such changes have been confirmed by research. For example in a 5-year study involving over 5000 hospitalized patients, it was concluded that most visceral disease appeared to influence more than one spinal region, and that the number of spinal segments involved seemed to be related to the duration of the disease. Kelso (1985) noted in this study that there was an increase in the number of superficial (soft tissue and skin) palpatory findings:

- in the cervical region in patients with sinusitis, tonsillitis, diseases of the esophagus and liver complaints

- in the region of T5–12 in patients with gastritis, duodenal ulceration, pyelonephritis, chronic appendicitis and cholycystitis.

Skin palpation might therefore usefully include:

- off-body scan (manual thermal diagnosis, MTD) which may offer evidence of variations in local circulation; trigger point activity is more likely in areas of greatest "difference" (Barral 1996)

- movement of skin on fascia – resistance indicates general locality of reflexogenic activity, a "hyperalgesic skin zone" such as a trigger point (Lewit 1992, 1999)

- local loss of skin elasticity – refines definition of the location (Lewit 1992, 1999)

- light stroke, seeking "drag" sensation (increased hydrosis), offers pinpoint accuracy of location (Lewit 1992, 1999).

Palpation exercises in this chapter focus on just such changes.

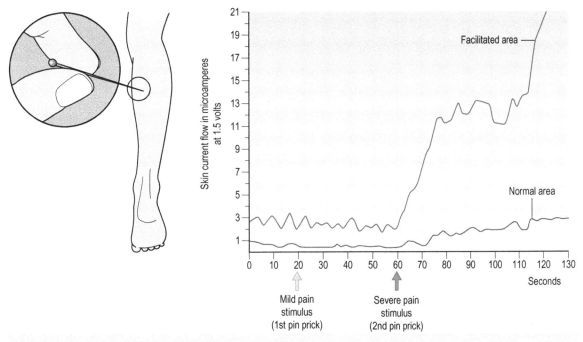

Figure 4.1
Pain stimuli produce a marked reaction in the facilitated area (red line) and little reaction in normal area (gray line).

The skin contains nearly 750,000 sensory receptors that vary in the density of their presence in different regions, from 7 to 135 per square cm. However, it is not neural endings that receive most attention from these researchers; rather, they focus much of their attention onto the characteristics of human skin that derive from the activities of atrichial sweat glands. These secretions, apart from playing a role in temperature control, influence "the energy and mass transfer characteristics of skin, as well as altering its properties by establishing different levels of epidermal hydration and salinisation" (Adams et al. 1982). They ask us to make a clear distinction between *epitrichial* and *atrichial* sweat glands, the former being associated with hair shafts, and the latter emptying directly on the skin, and thus directly influencing the important phenomena of skin friction and heat transfer properties.

Atrichial (sweat) activity influences on palpation

- The atrichial glands on the palmar surface of the hand (and the soles of the feet) have only a small potential for influencing heat loss but are important in being capable of modifying skin friction and pliability.

- The atrichial sweat glands are totally controlled by the sympathetic division of the autonomic nervous system, and this means that any palpable changes resulting from sweat production may be influenced by reflex activity, such as occurs when trigger points are active, and when emotional or stress factors are operating.

- The chemical mediator between the motor nerve and the secretory tubule of atrichial sweat glands is acetylcholine, a neurotransmitter that increases the tendency for muscles to contract.

- The complexities of water movement through the skin need not concern us, apart from a need to emphasize that the mechanical, electrical, and heat transfer properties, and characteristics, of the skin are altered by this process.

- As sweating occurs, liquid is not only passed through the tubule, but diffuses laterally into surrounding peritubular drier skin areas.

- Even when there is no obvious moisture on the skin surface, sweat gland activity in the underlying skin continues, with some of the water that spreads into surrounding skin being reabsorbed.

- This mechanism can be compared with the way kidney tubules deal with sugar in the urine.

- It is therefore incorrect to conclude that the sweat glands are inactive simply because there is no water on the skin surface (Adams et al. 1982).

- Low-level sweat gland activity has the effect of altering the degree of skin friction.

- Friction is low when the skin is dry, and higher as it becomes moist, decreasing again when sweating becomes very intense. It is hard to turn a page with a dry finger, but moisten it slightly and the task is easier, while a very sweaty hand cannot grasp anything easily.

- We can conclude that there is a narrow range of epidermal water content that produces maximum frictional contact at the skin surface.

Glabrous and non-glabrous skin

The palm of the hand and the sole of the foot contain a tough sheet of dense connective tissue that protects underlying vessels and nerves from the pressure associated with grip or body weight.

Both are firmly attached to the thick skin overlying them, to limit movement. (Benjamin 2009)

It is easy to rapidly feel the difference between "normal" and glabrous skin by sliding the skin on the dorsum of your hand in various directions – and then trying to do the same on the palmar surface (or the sole and the dorsum of the foot).

- Note the differences in the sliding facility in these different types of skin and the association with underlying connective tissue.

The skin drag phenomenon

Understanding these basic features of sweat behavior helps explain some of the reasons for regional variations in skin friction ("skin drag") noted on palpation. Adams and his colleagues (1982) ask:

Is it possible that regional differences in "skin drag" perceived by the examining physician are related to segmentally active, autonomic reflexes that trigger chronic, low level, atrichial sweat gland activity, which in turn increases local epidermal hydration and skin friction at a defined body site? Do these reflexes produce, through chronic sweat gland activity, changes in the mechanical properties of the skin's surface, similar to those you might detect on the wrist skin surface when a watchband is initially removed?

Initially, after removing a watch strap (or bracelet), when the skin under it is lightly stroked, there will be a high level of epidermal water that makes the friction level high, with a great deal of *skin drag*. After a while this is lost and the degree of drag will be similar to the surrounding skin characteristics.

The more fluid (sweat) there is in the tissues the stiffer, less elastic, they become. This explains why Karel Lewit (1999) is able to identify trigger point activity (or any other active reflex activity) simply by assessing the degree of elasticity (i.e., stretchability – see Exercise 4.8 for example) in the overlying skin, and comparing it with neighboring tissue. Lewit terms local skin areas of this type "hyperalgesic skin zones."

The increased presence of fluid in hyperalgesic, hypertonic areas explains why, prior to the introduction of methods of electrical detection of acupuncture points, any skilled acupuncturist could rapidly identify active points by palpation and also why measurement of the electrical resistance of the skin can now do this even more quickly (i.e., when skin is moist it conducts electricity more efficiently than when dry!).

We will examine more of Lewit's thoughts later in this chapter. We now need to examine how the degree of epidermal hydration (sweat) influences perception of temperature in the tissues being palpated, and how the condition of the skin of the person performing palpation, influences the process.

First, however, there is discussion of palpation without touch, scanning off the body in order to evaluate differences in perceived hot and cooler areas.

Thermography in bodywork

Various forms of thermal assessment, including infrared, electrical, and liquid crystal methods (Baldry 1993), as well as manual thermal diagnosis (MTD), are used clinically to identify trigger point activity and other forms of dysfunction (Barral 1996).

Swerdlow and Dieter (1992) found, after examining 365 patients with demonstrable trigger points in the upper back, that "although thermographic 'hot-spots' are present in the majority, the sites are not necessarily where the trigger points are located." Is it possible that "old" trigger points lie in ischemic, possibly fibrotic tissue, leading to "cold-spots" in the tissues involved?

Simons (1987) suggests that while hot-spots may commonly represent trigger point sites, some triggers may exist in "normal" temperature regions, and that hot-spots can exist for reasons other than the presence of trigger points.

Thermal examination of the reference zone (target area) to which a trigger point refers, or radiates, usually shows skin temperature raised, but not always. Simons attributes this anomaly to the different effects trigger points have on the autonomic nervous system. Simons (1993) explains:

> Depending upon the degree and manner in which the trigger point is modulating sympathetic control of skin circulation, the reference zone initially may be warmer, isothermic or cooler than unaffected skin. Painful pressure on the trigger point consistently and significantly reduced the temperature in the region of the referred pain and beyond.

Scanning accuracy : Barral's evidence

A "scan" of the tissues being investigated, keeping the hand approximately 2.5 cm (about 1 inch) from the skin surface, is used by some practitioners as a means of establishing areas that apparently differ from each other in temperature. But how accurate is this?

Using sophisticated equipment, French osteopath Jean-Pierre Barral has established that areas that scan (non-touching, see Exercise 4.5) as "hot" are only truly warmer/hotter than surrounding areas in 75% of instances. It seems that scanning for hot and cold areas results in the perception of greater heat whenever a major difference occurs in one area compared to a neighbouring one. This means that scanning over a "normal" and then a cooler area will often (usually) result in a perception that greater heat is being sensed. This does not nullify the usefulness of such scanning methods, but does mean that what seems "hot" may actually be "cold" (ischemic?) (Barral 1996).

Apparently when scanning manually for heat, any area that is markedly different from surrounding tissues in temperature terms is considered "hot" by the brain. Manual scanning for heat is therefore a relatively accurate way of assessing "differences" between tissues but not their actual thermal status.

Learning to measure skin temperature by touch

Exercises 4.1–4.9 are designed to help you to establish the basic palpation skills needed to determine heat variations in the objects and tissues being evaluated, as well as introducing you to the phenomenon of "drag," an extremely useful palpation tool.

Exercise 4.1 *Temperature Discrimination Using Inanimate Objects*

Time suggested **5–10 seconds per object palpated**

- Assemble in front of you small objects made of wood, plastic, metal, china, rough-textured ceramic and paper.
- If possible, have several different items made of each substance.

Make sure that they have all been in the same place, in the room in which you are carrying out this exercise, for at least an hour before you start. We can presume that the ambient temperature is uniform in this part of the room.

Palpate each of the items individually with each hand, sensing the relative feeling of warmth or coolness that it imparts when in your hands.

Were the objects to be measured with a thermocouple they would show almost exactly the same reading, and yet you will have noted that there is a distinct difference in temperature as you feel them.

Why do you think this is?

The answer will be found as you work your way through this chapter.

Exercise 4.2 *Temperature Discrimination*

Time suggested: **15 seconds**

Stand barefoot on a cold ceramic tile, piece of marble, or sheet of plastic.

Rest one foot on the tile, and the other on a rug or towel that has been in the room for some time.

One foot feels cooler than the other, and yet the temperature of the tile, and the rug, are almost certainly the same.

What is the reason for the perceived difference?

Does this raise any questions in your mind as to the accuracy of what temperature variations we *think* we can "feel" when we are palpating/touching something or someone?

Record your thoughts in your journal.

Discussion regarding Exercises 4.1 and 4.2

The variables that influence heat flow from an object we are feeling to the surface of the tissues we are using to feel with (fingertips, hand, foot) relate to the thermal properties of these two "exchanging surfaces" (see below, Fig. 4.2). These thermal properties include:

the surface areas of the exchanging surfaces

the differences in temperature between the exchanging surfaces

the distance over which heat is being transferred

the intrinsic properties of heat conduction associated with the object being palpated and the palpatory unit (your hand or fingers).

A characteristic of this process, called the "thermal conducting coefficient" (TCC), requires explanation. The TCC of a tiled floor is greater than that of a rug or carpet, and this causes the thermoreceptors in your foot on the tile to be more rapidly cooled than the other foot. Your perception of one foot being "cooler" than the other is accurate, but it does not relate to any differences in the temperature of the surfaces on which you are standing.

If it can be independently verified that two objects *that feel as though they have different temperatures* are actually at the same temperature, then the difference sensed by your thermoreceptors (the neural receptors that transmit messages relating to heat and cold to your brain) can be attributed to a difference in thermal conductivity or some other heat transfer property of the object(s) being examined, but not to a difference in temperature. This is clearly of significance when it comes to making clinical judgments as to how warm or cool an area of skin feels when you are palpating it.

A further complication becomes apparent when we examine the influence of the degree of epidermal hydration (sweat), both in and on the palpated tissues and the palpating hand. Let us try to discover the effect of sweat on your judgment of the temperature of the tissues you are palpating.

Exercise 4.3 *Thermal Conductivity and The Influence of Moisture*

Time suggested **10–15 seconds per object, per test**

Take any two of the objects that you have previously palpated for temperature difference, say a pencil and a metal key or other metal object.

Once again, palpate these by hand and sense the difference in thermal sensation reaching the thermoreceptors in your hand.

- Use the same part of your hand (palm, dorsum, fingertip, etc.) to palpate each object.

- Try this first with your hands dry and then moisten the fingertips (or whatever part of the hand is being used) and repalpate the objects.

- Do this exercise with each hand.

- Do you notice any difference in what you sense in terms of temperature when the dry hand/fingers and then the moist hand/fingers are in touch with the object?

- If so, what is the difference?

- Record your findings.

Exercise 4.4 *Testing Different Regions for Thermal Sensitivity*

Time suggested **10–15 seconds per object, per test**

- Next, try to see whether the thermal sensitivity of the dorsal aspect of your hand is greater than that of the palm or finger pad when assessing a wooden pencil and then a metal object.

- Are you more aware of temperature differences when palpating with one or other part of your hand?

- Or with one hand or the other?

- *Now test the same objects again, but this time use the tip of your tongue as your "palpating" organ.*

- Did you sense the apparent differences in temperature more clearly with the tip of your tongue? Yes/No

Discussion regarding Exercises 4.3 and 4.4

The thermoreceptors in the palmar surface of the hand are far more densely sited than on the dorsum of the hand and there are even more on the tip of the tongue (where they are close to the surface), making these regions more sensitive for palpation of heat. This means that despite the differences in epidermal thickness on the dorsum of the hand as compared with the palmar surface, the palm is *usually* a better place to make contact when seeking thermal information.

Test this out for yourself, since some people seem to be more sensitive where heat measurement is concerned when

using the dorsum of the hand, and you may be one of these. This may be due to sensitization of the palmar surface through repetitive manual contacts and the relative lack of contact of the dorsum with objects.

Note that the relative dampness, or otherwise, of the palpating surface influences perception of heat. This is because of better conduction when water (sweat, for example) is present, so that the temperature of the thermoreceptors is closer to that of the object being examined than it would be with a dry contact.

Variables

- Your own state of hydration

- Your peripheral circulatory efficiency

- Your sympathetic nervous system activity

- Recent physical activity

- Ambient humidity and temperature

… will all influence your thermal perception as you palpate.

Adams et al. (1982) summarize the problem of understanding the variables:

> The thermoreceptors in an examining finger are part of a complex heat exchange system. The temperature that is felt by the examiner is directly related to the rate of action potential formation on afferent, sensory nerves arising from thermoreceptors near the dermo-epidermal junction. Their temperature is strongly dependent on heat brought to the skin (or taken away from it) by the circulating blood.

The perceived temperature is also determined by the rate of heat transfer out of, or into, the examiner's skin, from the patient's skin. This is influenced by numerous factors, including:

- the size of the area of contact

- the thickness of skin in both examiner and patient

- the status of epidermal hydration in both

- heat transfer characteristics, including such factors as material trapped between the two skin surfaces – examiner and patient – including air, water, lotion, grease or oil, dirt, fabric and so on. All or any of these variables will be operating each time you palpate and, to some extent at least, their net effect needs to be taken into consideration. Some of the variables affecting thermal perception are illustrated in Fig. 4.2.

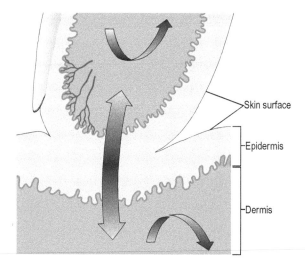

Figure 4.2
This diagram depicts some of the physical and physiologic factors that affect the thermoreceptor (TR) discharge rate and consequently the temperature sensed in an examiner's skin in contact with a patient's skin. The temperature and its rate of change of the examiner's thermoreceptors are functions of the net effects of the time that the tissues are in contact, their contact area (A), the temperatures (TBe and TBp) and volume flow rates (Ve and Vp) of blood perfusing the examiner's and patient's skin, epidermal thickness (Xe and Xp) and thermal conductivity (Ke and Kp) of both, dermal temperature (TDe and TDp) of both, as well of the net heat exchange rate (QH) between the two tissues. QH is strongly affected by the heat transfer properties of material trapped between the two skin surfaces, for example, air, water, oil, grease, hand lotion, dirt, tissue debris, fabric (Adams et al. 1982).

Palpating the skin for temperature and skin variations

Having established the need to be aware of possible misinterpretations of information gathered regarding apparent temperature differences due to some of the many variables discussed above, it's time to begin to try to make sense of the human body as you palpate for specific characteristics.

The objective of the next few exercises (4.5–4.8) is to highlight the importance of using the skin as a source of valuable information, that allows for the intelligent exploration of deeper tissues. Try to ensure that these four exercises are done sequentially, in the same study/palpation exercise session, so that the results of each can be compared with the others, with the results of the previous test being factored into the subsequent one, and also so that they can be learned as a routine that can be used clinically.

Notes

Ideally, Exercises 4.8–4.10 should be performed in sequence, at one training/class session. Similarly, Exercises 4.11–4.13 should be performed in sequence at another training/class session.

Exercise 4.5 *Off-Body Scanning for Temperature Differences*

Time suggested **2–3 minutes maximum**

- Stand at your palpation partner's waist level, with them lying prone on the treatment table, exposed from the waist up.

- Hold your dominant hand, with palm down, close (1–3 inches/2.5–7.5 cm) to the surface of the back and make steady, deliberate sweeps of the hand to and fro, across the back, until all of it has been scanned.

- As you "scan" for temperature variations "off the body" in this way, keep the hand moving slowly.

- If the hand remains still or moves too slowly you have nothing to compare; if you move too fast you will not perceive the slight changes as the hand passes from one area to another.

- Approximately 4–5 inches (10–15 cm) should be scanned per second.

As previously discussed, different aspects and areas of your hand may be more sensitive than others, so test whether your sensitivity is greater in the palm, near the wrist or on the dorsum of the hand, as you evaluate areas that feel warmer or cooler than others. These should be charted.

Focus on the areas that appear to you to be "warmest" during subsequent tests in this sequence, because these are the areas of greatest potential interest. Remember Barral's (1996) evidence, outlined earlier in this chapter, that the actual temperature of such areas may be cooler, and that your brain will commonly interpret areas that are different from each other, as warmer.

- Does your experience agree with the suggestion that the palmar surface is more sensitive than the dorsal surface of the hand?

- Record your findings.

Viola Frymann (1963) states:

> Even passing the hand a quarter of an inch above the skin provides information on the surface temperature. An acute lesion area will be unusually warm, an area of long-standing, chronic lesion may be unusually cold as compared with the skin in other areas.

Exercise 4.6 *Direct Palpation for Temperature Differences*

Time suggested **3–4 minutes for each segment of this exercise (A, B, and C)**

Your palpation partner should be lying prone, as in the previous exercise, with the back exposed.

You should now apply hand or finger contact, without pressure, to the tissues being evaluated. Choose areas that both tested as "warm" in the previous (scan) exercise, as well as those which did not.

Do not rub or press the tissues, merely mold your hand(s) to the skin surface for a few seconds, before moving to an adjacent area. In this way, slowly and carefully palpate the back for variations of skin temperature, using both hands, one at a time or both at the same time:

A. when the "patient" has been lying still for some minutes in a room of normal temperature/humidity

B. when the "patient" has actively skipped, jogged, danced, or performed some other exercise for several minutes

C. when you have performed similar exercise for some minutes.

Do you note any differences between A, B, and C?

- Vary your contact so that sometimes you use the palmar and sometimes the dorsal surface of the hands for this assessment, under similarly variable conditions.

- Is one hand more sensitive than the other?

- Is one palpation contact more accurate than the other?

- Do you sense differences in temperature from one area to another of the body surface, and if so, how does this relate to the findings of the off-the-body scan in the previous exercise?

- How does your, or your partner's, degree of hydration/sweating influence what you feel?

- Record your findings.

Exercise 4.7 *Evaluating Skin on Fascia Resistance*

Time suggested **3–5 minutes**

This palpation is based on German connective tissue massage (*Bindegewebsmassage*) named by physical therapist Elizabeth Dicke (1954). For a discussion on this method see Box 4.2.

The subsequent treatment methods used involve patterns of repetitive dry-contact, strong friction strokes aimed at evoking reflex responses. These should not concern us in this text; however, the diagnostic methods used to identify areas (zones) suitable for treatment are useful to our palpation skills task.

Dicke's method of diagnosis was discussed by Bischof and Elmiger (1960).

- The subject is seated or lying prone (Fig. 4.3).

- Both hands (or finger pads), using a flat contact, displace the subcutaneous tissues simultaneously against the fascia, with small to-and-fro pushes.

- The degree of displacement possible will depend upon tension of the tissues.

- It is important that symmetrical areas (i.e., both sides of the body) be examined simultaneously.

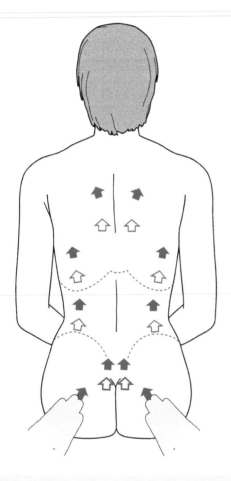

Figure 4.3
Testing tissue mobility by bilaterally "pushing" skin with fingerpads.

- With your fingers lightly flexed and using only enough pressure to produce adherence between the fingerpads and the skin (do not slide on the skin, instead slide the skin on the underlying fascia), make a series of short, deliberate, pushing motions, simultaneously with both hands, which eases the tissues (skin on fascia) to the elastic barrier on each side (see Fig. 4.3).

- Pay particular attention to comparing areas where "heat" was sensed during the scan exercise.

- The pattern of testing should be performed from inferior to superior, moving the tissues either superiorly or bilaterally in an obliquely diagonal direction toward the spine.

- Whether your partner is prone or seated, tissues from the buttocks to the shoulders may be tested, always comparing the sides for symmetry.

As a palpation exercise try to identify local areas where your "push" of skin on connective tissue reveals restriction as compared with its opposite side.

Dicke also suggests (Bischof & Elmiger 1960):

> By pulling away a skinfold from the fascia [see Fig. 4.3], the degree of tissue tension and displacement may be determined.

> Three different levels of displacement are distinguished:

> - the most superficial displacement occurs between skin and subcutaneous tissues and is easier to find in children and in old people because the displacement is slight

> - the main displacement occurs between the subcutaneous tissue and the fascia

> - the deepest displacement layer is between the fascia and the interstitial connective tissue. The movement is most evident upon large, flat areas such as the lumbosacral area, on the sacrum, and in regions of the tensor fascia lata.

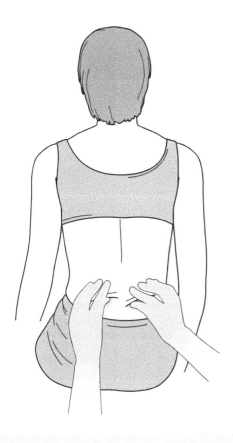

Figure 4.4
Assessing bilateral elasticity of skin by lifting it in folds or "rolling" it.

- By gently grasping and lifting bilateral skinfolds (Fig. 4.4), see whether you can make any judgements using Dicke's comments.

- Compare your findings using this method with those achieved by "skin on fascia pushes" as described above.

Box 4.2 Connective tissue massage (CTM) concepts

Apart from the diagnostic methods described in Exercise 4.7 (skin on fascia resistance), CTM uses a further "diagnostic stroke" that employs a two-finger contact (patient seated, as a rule) that runs longitudinally, paravertebrally, starting at the level of L5 up to the level of the seventh cervical spinous process. As the stroke (pull) starts, the upper layers of tissue displacement are superficial and gentle; but they are followed by a slower, deeper stroke that pulls on subcutaneous tissue and fascia. Displacement of the deeper tissue, as well as interstitial tissue, is accomplished by a deep and slow pull along the same "track."

This highlights the important point that the desired depth-effect is obtained by the *speed* of the stroke, as well as the amount of *pressure* used.

Notes

Compare the tip in the final sentence of Box 4.2 with advice on Neuromuscular Technique pressure – as described in Chapter 5.

Slow down – palpation should not be hurried.

What should such deliberate strokes show?

- Healthy tissue elevates or "mounds" ahead of the stroking digits (2–3 cm/1 inch ahead).

- When an area of resistance is reached, increased tension is felt, and further displacement of the skin becomes difficult or impossible.

- Folds of skin will be formed in front of the advancing stroke in such areas, and the mass will become larger.

- The progress of the stroke will also become slower, as compared with the stroke across healthy tissue.

- Factors such as the age of the patient, constitutional state, posture, and the area being tested may all alter the anticipated findings.

- It is easier to displace skin against underlying tissue in slim individuals, with little fatty tissue.

- Obese individuals have a higher subcutaneous fat and water content, making displacement more difficult.

Dicke pointed out that even before use of the diagnostic stroke, it is often possible to see reflex areas, characterized by being retracted or elevated, for example:

- Retracted bands of tissue are commonly seen in areas such as the neck, lower thoracic border, and over the pelvic and gluteal areas.

- Depressed or flattened areas are seen over the thorax, the scapulae, and between the thoracic spine and the scapulae, as well as over the upper iliac tissues and the sacrum.

- Flat elevations are visible, in many cases, around the seventh cervical spinous process, on the outer border of the scapulae, or around the sacrum.

- These raised or depressed tissue areas are not amenable to dissipation by massage and represent chronic reflex activity. They are considered to be viscerocutaneous reflexes (viscerosomatic in other words) resulting from altered blood supply, leading to colloidal changes in the cells and tissues.

What is revealed by these diagnostic strokes is an altered vascular skin reaction, tissue tension, tissue density, tissue sensitivity, and often tissue displacement. Valuable clinical evidence can be gathered using these strokes and "pushes."

For a deeper understanding of this system, Dicke's work should be studied in depth. Fortunately this system is now taught worldwide by her followers and is much used by physical therapists, massage therapists and some doctors, osteopaths and chiropractors who employ soft tissue methods.

Lewit's methods of skin evaluation

Karel Lewit has compiled a treasure-house of information (Lewit 1992, 1999). His discussion of the importance of skin palpation is worth examining in some detail (Box 4.3).

Box 4.3 Lewit's hyperalgesic skin zones (HSZ)

Lewit (1992, 1999) points out that it was late in the 19th century that Head first reported on increased sensitivity to pinprick sensations in particular zones involved in reflex activity. Unfortunately, such a subjective symptom meant that the practitioner was dependent upon accurate feedback from the patient, for whom it was a slow and not particularly comfortable experience.

Lewit also discusses the technique of "skin rolling," in which a skinfold is lifted and rolled forwards between the fingers. Increased resistance is easily noted by the practitioner, as is the fact that, wherever reflex activity is operating, these folds of skin will also be "thicker" (see Fig. 4.4). Unfortunately, this technique may be painful to the patient and is also difficult to perform on areas where skin is tightly adherent to underlying tissue.

In the German system of connective tissue massage (CTM, see Box 4.2), a variation on this assessment method involves the skin being lightly stretched over the underlying fascia by pressing with the fingertips in a direction away from the operator. As described in Exercise 4.7 (see Fig. 4.3), this is usually performed bilaterally, so that variations in the degree of elasticity can be compared from one side of the body to the other, so producing evidence of reflex activity if there is a reduced degree of "stretchability" when the two sides are compared.

The disadvantages of these methods lie in their fairly general indications, although this matters little to those using CTM, since they are usually attempting to identify large reflex zones that relate to organ or system dysfunction, rather than small localized areas of reflex activity required to identify, for example, myofascial trigger points.

Lewit reports that he has developed a painless and effective method that is more reliable diagnostically than those mentioned above and which transforms from diagnostic evaluation to therapeutic treatment if the process is prolonged (see Exercise 4.8). He calls the method "skin stretching."

Lewit first stretches the skin with the minimum of force in order to take up the available slack and then takes

Box 4.3 *continued*

the stretch to its end-range, without force, where a slight "springing" of the skin is introduced. He performs a similar stretch in various directions over the area being assessed.

If a hyperalgesic skin zone (HSZ) exists, due to reflex input to the area, a "stiff" resistance is felt after the slack is taken up, rather than an elastic "end-feel."

Like has to be compared with like, and it is little use comparing the degree of elasticity available in skin overlying, say, the lumbar paraspinal muscles with that overlying the dorsal paraspinal tissues. The first would usually be relatively "loose" and the other fairly "tight," as a natural matter of course. However, if one area of dorsal paraspinal skin elasticity is compared with another area of dorsal paraspinal skin elasticity, and one of these is significantly less elastic than the other, this suggests that reflex activity may exist below the "tighter" skin area.

Treatment of such areas, aimed at initiating a degree of normalization of the reflex activity which created them, is achieved by maintaining the degree of stretch for a further 10 seconds or so.

According to Lewit:

> *If the therapist then holds the stretched skin in end-position [around 10 seconds is usual] resistance is felt to weaken until normal springing is restored. The hyperalgesic skin zone can then as a rule no longer be detected. If pain is due to this hyperalgesic skin zone this method is quite as effective as needling, electrostimulation and other similar methods.*

Lewit suggests that this method allows us to diagnose (and treat) even very small reflex areas (HSZ) lying in inaccessible or potentially painful places, such as between the toes, over bony prominences and around scars.

Just what is going on in these HSZs? They sometimes overlie areas affected by viscerosomatic reflex activity or areas of segmental facilitation (sensitization) in which the neural structures in any spinal region may respond to repetitive stress factors of varying types by becoming hyperreactive. This produces undesirable consequences, both locally and in the areas supplied by nerves from that spinal level.

Palpation methods for identifying levels of spinal segmental facilitation (other than HSZ) are discussed in the context of muscular palpation in Chapter 5.

Localized myofascial facilitation also takes place in relation to the development of trigger points. Such localized areas of soft tissue disruption have the ability to bombard distant tissues with aberrant neural impulses, often of a painful nature. HSZ will be found overlying active (and also "embryonic" and dormant) trigger points, as well as over the target zone that the trigger point influences.

Therapists who are interested in the acupuncture model of treatment will be aware that active points in the meridian system have an area of lowered electrical resistance in the skin overlying them. The location of these areas is easily identified by means of Lewit's method of skin stretching – and by drag palpation (see Exercise 4.14). According to Lewit these areas respond therapeutically to further stretching, as well as to needling.

More detail on the trigger point phenomenon is given in Chapter 5, including a summary of methods for identifying these common troublemakers, as well as a reminder of Lewit's methods. See also Special topic 4.

Positional release and the skin

Evaluating "ease" in skin and superficial tissues is a useful and important step in understanding ways in which soft tissues can respond to mechanical positioning in clinical settings (Box 4.4).

Box 4.4 Positional release experiment

Locate an area of skin that tested as "tight" when evaluated using skin rolling or connective tissue "pushing" (Exercise 4.7), or Lewit's skin-stretch methods (Exercises 4.8–4.13).

- Place two or three finger pads onto the skin and slide it superiorly and then inferiorly on the underlying fascia.

- In which direction does the skin slide most easily?

- Slide the skin in that direction and, holding it there, now test the preference of the skin to slide medially and laterally.

- Which of these is the easiest direction?

- Slide the tissue toward this second position of ease.

- Now introduce a slight clockwise and anticlockwise twist to these tissues that are already being held ("stacked") in two directions of ease.

- Which way does the skin feel most comfortable as it rotates?

- Take it in that direction, so that you are now holding the skin in three directions/positions of ease.

- Hold this for not less than 20 seconds.

- Gently release the skin and retest; it should now display a far more symmetrical preference in all the directions that were previously "tight."

You have already established that holding skin *towards* its barrier (unforced) changes its function as the skin releases (see Exercise 4.12) and you should now have observed that moving tissues *away* from the barrier, into ease, can also achieve a release. This is an example of a functional positional release technique (Chaitow 2015).

Exercise 4.8 *Lewit's Skin-Stretching Palpation (A)*

Time suggested 5–10 minutes

At first, it is necessary to practice this method slowly. Eventually it should be possible to move fairly rapidly over an area that is being searched for evidence of reflex activity (or acupuncture points).

- Your palpation partner should be lying prone, as in the previous few exercises.

- Choose two regions to be assessed, ideally areas that were "different" on scanning and that also showed an abnormal degree of skin-on-fascia adherence in previous exercises.

- If possible, select an area 7.5 × 7.5 cm (3 inches × 3 inches) to the side of the dorsal spine, covering the muscular paraspinal region as well as some of the skin over the scapula and/or ribs.

- A second area should be of a similar size, in the low back/buttock area, involving far more elastic, "loosely fitting" skin.

- Mark these areas with a skin pencil or felt-tip pen and begin the search.

- Place your two index fingers adjacent to each other on the skin, side by side or pointing towards each other, with no pressure at all onto the skin, just a contact touch (Fig. 4.5A).

- Lightly and slowly separate your fingers, feeling the skin stretch as you do so (Fig. 4.5B).

- Take the stretch to its "easy" limit. In other words, do not forcibly stretch the skin but just take it to the point where resistance is first noted. This is the "barrier of resistance" and it should be easily possible, with a little more effort, to "spring" the skin further apart, to its absolute elastic limit.

- Release this stretch and move both fingers 0.5 cm to one side of this first test site and test again in the same way, and in the same direction of pull, separating the fingers.

- Perform exactly the same sequence over and over again until the entire area of tissue has been searched.

- When performing the series of stretches, ensure that the rhythm you adopt is not too slow (it is usually impossible

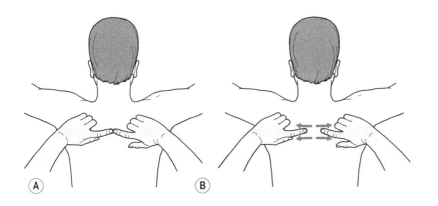

Figure 4.5
(A) Fingers touch each other directly over skin to be tested – very light skin contact only.
(B) Pull apart to assess degree of skin elasticity – compare with neighbouring skin area.

to retain the subtle proprioceptive memory of the previous stretch if there is too long a gap between stretches).

- On the other hand, if the series of stretches is performed too rapidly the individual stretch is unlikely to be to the true elastic barrier which is being assessed.

- My recommendation is that one stretch per second be performed, if possible.

- In some local areas you may sense that the skin is not as elastic as it was on the previous stretch. This is a potential hyperalgesic skin zone (HSZ). Mark it with a skin pencil or felt-tip pen, for future attention.

- If you were to apply light finger pressure to the center of that small zone, you would almost always locate a sensitive contracture, which on sustained pressure may radiate sensations to a distant site (meaning that it is a trigger point, in which case add to your marking on the skin – or a record card – the direction of the radiating sensation) or may not radiate (meaning that it is either an active acupuncture point, a latent or an embryonic trigger point, or some other reflex manifestation).

- Record your findings.

Exercise 4.9 *Lewit's Skin-Stretching Palpation (B)*

Time suggested **5–10 minutes**

- Now reassess precisely the same skin areas as in the previous exercise, but this time make the direction of each stretch different, perhaps going parallel to the spine rather than vertical to it, for example.

- See whether you identify the same reflex areas/trigger points (HSZs) this time.

- Using a skin pencil or felt-tip pen, mark one or two particularly "tight" areas (HSZs).

- Record your findings.

Exercise 4.10 *Lewit's Skin-Stretching Palpation (C)*

Time suggested **10 minutes**

Having satisfied yourself that you can utilize skin stretching effectively to identify localized areas of dysfunction, as described in the previous two exercises, perform a search of other spinal areas and note:

- the difference in elasticity that is available between skin overlying the dorsal area and the lumbar/gluteal area

- how it is possible to vary the direction of stretch as you move your finger contacts around the area and still be able to discriminate between elastic and less elastic skin areas

- how it is possible to begin to speed up the process, so that what took you 5 minutes of painstakingly careful stretch, followed by stretch, can now be achieved in 1 or 2 minutes, without loss of accuracy.

- Record your findings.

Exercise 4.11 *Lewit's Skin-Stretching Palpation (D)*

Time suggested **12 minutes**

In order to develop your skills in using skin stretching diagnostically, you should now try to assess for variations in the elasticity of skin in difficult areas such as:

- the sternum/xiphoid process
- over the spinous processes
- in the webbing between the toes or fingers.

If you have no available palpation partner, perform as many of the above exercises as you can on yourself.

Using a skin pencil or felt-tip pen, mark one or two particularly "tight" areas (HSZs).

Remember that no lubricant should be used during any of these assessments; they are best and most accurately performed "dry."

Be careful on hairy areas, as this could obviously cause discomfort.

Note the variations in degree of skin elasticity as you assess first one and then another anatomical site.

Exercise 4.12 *Lewit's Sustained Skin Stretch of HSZs*

Time suggested **3–5 minutes**

- Now go back to a marked hyperalgesic skin zone identified in one of the previous exercises.
- Gently stretch the skin to its elastic barrier and hold it there for at least 10–15 seconds, without force.
- Do you then feel the skin tightness gradually release so that, as you hold the elastic barrier, your fingers actually separate further?
- Hold the skin in its new stretched position, at its new barrier of resistance, for a few seconds longer and then do the same to other HSZs that you identified and noted in previous assessments.

- Now go back and retest the areas you have "released" in this way and see whether these areas, which previously demonstrated reflexively restricted skin, have regained comparative elasticity.
- Record your findings.

Exercise 4.13 *Lewit's Large Skin Area Assessment/Palpation*

Time suggested **2–4 minutes**

Lewit (1999) describes a contact in which the ulnar borders of the cross-hands are used to assess large skin areas (such as the low back) in much the same way as the small areas were assessed by fingerpad-induced stretching of the skin in previous exercises.

- Place the palms of the hands together and then, using a firm contact, place the full length of the sides of both hands, from the little fingers to the wrist, onto an area of skin on the low back (as an example).
- Separate the hands slowly, stretching the skin with which they are in contact, until an elastic barrier is reached.
- Move to an immediately adjacent area of skin, place the hands and test as above, comparing the distance the skin stretches with the previous effort.
- Do this sequentially, stretch following stretch, so that an area such as the back or thigh is covered.
- Identify and mark those stretches in which there seems to be restriction as compared to areas where skin elasticity was more normal.
- This exercise may reveal large reflexively active zones that could relate to organ dysfunction or other neurological involvement.
- Practice "releasing" these restrictions, as in the example in Exercise 4.12, by holding the stretch at the barrier or resistance, without force, for 15–20 seconds, or until an easing of tone, release of tightness, is experienced.
- Retest to see whether this has indeed made a difference to the elasticity of the area compared with neighboring areas.
- Record your findings.

Discussion regarding Exercises 4.8 to 4.13

The causes of reflex activities that manifest as hyperalgesic skin zones may involve organic, systemic, or structural dysfunction and may be local or global in their influences. They may be acute or chronic.

Thus, while identifying HSZs offers evidence of *where* reflexive activity may be operating, and while releasing skin tension in the manner described by Lewit may have some input in normalizing function, this is likely to be of only temporary duration unless *underlying causes* are also dealt with.

The methods described above are therefore useful in identifying and localizing tissues involved in reflex activity but their value in therapeutic terms should be thought of as short term rather than long term.

General considerations

In this chapter some very important concepts regarding skin palpation have already been outlined. The significance of what is being noted during skin palpation has been addressed by a number of experts, for example Walton (1971), who says:

> *In superficial palpation, the operator [practitioner], using the pads of his fingers, strokes the skin gently, but firmly enough to allow perception, over the area to be examined. There are five types of change to be noted by superficial palpation in both acute and chronic lesions:*

- *skin changes*
- *temperature changes*
- *superficial muscle tensions*
- *tenderness and oedema.*

> *In acute lesions an actual increase in temperature may be felt in the skin overlaying it, but evidence is vague and extremely fleeting, and not much reliance should be placed on it. The skin overlaying the lesion will feel tense and relatively immobile owing to the congestive effect of the lesion below it. In the chronic lesion, temperature changes may or may not be present ... the skin overlaying a chronic lesion may be* either normal or reduced as a result of ischaemia of the underlying tissues. This is characteristic of chronic fibrotic change.

Differences of opinion

Byron Beal (1983) has researched common paraspinal palpatory findings (mainly involving upper thoracic facilitated segments) relating to patients with acute and chronic cardiovascular disease and seems to place less importance on the reliability of superficial evidence as compared to deeper palpated changes. Skin texture and temperature changes were, he reports, not apparent as consistent, strong findings, compared with the hypertonic state of the deep musculature.

John Upledger, however, does not agree with Beal as to skin evidence being unreliable in such diagnosis (Upledger 1983). He describes use of the skin in localized diagnosis using a "drag" palpation in precisely the areas in that Beal feels that deeper palpation is more reliable.

The difference of opinion between Beal and Upledger may have resulted from different palpatory methods or, more likely, simply because Beal finds the evidence from the muscles more reliable (see Exercise 5.1, Chapter 5). He does, after all, say that the skin evidence is not "as consistent" as the muscle evidence, not that skin evidence is not available or reliable.

In the next few exercises the phenomenon of increased hydrosis (sweat) and its effects on palpation are used to remarkable effect in what is known as "drag" palpation.

Drag palpation of the skin

Exercise 4.14 *Skin Drag Palpation*

Time suggested **5–7 minutes**

- Before performing this exercise do a scan of the tissues you intend to palpate, seeking apparent areas of increased warmth (as in Exercise 4.6).

- Also palpate directly the tissues where increased warmth was noted in the scan (as in Exercise 4.6A).

- Now palpate the same skin areas, this time assessing for variations in skin friction by lightly running a fingertip across the skin surface (*no lubricant should be used*), particularly comparing areas which scanned or palpated as warmer than surrounding tissues (Fig. 4.6).

- Perform this exercise with different fingers of each hand.

The degree of pressure required is minimal – skin touching skin is all that is necessary ("feather-light touch") (see Fig. 4.5).

- Movement of a single palpating digit should be purposeful, not too slow and certainly not very rapid. Around 3–5 cm (1–2 inches) per second is a satisfactory speed.

- Feel for any sense of "drag," which suggests a resistance to the easy, smooth passage of the finger across the skin surface.

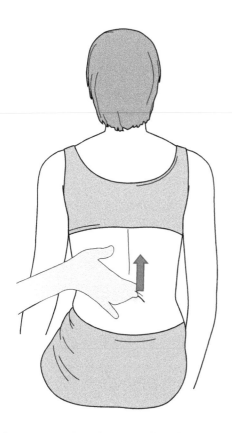

Figure 4.6
Assessing variations in skin friction (drag, resistance).

- A sense of "dryness," "sandpaper," a slightly harsh or rough texture may all indicate increased presence of sweat on, or increased fluid in, the tissues.

Variation of focus ("hills and valleys")

- While performing the drag palpation exercise, attempt to modify your focus.

- Using precisely the same single-digit stroke, instead of thinking about the sensation of drag, attempt to appreciate a subtle rising and falling of the stroking digit as it moves across the tissues.

- You are using an ancient Chinese palpation method that allowed acupuncturists to identify active acupuncture points.

- When an obvious sense of rise or fall ("hill" or "valley") was noted in the region of a known acupuncture point site it was considered that there was an excess of chi (hill) or a deficiency of chi (valley), and the point was treated accordingly.

- Perform a light stroke precisely where you previously noted "drag."

- Does the stroking finger seem to slightly rise or fall?

- Some practitioners prefer to evaluate using this focus rather than drag; however, both are equally effective if your discriminatory focus is applied to pick up the signals.

After physical exercise

- Once you have identified several areas of "drag," introduce the same variables as were used in Exercise 4.6B and C, in which either you or your palpation partner will have briefly but vigorously exercised, before you repeat the "drag" assessment.

- Note your results, especially if skin friction and temperature variation noted in previous exercises (scan and direct palpation, Exercises 4.5 and 4.6) have been identified in the same skin region.

- Make a note of the findings on a chart, especially any that indicate both local skin drag/friction characteristics and also greater warmth than surrounding tissue.

Exercise 4.15 *Skin Drag (Watch Strap) Palpation*

Time suggested **10 seconds**

- If you are even slightly confused as to what it is that you are trying to feel in the previous exercise (Exercise 4.14), remove your watch or bracelet (or have someone else remove their watch/bracelet) and lightly run a finger across the skin that was under the strap as well as over the adjacent skin.

- By running your palpating finger(s) over both "dry" and "moist" skin, you should easily be able to feel the difference in drag, friction, and resistance.

- Now wait for about 5 minutes and then, without having replaced the watch strap/bracelet, perform the exercise again.

- See how the drag on the skin that was under the strap is now absent, so that the previous site of "drag" now palpates as the same as the surrounding skin.

- On another occasion, study perceived temperature differences in the skin under a watch strap, first immediately after it is removed and then again 5–10 minutes later, compared with surrounding skin.

- Record your findings in your journal.

Discussion regarding Exercises 4.14 and 4.15

You need to ask yourself whether an area of skin that "feels" colder than surrounding skin is really colder (or warmer) or whether this actually relates to a higher thermal conductivity coefficient, which could be due to an increase in epidermal hydration (yours or the subject's) arising from a local or general increase in activity of the atrichial sweat glands. This in turn could be due to reflex activity, emotional distress, or some other phenomenon (air conditioning, central heating?) or, as you may have discovered, exercise (Lewit 1992, 1999).

If the same skin area that scans and palpates as having a different temperature from its surrounding tissue also displays increased skin friction characteristics (drag), the likelihood of this being due to increased atrichial sweat gland activity is strong (Barral 1996).

You also need to keep in mind your own state of physical and sympathetic activity as it relates to peripheral circulation and epidermal hydration when you palpate. Ask yourself:

- Are my hands sweating?

- Have they been sweating?

- Am I feeling anxious?

If your answer to any of these questions is in the affirmative, your thermoreceptors might be providing potentially inaccurate information as you palpate for temperature variables, a fact that would be compounded were the patient sweating, or if the relative ambient humidity or temperature was high.

You could also become confused in any attempt you might make to assess tissue texture changes (friction or "skin drag") were you not aware of the possibility that similar interacting influences (hydration, humidity, and so on) can alter "skin drag" characteristics.

The phenomenon of "drag" is commonly noted overlying active myofascial trigger points and areas of reflexogenic activity and is a superb assessment tool.

Overall palpation skill status

The successful completion of the exercises up to this point means that you should by now have established an ability to discern variations in:

- skin/surface temperature

- elastic qualities of skin

- skin's relation to underlying fascia.

And you should be able to use the "drag" phenomenon to locate areas of increased hydrosis.

If you are not satisfied with your degree of sensitivity in feeling temperature variations and "drag," then repeat the exercises at regular intervals, daily if possible but several times a week at least, until you are comfortable with both the concepts and the practice of these methods.

You should also have satisfied yourself that different aspects of your hand are more sensitive than others and that a number of variables can influence the potential accuracy of what it is that you think you feel.

In the end you need to be able to compute your palpation findings along with variables such as ambient temperature, patient's (and your own) level of hydrosis, previous activity, anxiety, etc., almost instantaneously, and to interpret findings according to the body of knowledge you have acquired, so that interpretation forms a part of your overall assessment of the patient's current status and requirements.

- Do you understand the physiology of the "drag" sensation?

- Do you feel that you can discern temperature variations by means of scanning from off the body and also by direct palpation?

- Do you feel that you understand what these palpated phenomena indicate?

Review appropriate texts and note your current level of awareness relating to these topics in your journal.

Scars

Karel Lewit (1999) brings into focus yet another skin phenomenon that is all too often overlooked – the scar. In his discussion of conditions resistant to treatment, or where symptoms do not seem to be explained by findings, he suggests we look for scar tissue:

> *The German literature uses the term storungsfeld –* *"focus of disturbance". This is frequently an old scar after injury or operation, often a tonsillectomy scar. This focus-scar is usually tender on examination, with pain spots embedded, or alongside, and surrounded by a hyperalgesic [skin] zone [HSZ].*

Changes of skin behavior can cause functional changes in other systems, for example the respiratory system (Petrů 2003), lymphatic (Wald et al. 1999), and neuromuscular system (Lewit 2003).

A large scar changes the mechanical behavior of the skin, because of disturbances in the natural tissue morphology, its nature and texture (Cerda 2005). From the histological point of view skin with a scar has a different architecture of collagen fibers in the dermis compared with healthy skin (van Zuijlen et al. 2002).

Such scars may act as "saboteurs," Lewit believes, requiring special attention. Lewit (1999) suggests deep palpation for pain spots near scars, assessing for increased resistance ("adhesions"), as well as for HSZ, by skin stretching.

If release of the skin by stretching (as in Exercise 4.12) fails to resolve the situation, needling (into pain spots), or local infiltration injections may be called for. When treatment has been successful, the local skin resistance and the pain spots should vanish, and the patient's symptoms should start improving.

Upledger and Vredevoogd (1983) discuss scar tissue, illustrating its importance with the example of a patient with chronic migraine headaches which resulted from chronic fascial drag, produced by an appendectomy scar. "Deep pressure medially on the scar produced the headache; deep pressure laterally caused relief of the headache. Mobilization of the scar was performed by sustained and deep but gentle pressure." This resulted in freedom from headaches, according to these respected authors, who add: "Spontaneous relief of low back pain, menstrual disorders and chronic and recurrent cervical somatic dysfunction also occurred following cicatrix [scar] mobilisation."

Valouchová and Lewit (2008) report that among the clinical symptoms caused by active scars in the abdominal region, back pain is very frequent. They report:

> *In patients with an active scar in the hypogastrium on one side, there was increased asymmetry of surface electromyography (SEMG) activity in the rectus abdominis between the two sides. This asymmetry diminished immediately after treatment by soft tissue techniques. In about half the cases the SEMG activity on the side of the scar was higher during thoracic flexion, yet on palpation there was hypotonus. This discrepancy is due to the hypotonus of the overlying soft scar tissue, producing a palpatory illusion. The immediate decrease in asymmetry, and decrease of back pain, after scar treatment indicates a reflex mechanism, whereby active scars can produce clinical symptoms.*

The influence of fascia on soft tissue function and dysfunction will be considered in the next chapter.

Exercise 4.16 *Scar Palpation*

Time suggested *3 minutes*

- Palpate a scar.
- Feel the scar tissue itself and see how the surrounding tissue associates with it.
- Is there a sense of tethering, or does the scar "float" in reasonable supple, elastic, local tissues?
- If possible, palpate a recent and also a very old scar and compare their characteristics.
- See if local tenderness exists around the scar.
- See how the skin elasticity varies when this is the case.
- Can you release the skin by sustained painless stretching, and if so does this change the degree of tenderness?

Record your findings relating to the feel of as many scars as you come across, recent and of long standing.

Exercise 4.17 *Combined Skin Palpation Exercise*

Time suggested **20–30 minutes**

You should have now practiced the various exercises involved in assessing temperature variations, both by scanning and directly, as well as Dicke's connective tissue method (skin on fascia "pushes"), together with Lewit's method for identification of hyperalgesic skin zones using skin stretching, and "skin drag." You should therefore now be ready to attempt an assessment in which you compare the reliability and accuracy of all these methods with each other, on one individual.

Obviously, such comparisons will only have validity if you use the same palpation partner. Try to ensure that you use all the skin assessment variations described on the same subject and compare results as you use the following palpation methods, in the following sequence:

1. Perform an off-body scan for temperature variations (remembering that cold may suggest ischemia, hot may indicate irritation/inflammation). Note areas that are "different."

2. Now palpate directly, molding your hands lightly to the tissues, to assess for temperature differences. Avoid lengthy hand contact or you will change the status of whatever you are palpating. A few seconds should be adequate.

3. Paying particular attention to those "different" areas (from scan palpation), evaluate skin adherence to underlying fascia (using light or firm "pushing" of assessed structures and/or skin rolling and/or tissue-lifting methods). Do such areas correspond with information gained from the scanning and palpation assessments?

4. Using those areas where dysfunction has been indicated by previous assessments (1, 2 and 3 above), look for variations in local skin elasticity (Lewit's "skin stretch"). Loss of elastic quality indicates a possible hyperalgesic zone and probable deeper dysfunction (e.g., trigger point) or pathology.

5. Finally, attempt to identify reflexively active areas (triggers, etc.) by means of very light single-digit palpation, seeking the phenomenon of "drag" (and/or "hills and valleys"). Do these findings agree with each other? They should. If not, try again and again.

Incorporate as many of those methods that seem accurate to you, and with which you are comfortable, into your usual pattern of assessment.

Testing skin-palpation skills of reflex areas

The soft tissue changes associated with various forms of dysfunction are usually palpable, both superficially – using drag palpation – and by means of the other methods that have been described in this chapter.

A number of other systems, where local superficial, palpable areas of tissue change are found, are described in Chapter 5, including trigger points (Travell & Simons 1992, 1999), but in the next exercise in this chapter your ability to discriminate between localized, normal and potentially reflexively active areas ("points") may be evaluated.

Chapman's neurolymphatic reflex points

In the 1930s, Chapman and Owens charted a group of palpable reflex changes that they termed neurolymphatic reflexes. Owens (1963) described the palpable changes, consistently associated with the same viscera, which are found in the fascia:

These extremely localised tissue changes (gangli-form contractions) are located anteriorly in the inter-costal spaces near the sternum. They may vary in size from one half the size of a shotgun pellet to that of a small bean, and occasionally are multiple. This type of change is apparent in some of the reflexes found on the pelvis, but the ones found on the lower extrem-ity (colon, broad ligament and prostate) vary in char-acter. Here there may be areas of "amorphous shotty plaques" or "stringy masses."

Patriquin (1997) described the characteristics of Chap-man's reflexes as: "small, smooth, firm, discretely palpable, approximately 2–3 mm in diameter. Sometimes described as feeling like small pearls of tapioca, lying, partially fixed, on the deep aponeurosis or fascia."

In recent years, in osteopathic practice, anterior Chap-man points have been found to be especially useful in viscerosomatic diagnosis (Fossum et al. 2011). The varia-tions in tissue texture probably result from a combination of both the nature and severity of the associated visceral involvement and the constitution of the patient.

- The degree of tenderness noted on palpation differenti-ates these from what Chapman terms "fat globules."

- In some areas, such as in the rectus femoris muscle, reflexes (from the suprarenal gland) have the feel of acute contraction.

- Posterior reflexes are found mainly between the spinous processes and the tips of the transverse processes, where they have more of an edematous, swollen feel and some-times are "stringy" in nature, on deeper palpation.

Arbuckle (1977) discussed Chapman's initial discovery of these reflexes in her collection *Selected Writings of Beryl Arbuckle*:

Chapman found highly congested points, in differ-ent regions of the fascia, and with certain very definite groupings he found to exist a definite entity of disease or, reversely, with a particular disease he always found a definite pattern in these regions. These findings led him to conclude that the states of hypercongestion were due to a lymph stasis, in viscus, or gland, which was manifested by soreness or tenderness at the distal ends of the spinal nerves. To understand this reasoning one

must have a knowledge of the lymphatic system, the autonomic nervous system, and the interrelation of the endocrine glands, and the embryologic segmentation of the body.

Arbuckle cites Speransky (1944) in support of Chapman's concepts. Speransky demonstrated that CSF travels through the lymphatic structures to all areas of the body. This fact, reinforced by Erlinghauser's (1959) research into CSF circu-lation through tubular connective tissue fibrils (described in Chapter 13), combined with knowledge of the many nutrient substances carried by nerve axons, strongly supports Chap-man's concept of neurolymphatic reflexes (Korr 1967).

Validating study (Snider et al. 2016)

Recent research has validated the existance and usefulness of assessment of Chapman's reflexes :

Statistically significant positive associations were found between specific vertebral [palpation] findings and abnormalities of the esophagus, gastroesophageal junction, pylorus, ascending colon, and sigmoid colon; specific Chapman reflex point tenderness and abnor-malities of the esophagus, gastroesophageal junction, pylorus, ascending colon, descending colon, sigmoid colon, and rectum; and specific visceral sphincter ten-derness and abnormalities of the duodenum, ascend-ing colon, and sigmoid colon.

Notes

Charts and details for the manual treatment of these reflexes are to be found in:

An endocrine interpretation of Chapman's reflexes (Owens 1963)

Modern Neuromuscular Techniques (Chaitow 2002).

Notes

The illustrations in this chapter, and the accompany-ing tables *located in the Appendix,* are intended to be used for palpation purposes only.

How difficult is it to find these reflexes?

Arbuckle comments on the palpation requirements for locating these reflexes: "Trained, seeing, sensing, feeling fingers … are able to 'open some of the windows and doors' for the correction of perverted circulation of fluids."

How easy is it to achieve this? Owens says:

> *You may not at first be able readily to locate the gangliform contractions with ease, but with practice you will acquire a readiness of tactile perception that will greatly facilitate your work. Do not use excessive pressure on either anterior or posterior.*

Possible clinical value of neurolymphatic reflexes

Since the location of these palpable tissue changes is relatively constant in relation to specific viscera, it may be possible to establish the location of pathology without knowing its nature.

The value of these reflexes is threefold:

1. They are valuable as diagnostic aids. Patriquin (1997) points out that some of the reflexes, such as that for the appendix (tip of 12th rib on the right – see Fig. 4.8, point 38) are invaluable in helping with differential diagnosis when faced with right lower abdominal pain. "Today, Chapman's reflexes are more likely to be used as an integral part of [osteopathic] physical examination, than as a specific therapeutic intervention."

2. They can be used to influence the motion of lymph.

3. Visceral function may be influenced via the nervous system.

> *[The] reflexes can be clinically manipulated to specifically reduce adverse sympathetic influence on a particular organ or visceral system … patients with frequent bowel movements from the effects of IBS report they have normal or near normal function for days to months after soft tissue treatment over the iliotibial bands and/or the lumbosacral paraspinal tissues and associated Chapman's reflexes. (Patriquin 1997)*

For our purposes these possible uses of the reflexes are less important than establishing whether you are able to identify localized changes as descibed.

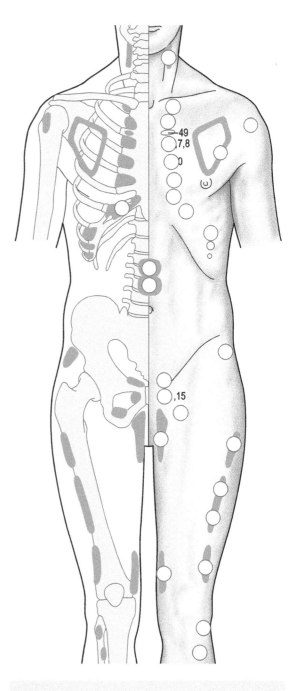

Figure 4.7

Chapman's neurolymphatic reflexes – anterior surface. See the tables in the Appendix (pp. 373–375).

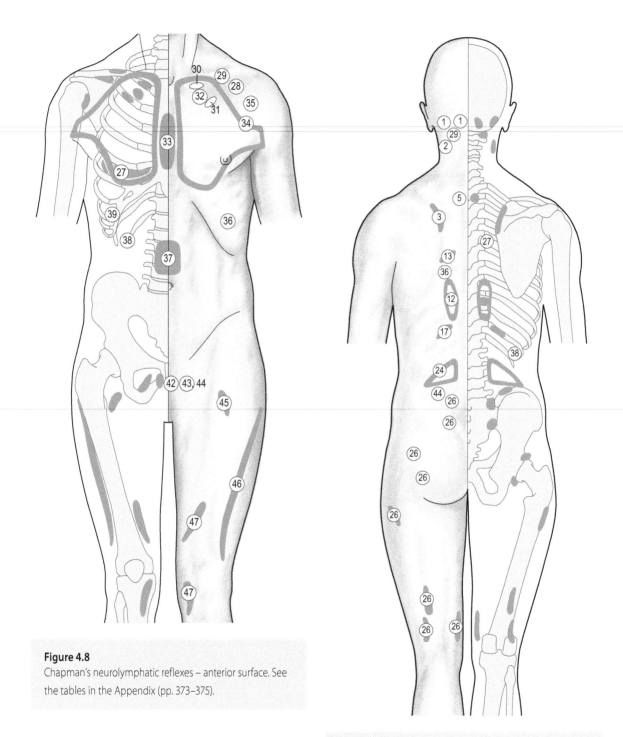

Figure 4.8
Chapman's neurolymphatic reflexes – anterior surface. See the tables in the Appendix (pp. 373–375).

Figure 4.9
Chapman's neurolymphatic reflexes – posterior surface. See the tables in the Appendix (pp. 373–375).

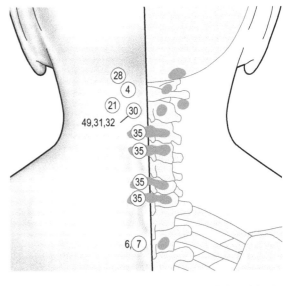

Figure 4.11
Chapman's neurolymphatic reflexes – posterior cervical
surface. See the tables in the Appendix (pp. 373–375).

Chapman, Owens, and Arbuckle suggest that these points are only active – and therefore of use for treatment purposes – when both the anterior and posterior points of a pair are active, as evidenced by both being at the same time palpable and sensitive.

The degree of sensitivity of the anterior of the pair is suggested to indicate the degree of associated lymphatic congestion.

Sequence

The palpation sequence suggested by these researchers is as follows:

- Start by palpating the anterior reflexes.

- If any are found to be active (i.e., they are easily palpated/located and are sensitive), the pair of this reflex should then be examined on the posterior aspect of the body.

- If this is also easily palpable and sensitive, treatment commences on the anterior reflex point.

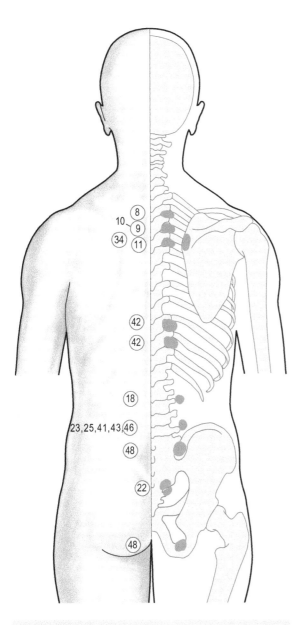

Figure 4.10
Chapman's neurolymphatic reflexes – posterior surface.
See the tables in the Appendix (pp. 373–375).

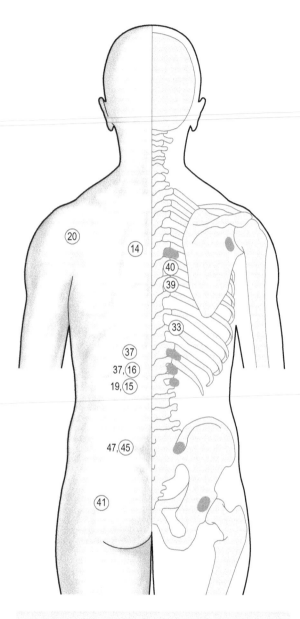

Figure 4.12
Chapman's neurolymphatic reflexes – posterior surface.
See the tables in the Appendix (pp. 373–375).

- Gentle rotary pressure is used in the treatment phase, "dosage" being determined by palpation.

- The aim is to decrease palpated edema, as well as an easing of the gangliform contracture in the deep fascia, together with reduction of tenderness in the anterior reflex areas.

- The actual time involved in treating a point may be from 20 seconds to 2 minutes.

- Rechecking for sensitivity by gentle palpation is suggested after treatment.

Notes

These points may also be searched for by using skin stretching, "drag" palpation, or via a systematic soft tissue assessment, as advocated in Lief's NMT evaluation described in the next chapter.

Exercise 4.18 *Palpating Chapman's Reflex Areas/Points*

Time suggested **4–6 minutes to evaluate and "treat" a pair of reflex points**

- If this system interests you, spend some time palpating (using all or any of the evaluation methods outlined in this chapter) for pairs of neurolymphatic points as illustrated (see Figs 4.7–4.12) and described above.

- See the tables in the Appendix (pp. 373–375) for captions/legends relating to these figures.

- Record your findings.

Next

In the next chapter, palpation and assessment of muscle is the focus. Before that, Special topic 5 discusses the connection between acupuncture points and the soft tissues (skin, fascia etc).

Skilled skin palpation allows you to target areas of dysfunction below the surface and it is towards the structural information lying in the superficial tissues and muscles themselves that our attention will next be focused.

References

Adams T, Steinmetz J, Heisey R et al. (1982) Physiologic basis for skin properties in palpatory physical diagnosis. Journal of the American Osteopathic Association 81 (6): 366–377.

Arbuckle B (1977) Selected writings of Beryl Arbuckle. Chicago, IL: National Osteopathic Institute.

Baldry P (1993) Acupuncture, trigger points and musculoskeletal pain. Edinburgh: Churchill Livingstone.

Barral J-P (1996) Manual-thermal diagnosis. Seattle: Eastland Press.

Beal M (1983) Palpatory testing of somatic dysfunction in patients with cardiovascular disease. Journal of the American Osteopathic Association 82 (July): 822–831.

Beal M (1985) Viscerosomatic reflexes: A review. Journal of the American Osteopathic Association 85 (12): 786–801.

Benjamin M (2009) The fascia of the limbs and back – a review. Journal of Anatomy 214: 1–18.

Bischof I and Elmiger G (1960) Connective tissue massage, in Licht S (ed) Massage, Manipulation and Traction. New Haven, CT: Licht.

Brugger A (1962) Pseudoradikulare syndrome. Acta Rheumatologica 19: 1.

Cerda E (2005) Mechanics of scars. Journal of Biomechanics 38: 1598–1603.

Chaitow L (2002) Modern neuromuscular techniques. Edinburgh: Elsevier.

Chaitow L (2015) Positional release techniques, 4th edn. Edinburgh: Elsevier.

Dicke E (1954) Meine Bindegewebsmassage. Stuttgart: Hippokrates.

Dvorak J and Dvorak V (1984) Manual medicine diagnostics. Stuttgart: Georg Thieme Verlag.

Erlinghauser R (1959) The circulation of CSF through the connective tissue system. Newark, OH: Yearbook of the Academy of Applied Osteopathy.

Fossum C, Kuchera ML, Devine WH et al. (2011) Chapman's reflexes, in Chila AG (ed) Foundations for Osteopathic Medicine, 3rd edn. Baltimore: Lippincott, Williams and Wilkins, pp 853–865.

Frymann V (1963) Palpation – its study in the workshop. Newark: Yearbook of the American Academy of Osteopathy, pp 16–30.

Gutstein R (1944) A review of myodysneuria (fibrositis). American Practitioner and Digest of Treatments 6 (4): 114–124.

Juhan D (1987) Job's body. New York: Station Hill Press.

Kelso AF (1985) Viscerosomatic reflexes: A review. Journal of the American Osteopathic Association 85 (12): 786–801.

Korr I (1967) Axonal delivery of neuroplasmic components to muscle cells. Science 155: 342–345.

Korr I (1970) Physiological basis of osteopathic medicine. New York: Postgraduate Institute of Osteopathic Medicine and Surgery.

Korr I (1975) Proprioceptors and somatic dysfunction. Journal of the American Osteopathic Association 74: 638.

Korr I (1976) Spinal cord as organiser of disease process. Newark, OH: Academy of Applied Osteopathy Yearbook.

Korr I (ed) (1977) Neurobiological mechanisms in manipulation. New York: Plenum Press.

Lewit K (1992) Manipulative therapy in rehabilitation of the locomotor system, 2nd edn. London: Butterworths.

Lewit K (1999) Manipulative therapy in rehabilitation of the locomotor system, 3rd edn. London: Butterworths.

Lewit K (2003) Manipulační léčba v myoskeletální medicíně. Prague: Nakl. Sdělovací technika s.r.o, p 411.

Owens C (1963) An endocrine interpretation of Chapman's reflexes, 2nd edn. Carmel, CA: Academy of Applied Osteopathy.

Patriquin D (1997) Chapman's reflexes, in Ward R (ed) Foundations for Osteopathic Medicine. Baltimore: Williams and Wilkins.

Petrů V (2003) Ovlivnění ventilace u žen po ablaci prsu pomocí měkkých technik na hrudníku. Prague: Thsis FTVS UK, p 82.

Simons D (1987) Myofascial pain due to trigger points. International Rehabilitation Medicine Association, IRMA Monograph Series Number 1, pp 22–26.

Simons D (1993) Myofascial pain and dysfunction review. Journal of Musculoskeletal Pain 1 (2): 131.

Snider KT, Schneider RP, Sinder EJ et al (2016) Correlation of somatic dysfunction with gastrointestinal endoscopic findings: an observational study. Journal of the American Osteopathic Association 116: 358–369.

Speransky AD (1944) A basis for the theory of medicine. New York: International Publisher.

Swerdlow B and Dieter N (1992) Evaluation of thermography. Pain 48: 205–213.

Travell J and Simons D (1992, 1992) Myofascial pain and dysfunction, vols 1 and 2. Baltimore: Williams and Wilkins.

Upledger J (1983) Craniosacral therapy – beyond the dura. Seattle: Eastland Press.

Upledger J and Vredevoogd W (1983) Craniosacral therapy. Seattle: Eastland Press.

Valouchová P and Lewit K (2008) Surface electromyography of abdominal and back muscles in patients with active scars. Journal of Bodywork and Movement Therapies 13 (3): 262–267.

van Zuijlen PP, de Vries HJ, Lamme HM et al. (2002) Morphometry of dermal collagen orientation by Fourier analysis is superior to multi-observer assessment. Journal of Pathology 198 (3): 284–291.

Wald M, Křížová H, Prausová J et al. (1999) Sekundární lymfedém po lymfadenektomiích. Praktický lékař 79: 665–716.

Walton W (1971) Palpatory diagnosis of the osteopathic lesion. Journal of the American Osteopathic Association 71: 117–131.

Special topic 4

Source of pain: is it reflex or local?
Leon Chaitow

If someone is experiencing pain that is referred from a distant site, then palpation of that area will seldom increase the discomfort being experienced. In contrast, when pain is actually arising from the tissues being palpated, the process of applied pressure (even light) to these tissues will commonly increase the discomfort being experienced.

But where might referred pain be coming from? A Norwegian study involving over 3000 people showed that localized musculoskeletal pain is relatively rare, and that musculoskeletal pain usually coexists with pain in other parts of the body (Kamaleri et al. 2008).

Knowledge of the patterns of distribution of trigger point symptoms/pain allows for a swift focusing on suitable sites in which to search for an offending trigger (if the pain is indeed related to a myofascial trigger point).

Alternatively, the discomfort could be a radicular symptom, deriving from the spine. Grieve (1984) reports: "When pain is being referred into a limb due to a spinal problem, the greater the pain distally from the source, the greater the index of difficulty in successfully treating it" (i.e., the further distal the pain is from the cause, the greater the difficulty).

Dvorak and Dvorak (1984) observe: "For patients with acute radicular syndrome there is little diagnostic difficulty, which is not the case for patients with chronic back pain, some differentiation for further therapy is especially important, although not always simple.

> **Notes**
>
> Note: The term "referred pain" includes other sensations including numbness and tingling. The functional limitations caused by trigger points include muscle weakness, poor co-ordination of movement, fatigue with activity, decreased work tolerance, lack of endurance, and joint stiffness, as well as limitations in active and passive range of motion (Dommerholt & Issa 2009).

Noting that a mixed clinical picture is common, Dvorak and Dvorak then say: "When testing for the radicular syndrome, particular attention is to be paid to the motor disturbances and the deep tendon reflexes. When examining sensory radicular disorders, the attention should be towards the algesias."

However, the referred pain may not be from either a trigger point, or the spine. Kellgren (1938, 1939) showed that:

The superficial fascia of the back, the spinous processes and the supraspinous ligaments, induce local pain upon stimulation, while stimulation of the superficial portions of the interspinous ligaments and the superficial muscles, results in a diffused (more widespread) type of pain.

Mense and Simons (2001) give clear guidelines as to what the practitioner needs to be aware of when seeking the source of muscular pain: "Because muscle pain and tenderness can be referred from trigger points, articular dysfunctions, and enthesitis [inflammation associated with musculotendinous junctions], the examiner must examine these sites for evidence of a condition that would cause referred muscle pain and tenderness."

Mense and Simons maintain that "local pain and tenderness in muscle is commonly caused by trigger points," but suggest that it is necessary to separate such local pain from other possible sources, including projected, referred and central sources:

- "projected pain" (deriving from "peripheral nerve irritation that initiates sensory action potentials at the site of irritation," e.g., the lightning pain felt when the ulnar nerve at the elbow is bumped)

- "referred pain", which commonly has a "diffuse aching quality". However, at times there may be a sharper "projected pain," deriving from a nerve lesion.

Visceral factors and "imposter" symptoms

Grieve (1984) has described "imposter" symptoms deriving from conditions other than musculoskeletal ones. He suggests that we need an awareness of when manual or other physical therapy may be unsuitable – and perhaps foolish – when sources of pain masquerade as musculoskeletal symptoms. He suggests that we should be suspicious of symptoms which present as musculoskeletal if:

- the symptoms as presented do not seem "quite right"; for example, if there is a discrepancy between the patient's story and the presenting symptoms

- the patient reports patterns of activity which aggravate or ease the symptoms that are unusual in the practitioner's experience.

Grieve cautions that practitioners should remain alert to the fact that symptoms that arise from sinister causes (e.g., neoplasms) may closely mimic musculoskeletal symptoms or may coexist with actual musculoskeletal dysfunction. If a treatment plan is not working out, if there is lack of progress in the resolution of symptoms, or if there are unusual responses to treatment the practitioner should urgently review the situation.

Additionally visceral lesions may refer pain into muscle, such as in the pain noted in the lower left abdomen with appendicitis, which is very much the same type of pain noted when trigger points are present in that region.

Central pain derives from sources such as a spinal cord injury, surgery involving the CNS, or a peripheral injury that interrupts the connection to the CNS, such as occurs in amputation and subsequent phantom limb pain. Mense and Simons (2001) report that: "apparently, a peripheral pain experience can produce a central imprint that can serve as a central source of pain and also modifies peripheral referral patterns."

Pain can also be referred to a muscle from:

- unknown sensitive locations other than trigger points. For example, pressure on areas several inches from active and latent trigger points can produce referred pain. Mense and Simons (2001) state that "the reason for this spot sensitivity in normal muscle is unexplored."

- joints, particularly the capsules, zygapophyseal (facet) joints. This can lead to confusion when local trigger points produce similar patterns of pain. Mense and Simons (2001) report that "the muscles crossing involved [blocked] joints are … likely to develop trigger points producing secondary muscle-induced pain because of the joint problem."

Thus, ligaments and fascia must be considered as sources of referred pain, and this is made clearer by Brugger (1960), who describes a number of syndromes in which altered arthromuscular components produce reflexogenic pain. These are attributed to painfully stimulated tissues (origins of tendons, joint capsules and so on) producing pain in muscles, tendons and overlying skin.

Anterior thorax

As an example, irritation and increased sensitivity in the region of the sternum, clavicles, and rib attachments to the sternum, through occupational or postural stresses, will influence or cause painful intercostal muscles, scalenes, sternomastoid, pectoralis major and cervical muscles. The increased tone in these muscles, and the resultant stresses that they produce, may lead to spondylogenic problems in the cervical region, with further spread of symptoms. Overall, this syndrome can produce chronic pain in the neck, head, chest wall, arm, and hand (even mimicking heart disease).

Dvorak and Dvorak (1984) have charted a multitude of what they term "spondylogenic reflexes" that derive from (in the main) intervertebral joints. The palpated changes are characterized as:

Painful swellings, tender upon pressure and detachable with palpation, located in the musculofascial tissue in topographically well defined sites. The average size varies from 0.5 cm to 1 cm and the main characteristic is the absolutely timed and qualitative linkage to the extent of the functionally abnormal position (segmental dysfunction). As long as a disturbance exists, the zones of irritation can be identified, yet disappear immediately after the removal of the disturbance.

The Dvoraks also see altered mechanics in a vertebral unit as causing: "reflexogenic pathological change of the soft tissue, the most important being the 'myotendinoses,' which can be identified by palpation."

Some would argue that the soft tissue changes precede the altered vertebral states, at least in some instances (poor posture, overuse, misuse, abuse, trauma). Wherever you stand in this debate, this brief survey of some opinions as to "where the pain is coming from" shows clearly that we need to keep many possibilities in mind.

As we palpate and evaluate, the questions that we need to be asking ourselves almost constantly include: "which of this patient's symptoms, whether of pain or other forms of dysfunction, are the result of reflexogenic activity such as trigger points?"

In other words, what palpable, measurable, identifiable evidence is there that connects what we can observe, test and palpate to the symptoms (pain, restriction, fatigue, etc.) of this patient? And what, if anything, can be done to remedy or modify the situation, safely and effectively, and what can the person do (or be taught to do) to prevent recurrence?

References

Brugger A (1960) Pseudoradikulara syndrome. Acta Rheumatologica 18: 1.

Dommerholt J and Issa T (2009) Differential diagnosis of fibromyalgia, in Chaitow L (ed) Fibromyalgia syndrome: A practitioner's guide to treatment, 3rd edn. Edinburgh: Elsevier.

Dvorak J and Dvorak V (1984) Manual medicine: diagnostics. New York: George Thieme Verlag.

Grieve G (1984) Mobilisation of the spine. Churchill Livingstone, Edinburgh.

Kamaleri Y, Natvig B, Ihlebaek CM, Benth JS and Bruusgaard D (2008). Number of pain sites is associated with demographic, lifestyle, and health-related factors in the general population. European Journal of Pain 12 (6): 742–748.

Kellgren J (1938) Observation of referred pain arising from muscles. Clinical Science 3: 175.

Kellgren J (1939) On the distribution of pain arising from deep somatic strictures. Clinical Science 4: 35.

Mense S, Simons D (2001) Muscle pain. Philadelphia: Williams and Wilkins.

Special topic 5

The morphology of reflex and acupuncture points
Leon Chaitow

Pain researchers have demonstrated that approximately 75% of trigger points are located where acupuncture points are shown on traditional meridian maps (Melzack & Wall 1988; Wall & Melzack 1989). The remainder may be thought of as "honorary" acupuncture points since, according to Traditional Chinese Medicine (TCM), all spontaneously tender areas (whether or not they are on the meridian maps) are suitable for acupuncture (or acupressure) treatment – and a trigger point is nothing if it is not spontaneously tender!

Using delicate measuring techniques, Ward (1996) examined 12 acupuncture sites that are also common trigger point sites, in the trapezius and infraspinatus muscles. He found precisely the "spike" of electrical activity characteristic of an active trigger point in all of these.

Mense and Simons (2001) are less definite: "Frequently the acupuncture point selected for the treatment of pain is also a trigger point, but sometimes it is not."

However, if they usually lie in the same place as acupuncture points, what tissues are involved?

Bossy (1984) examined the associated tissues extensively and reported that all motor points of medical electrology are also acupuncture points (which he calls "privileged loci of the organism that allow exchanges between the inner body and the environment"). The skin manifestation is, he says, "easier to feel than to see. The most superficial morphological expression is a cupule" (see the "hills and valleys" palpation section in Chapter 4).

Under the skin (which is a little thinner than surrounding skin) covering these "privileged loci" there are common features:

- Neurovascular bundles are commonly found.
- Connective tissue is always a feature.
- Fatty tissue is sometimes present.
- Vessels and nerves seem to be important common features, although their stimulation during treatment is usually indirect, as the result of deformation of connective tissue and consequent traction.
- In some instances, tendons, periarticular structures, or muscle tissues are involved, as part of the acupuncture/trigger point morphology.

After extensive dissection, Bossy states that "fat and connective tissue are determinants for the appearance of the acupuncture sensation."

Bossy's research has been validated by subsequent investigation – most notably by Langevin and Yandow (2002), as described below.

Acupuncture points and fascia

Staubesand and Li (1997) studied human fascia using electron photomicroscopy and found smooth muscle cells embedded within collagen fibers. This research also showed that there are a great many perforations of the superficial fascial layer, characterized by penetration through the fascia of venous, arterial and neural structures (mainly unmyelinated vegetative nerves).

Heine (1995), who also documented the existence of these perforations in the superficial fascia, was additionally involved in the study of acupuncture, and established that the majority (82%) of these perforation points are topographically identical with traditional Chinese acupuncture points.

Langevin and Yandow (2002) noted that acupuncture meridians were traditionally believed to constitute channels, connecting the surface of the body to internal organs. Langevin and colleagues hypothesized that the network of acupuncture points and meridians can be viewed as a representation of the network formed by interstitial connective tissue. This hypothesis is supported by ultrasound images showing connective tissue cleavage planes at acupuncture points in normal human subjects. She mapped acupuncture points in serial gross anatomical sections through the human arm, and found "an 80% correspondence between the sites of acupuncture points and the location of intermuscular or intramuscular connective tissue planes in postmortem tissue sections."

This sort of research into the behavior and morphology of acupuncture (and other reflex) points helps to explain some of the common findings noted on palpation. For example, a slight "cupule" or depression, overlaid with slightly thinner skin tissue, can usually be felt, indicating the presence of an acupuncture point (which if sensitive is "active" and quite likely to be also a trigger point).

Shang (2009) explains the "cupule" phenomenon as follows: "Many acupuncture points are located at transition points, or boundaries, between different body domains or muscles, coinciding with the fascia and connective tissue planes."

As was noted in Chapter 4, other palpatory signs exist, skin "drag" and loss of elastic qualities being the most important palpatory indications.

References

Bossy J (1984) Morphological data concerning acupuncture points and channel networks. Acupuncture and ElectroTherapeutics Research International Journal 9 (2): 79–106.

Heine H (1995) Functional anatomy of traditional Chinese acupuncture points. Acta Anatomica 152: 293.

Langevin H and Yandow J (2002) Relationship of acupuncture points and meridians to connective tissue planes. Anatomical Record 269: 257–265.

Melzack R and Wall P (1988) The challenge of pain. Harmondsworth: Penguin Books.

Mense S and Simons D (2001) Muscle pain. Philadelphia: Lippincott Williams and Wilkins.

Shang C (2009) Prospective tests on biological models of acupuncture. Evidence-based Complementary and Alternative Medicine 6 (1): 31–39.

Staubesand J and Li Y (1997) Begriff und Substrat der Fazienssklerose bei chronisch-ven'ser Insuffizienz. Phlebologie 26: 72–79.

Wall P and Melzack R (1989) Textbook of pain, 2nd edn. London: Churchill Livingstone.

Ward A (1996) Spontaneous electrical activity at combined acupuncture and myofascial trigger point sites. Acupuncture Medicine 14 (2): 75–79.

Special topic 6

Is it a muscle or a joint problem?
Leon Chaitow

Is the patient's pain a soft tissue or a joint problem? And how can we rapidly make this differentiation?

There are several simple screening tests to apply in answer to these questions, based on the work of Kaltenborn (1980):

1. Does passive stretching (traction) of the painful area increase the level of pain? If so, it is probably of soft tissue origin (extra-articular).

2. Does compression of the painful area increase the pain? If so, it is probably of joint origin (intra-articular), involving tissues belonging to that joint.

3. If active (controlled by the patient) movement in one direction produces pain (and/or is restricted), while passive (controlled by the therapist) movement in the opposite direction also produces pain (and/or is restricted), the contractile tissues (muscle, ligament, etc.) are implicated. This can be confirmed by resisted tests, described below.

4. If active movement and passive movement in the *same* direction produce pain (and/or restriction), joint dysfunction is probable. This can be confirmed by the use of traction and compression (and gliding) tests of the joint (see Special topic 9 on joint play/"end-feel").

Resisted tests are used to assess both strength and painful responses to muscle contraction, either from the muscle or its tendinous attachment. This involves producing a maximal contraction of the suspected muscle while the joint is kept immobile, somewhere near the midrange position. No joint motion should be allowed to occur. This is done following test 3 above, to confirm a soft tissue dysfunction rather than a joint involvement. Before doing the resisted test it is wise to perform the compression test to clear any suspicion of joint involvement.

Cyriax's "strength" tests

- If on resisted testing (Cyriax 1962) the muscle seems *strong, and also painful,* there is no more than a minor lesion/dysfunction of the muscle or its tendon.

- If the muscle is *weak and painful,* there is a more serious lesion/dysfunction of the muscle or tendon.

- If it is *weak and painless,* there may be a neurological lesion or the tendon has ruptured. A normal muscle tests strong and pain free.

- It is suggested that you test all these statements on painful conditions of known origin.

- Obviously, in many instances, soft tissue dysfunction will accompany (precede, or follow on from) joint dysfunction.

- Joint involvement is less likely in the early stages of soft tissue dysfunction than (for example) in the chronic stages of muscle shortening.

- There are few joint conditions, acute or chronic, without some etiological – or maintaining – soft tissue involvement.

The tests described above will give a strong indication, though, as to whether the major involvement in such a situation is primarily of soft or osseous structures.

Compression – pain provocation

An example of a joint assessment involving compression would be that described by Blower and Griffin (1984) for sacroiliac dysfunction.

- This showed that pressure applied over the lower half of the sacrum, or over the anterior superior iliac spines, was diagnostic of sacroiliac problems (possibly indicating ankylosing spondylitis) *if pain is produced in the sacrum and buttocks.*

- Soft tissue dysfunction would not produce painful responses with this type of compression test.

Notes

Lumbar pain is not thought to be significant if it occurs on sacral pressure, as this action causes movement of the lumbosacral joint as well as some motion throughout the whole lumbar spine.

Joint or muscle dysfunction – which is primary?

Janda (1988) answers this question when he says that it is not known whether dysfunction of muscles causes joint dysfunction or vice versa. He points out, however, that since clinical evidence abounds that joint mobilization (thrust or gentle mobilization) influences the muscles that are in anatomical or functional relationships with a joint, it may well be that normalization of the muscles' excessive tone is what is providing the benefit and that, by implication, normalization of the muscle tone by other means (such as MET) would produce a beneficial outcome and joint normalization. Since reduction in muscle spasm/contraction commonly results in a reduction in joint pain, the answer to many such problems would seem to lie in appropriate soft tissue attention.

Liebenson (1990) takes a view with a chiropractic bias:

The chief abnormalities of (musculoskeletal) function include muscular hypertonicity and joint blockage. Since these abnormalities are functional rather than structural they are reversible in nature. Once a particular [spinal] joint has lost its normal range of motion, the muscles around that joint will attempt to minimise stress at the involved segment.

After describing the processes of progressive compensation, as some muscles become hypertonic while inhibiting their antagonists, he continues:

What may begin as a simple restriction of movement in a joint can lead to the development of muscular imbalances and postural change. This chain of events is an example of what we try to prevent through adjustments of subluxations.

We are left, then, with views that suggest that muscle release will frequently normalize joint restrictions, and also that joint normalization sorts out soft tissue problems.

Can both views be correct?

Absolutely, say Kappler and Jones (2003), describing what is perceived as a restricted joint being taken towards its end of range (as noted in Chapter 8):

As the barrier is engaged, increasing amounts of force are necessary and the distance decreases. The term barrier may be misleading if it is interpreted as a wall or rigid obstacle to be overcome with a push. As the joint reaches the barrier, restraints in the form of tight muscles and fascia, serve to inhibit further motion. We are **pulling** *against restraints rather than* **pushing** *against some anatomic structure.*

It is likely that both views are correct; however, the clinical certainty is that what is required is usually anything but a purely local focus, as Janda helps us to understand (see Chapter 5).

Special topic Exercise 6.1 Evaluating Soft Tissue and Joint Involvement

Time suggested: 5–10 minutes

You will require palpation partners with known soft tissue and joint dysfunction to perform this evaluation adequately.

- Test the various guidelines described above (i.e., performing active and passive movement in the same and in different directions as well as compression–distraction) to establish whether what you are dealing with is purely of joint or purely of soft tissue origin.

- Decide whether these assessment methods are accurate.

- Remember that it is common for both a joint and associated soft tissues to be distressed simultaneously, which might provide you with conflicting evidence (i.e., both joint and soft tissue involvement).

- If this is the case, knowledge that there is joint involvement may influence your therapeutic approaches.

References

Blower PW and Griffin AJ (1984) Clinical sacroiliac tests in ankylosing spondylitis and other causes of low back pain – 2 studies. Annals of Rheumatic Disease 43: 192–195.

Cyriax J (1962) Textbook of orthopaedic medicine. London: Cassell.

Janda V (1988) Muscles and cervicogenic pain syndromes, in Grant R (ed) Physical therapy of the cervical and thoracic spine. New York: Churchill Livingstone, pp 153–166.

Kappler RE and Jones JM (2003) Thrust (high-velocity/low-amplitude) techniques, in Ward RC (ed) Foundations for osteopathic medicine, 2nd edn. Philadelphia: Lippincott, Williams and Wilkins, pp 852–880.

Kaltenborn F (1980) Mobilization of the extremity joints. Oslo: Olaf Novlis Bokhandel.

Liebenson C (1990) AMRT, pt.1. Journal of Manipulative and Physiological Therapeutics 13 (1): 2–6.

Where does muscle end and connective tissue begin?

It is important that we establish what is meant in this text by the word "muscle."

> *Skeletal muscles comprise contractile tissue intricately woven together by fibrous connective tissue that gradually blends into tendons … made of fibrous connective tissue [that] attach the muscle to bone. Although contractile tissue and tendons are sometimes evaluated separately for research purposes, they cannot be separated during routine clinical testing and stretching procedures, nor during functional activity. For these reasons, the term "muscle" is used to indicate the entire skeletal muscle, including the contractile tissue and tendon components.* (Weppler & Magnusson 2010)

This definition needs to be kept in mind, in relation to palpation assessment of "muscles."

How do you feel?

Unlike the skin, which is there for us to see as well as touch, when we begin to explore below the surface to gather clinically useful information, far greater skills are required. Guidance can be given as to what superficial muscular tissues *should* feel like, under given conditions, in order to read such information by gentle palpation. This gives the phrase: "How do you feel?" a whole new meaning, because "how" you feel/touch/palpate will determine "what" you feel – after which interpretation of that information becomes necessary.

It is not just the relative state of tone, tension, contraction, flaccidity, and so on, that we need to be aware of, important though these factors are; there are also fluid fluctuations through connective tissue and other rhythmic patterns that may help to indicate the degree of normality, or otherwise, of the soft tissues.

In order to make sense of these fluid movements when it comes to palpating at greater depth, or understanding more subtle sensations, fairly refined skills are required.

Some of these have been well explored and explained, for example by Upledger (1987), Becker (1963, 1964, 1965), and Fritz Smith (1986), as discussed in Chapter 15, as well as by Stanley Lief, the prime developer of neuromuscular technique (see later in this chapter; Chaitow 1988, 2002; Chaitow & DeLany 2008).

In this chapter methods aimed at determining structural changes in the soft tissues (increased tone, shortening, fibrous development, periosteal pain points, trigger points and so on) are reviewed.

Overuse, misuse, and abuse of the soft tissues

Before we delve into methods of soft tissue palpation, we should briefly review the reasons why the changes we are trying to evaluate occur.

A host of interacting factors have the ability to increase muscular tone, including stress responses, postural anomalies and overload, repetitive physical actions (sport, occupation, hobbies, and so on), emotional distress, trauma, structural factors (congenital short leg), visceral and other reflex activities.

These, and other influences, can be summarized as *overuse, misuse and abuse* of the musculoskeletal structures involving adaptive, compensatory changes.

A sequence

Hypertonicity has been defined as, literally, *too much muscle tone* (Ng et al. 1998; Simons & Mense 1998; Mense 2008). There are two types:

- *Intrinsic* hypertonicity is an abnormal increase in the resistance to stretch of a resting muscle.

- *Neuromotor* hypertonicity is an abnormal increase in the readiness with which the nervous system activates the muscle in response to stimuli (Ng et al. 1998).

Masi & Hannon (2008) note that localized (focal) areas of nodularity (as in the presence of trigger points) may occur following muscle injury or repetitive strains. A possible mechanism involves occurrence of a small area of ischemia and calcium release in contracted sarcomeric units (Simons 2008).

- This is supported by the finding that in chronic tension-type headache, spontaneous electromyographic (EMG) activity of muscles surrounding trigger points was found to be no greater than in healthy subjects (Couppé et al. 2007).

- In another study both muscle tenderness and objective "hardness" were found to be greater in trigger point areas than in the muscle as a whole (Ashina et al. 2005).

These findings suggest that trigger points, and surrounding muscle hypertonicity, are local manifestations (Simons & Mense 1998) – *not involving the whole muscle.*

Higham and Biewener (2011) have shown that "it is possible for a part of a muscle to exhibit very little strain, while another region undergoes a considerable amount of shortening or lengthening." These observations also suggest that when the tone of a muscle is increased for any length of time, a degree of local irritation may result, due to two factors:

1. local tissue hypoxia or ischemia (and subsequent repercussions such as calcium release and trigger point development), involving inadequate oxygenation of the tissues due to increases in tone and demand

2. relative inadequacy of drainage and removal of metabolic waste products.

This combination leads firstly to fatigue, then to irritation, and in some instances to inflammation, over time. This is the "acute" phase of the body's response to any persistent increase in tone (see Local adaptation syndrome, below). During this stage, discomfort is probable and pain possible, creating a cycle in which even greater tone, and therefore more pain, becomes likely. If these changes occur in response to a single or short-term adaptive demand (for example, playing tennis for the first time after a long break, digging the garden in the spring, or any one-off, unaccustomed effort), self-regulatory mechanisms ensure that the stiffness and soreness fade away after a few days.

However, if the adaptive demands are repeated, different effects are likely.

Local adaptation syndrome

This phase may be equated with the alarm stage in Selye's (1984) general adaptation syndrome (GAS). Indeed, all elements of the GAS can be scaled down to a local level (a single muscle or joint, for example) in which the same stages are passed through (alarm, adaptation, collapse). This is then referred to as the local adaptation syndrome (LAS).

As would be expected, according to both the GAS and LAS, after the acute phase comes the phase of adaptation. In the muscular sense this means that if increased tone is maintained for longer than a few weeks, a chronic stage evolves, characterized by structural changes in the supporting tissues.[1]

Some see these adaptive alterations as an "organizing" response, in which sustained tone is replaced by concrete, supportive bands. The body is seen to be adapting to the seemingly permanent demand for increased tone in the musculature (Lewit 1999).

The degree of relative ischemia, hypoxia, and toxic debris retention increases at this stage, varying from person to person (and region to region) in relation to features such as age, degree of exercise, nutritional status, and so on. Any pain experienced usually has a deep, aching quality. Palpation tends to reveal a fibrous, stringy texture, and possibly edema. And it is during this adaptation stage that early signs may be noted of myofascial trigger point development, in which discrete areas of the affected soft tissues evolve into localized areas of facilitation/sensitization (Kuchera et al. 1990; Norris 1998). Or, as Kline (2011) puts it:

> *Time does not necessarily heal all wounds. Repetitive motion injuries as well as single incident injuries may create confusing, seemingly unrelated symptoms in areas far from the original source of strain years after the fact [affecting] both the condition and the function of [soft tissues].*

---

1 Note: Selye's models are discussed in this text with an awareness that they are regarded by many as over-simplistic, and possibly "outdated" (McEwen & Wingfield 2010), and that there exist more sophisticated explanations of homeostasis, allostasis, and the way tissues and the body respond to stress. Nevertheless, Selye's model remains a useful, even if partial, way of understanding bodily responses to life-events. For an overview of current thinking regarding "stress" see Le Moal (2007).

Pavan et al. (2014) offer these thoughts on the fascial changes we may feel when palpating:

> *Diet, exercise, and overuse syndromes are able to modify the viscosity of loose connective tissue within fascia, causing densification, an alteration that is easily reversible. Trauma, surgery, diabetes, and aging alter the fibrous layers of fasciae, leading to fascial fibrosis.*

Highly sensitive, discrete, and palpable tissue changes result that are themselves capable of sending noxious impulses to distant target areas, where pain is sensed, and new "crops" of embryonic trigger points develop. Bands of stress fibers commonly become evident in the hypertonic tissues, and muscles affected in this way begin to place increasing degrees of tension on their tendons and their osseous attachments (Mense & Simons 2001; Simons et al 1999). (See also notes on connective tissue diagnostic methods in Chapter 6.) As the tendons begin to adapt, it is usually possible to palpate very tender periosteal pain points (PPP; discussed further in this chapter – see Exercise 5.11), or to note early signs of joint dysfunction (Lewit 2009).

The natural sequence in which tissues progress from an acute phase to an adaptation phase (which can last many years), and ultimately (when adaptive potential is exhausted), to the final phase of degeneration and disease, is a consequence of any unrelieved chronic hypertonicity. The end result could take the form of arthritic joint changes or chronic muscular or other soft tissue dysfunction (Lewit 2009; Murphy 2000; Ward 1997).

Palpation tasks

The palpating hand(s) needs to uncover the locality, nature, degree and – if possible – the age of soft tissue changes that take place in the sequence outlined above. As we palpate we need to ask:

- Is this palpable change acute or chronic (or, as is often the case, an acute phase of a chronic condition)?

- If acute, is inflammation associated with the changes?

- How do these palpable soft tissue changes relate to the patient's symptom pattern?

- Are these palpable changes part of a pattern of stress-induced change that can be mapped and understood?

- Are these soft tissue changes associated with pain, and if so, what is the nature of that pain?

- Are these palpable changes active reflexively, and if so, are active or latent trigger points involved (and if so, do they refer symptoms elsewhere, and does the patient recognize the perceived pain as part of their symptom picture)?

- Are the palpable changes the result of trigger points elsewhere, or of other reflex activity?

- Are these changes present in a postural or phasic muscle group?

- Are these palpable changes the result of joint restriction ("blockage," restriction, subluxation, lesion) or are they contributing to such dysfunction?

- Is there any pathology related to these palpable changes?

In other words, we need to ask ourselves: "What am I feeling, and what does it mean?"

Viola Frymann (1963) suggests the need for some thought as to how deeper palpation might be carried out, as we search for such changes, acute or chronic:

> *A slightly firmer approach brings the examiner into communication with the superficial muscles to determine their tone, their turgor, their metabolic state. Penetrating more deeply, similar study of the deeper muscle layers is possible [and] the state of the fascial sheaths and condensations may be noted.*

Light and variable touch needed

The words "firmer" and "penetrating more deeply," if taken too literally, could lead to "counterproductive" irritating palpation. If these recommendations were to involve a noticeable increase in applied pressure, two negative possibilities might occur:

- Firstly, there could be a defensive retraction of the palpated tissues, tensing superficial musculature, making assessment difficult, or its interpretation invalid.

- Secondly, there is likely to be a lessening of sensitivity, as pressure increases on the surface of the palpating digit or hand, especially if it is sustained for more than a short time, affecting the accuracy of perception.

Palpation solutions

Different solutions have been found to overcome these problems:

- In Lief's system of neuromuscular evaluation, outlined later in this chapter, these problems are largely overcome by use of what is termed "variable" pressure, in which the digital contact matches the resistance it meets from the tissues.

- Others have approached this problem differently, most notably Upledger (1987), with his suggestions of "melding" and synchronization that lead to the palpating hand or digits doing "exactly what the patient's body is doing and would otherwise be doing, even if you weren't there" (see Chapter 15).

- Rollin Becker (1963) used what he described as a "fulcrum" palpation technique, which increased perception of tissues at depth, without greatly increasing direct pressure on the skin surface (see Chapter 15).

- Fritz Smith (1986) makes his assessments in yet another way, using, among other methods, what he terms a "half-moon" vector contact (see Chapter 15).

The first section of this chapter looks at the palpation of structure. One aspect of identification of structural change is to observe its behavior, its function, and several examples of Janda's functional assessments have been incorporated into exercises in this chapter. These functional exercises, which, for example, evaluate the firing sequence of muscles, as normal movements are performed, are not to be confused with the palpation of function, which involves the assessment of subtle rhythmic fluctuations and pulses, as discussed and evaluated in Chapter 13.

The exercises in this chapter incorporate various ideas and recommendations for palpation of the soft tissues, derived from a number of prominent physicians and researchers from various schools and disciplines, including the Dvorak brothers, Janda, Magoun, Tilley, Lief, Nimmo, Lewit, and Beal. There is inevitably a degree of overlap in the concepts of these innovators of palpatory (and therapeutic) technique, but each has a unique insight into the needs of the practitioner who is trying to make sense of physical problems as they "read" the body.

A summary of recommended methods for a sequential assessment of shortened postural muscles is also explained. Interspersed amongst this are a number of exercises that can further enhance palpation sensitivity. It is suggested that *all* the methods outlined in this chapter be attempted, practiced and assessed for their individual degree of usefulness. Many therapists use all these methods (and others) in appropriate settings.

Palpation and assessment of structure

Rolf (1962) reminds us of the importance of keeping fascia in mind when we try to make sense of what we are palpating:

> Osteopathic manipulators have observed and recorded the extent to which all degenerative changes in the body, be they muscular, nervous, circulatory or organic, reflect in superficial fascia. Any degree of degeneration, however minor, changes the bulk of the fascia, modifies its thickness and draws it into ridges in areas overlying deeper tensions and rigidities.

Dvorak and Dvorak (1984) have outlined their basic requirements for sound palpation of the musculoskeletal system. They insist that a healthy anatomical structure cannot be differentiated from surrounding tissues, whereas "altered structure, can be exactly differentiated from the surrounding healthy tissue." Apart from starting to palpate from the site where the patient localizes the symptom (usually pain), the Dvoraks usefully emphasize that the therapist should have a "three-dimensional anatomical perception" of what is being palpated. They suggest that such knowledge leads to the application of "adequate pressure with regard to area, force and direction" as "the muscles, ligaments and other structures are located above and next to each other in the specific topographical region." They also suggest beginning palpation at the site of pain, localizing this, and then feeling precisely for hard, bony structures, and along tendons, for information about the attachments – making comparisons with "locations with the same anatomical arrangement and sites undergoing no changes" by use of stroking and pressing palpation, performed perpendicular to the direction of the fibers, until origins and insertions are reached.

It is suggested that you compare this description with Lief's neuromuscular technique palpation, and Nimmo's methods, as outlined later in this chapter (see Box 5.2), and decide which approach best suits the way you work.

The facilitated segment

Magoun (1948) made an important contribution to our understanding of the structural analysis of muscular tissues. Discussing what the searching practitioner will uncover, he asks: "What should palpation reveal?" Firstly Magoun notes that, if the soft tissues are abnormal, the practitioner must determine if the condition is a primary lesion (local) or a viscerosomatic reflex.

The primary lesion involves mainly the deep muscles, producing an inert and irregular rigor; if of long standing, the superficial tissues may be atonic or stringy. The hypersensitivity is usually limited to the deeper tissues … fibrous degeneration takes place, with overgrowth of connective tissue, calcification, thickening of the periosteum, and so on.

However, if the cause of tissue changes are of reflex (perhaps resulting from organ disease) origin there is likely to be: "a concentration of both superficial and deep tissues, both of which are hypersensitive to the same degree. *This continuous contraction, or exaggerated tone, makes the tissues hard and tense in a regular homogeneous manner*".

Beal (1983) directs attention to correction of viscerosomatic reflex activity by dealing with the causes of the dysfunction of the affected organ, which might involve nutritional, manipulative, or surgical interventions.

According to Lewit (1999), the first signs of viscerosomatic reflexive influences are vasomotor (increased skin temperature) and sudomotor (increased moisture of the skin) reactions, skin textural changes (e.g., thickening), increased subcutaneous fluid and increased contraction of muscle. Therefore the value of light skin palpation in identifying such areas of facilitation, as described in the previous chapter, cannot be too strongly emphasized.

A recent study has confirmed earlier reports of a direct link between visceral dysfunction and palpable changes in the paraspinal muscles (Snider et al. 2016). "The study found numerous associations between somatic dysfunction and abnormal endoscopic findings."

Tilley and Korr on the facilitated segment

McFarlane Tilley (1961) summarized aspects of digital palpation of the spine as follows:

1. light palpation to discover areas of increased moisture on the skin surface, indicating increased sweat gland activity (such as drag palpation described in Chapter 4)

2. moderate friction of the skin by heavier stroking to elicit "red reaction" (see Special topic 7)

3. deep palpation to elicit muscular tension and tenderness of tissues upon pressure.

Stress patterns may develop for any number of physical or emotional reasons, he states, as a result of which spinal nerve pathways and cord centers become facilitated (hyperreactive/sensitized). When this occurs, related spinal musculature becomes palpably altered; reflex relationships may be involved, including both viscerosomatic (organ to body tissues) and somaticovisceral (body tissues to organ) pathways.

Korr (1976) compared a facilitated area of the spine to a "neurological lens," in which stress factors involving body or mind are channeled through the facilitated segment, further focusing and intensifying activity through its neurological structures.

A simple diagnostic palpation method that suggests the presence of a facilitated segment, using "compressing" or "springing" of the paraspinal tissues, is outlined below (see Exercise 5.2).

Key palpatory features of the facilitated segment

- The common palpatory feature of segmental facilitation in the paraspinal musculature is a feeling of relative rigidity and tenderness when compared with the segments above and below.

- As a rule this will involve two or more adjacent segments, rather than just one local segment.

- There is likely to be both a loss of full range of motion involving the affected segment(s), as well as an asymmetry, with one side being more affected than the other.

● If the paraspinal rigidity results from visceral pathology, it will fail to respond – other than for a very short time – to any manual treatment applied to the muscles or joints involved.

● These rigid muscular states can, however, be a useful prognostic indicator of change, for better or worse, as treatment of the dysfunctioning organ proceeds.

● The palpation criteria discussed in Chapter 3 under the acronym "ARTT" will therefore apply: *asymmetry, restricted range of motion, tenderness and tissue changes.*

McFarlane Tilley (1961) lists the possible regional tissue implications of segmental facilitation, in various spinal regions, based on osteopathic clinical observations.

● Myocardial ischemia: rigid musculature in any two adjacent segments between T1 and T4 (usually left, but not essentially so).

● Cardiopulmonary pathology: any two adjacent segments of muscular paraspinal rigidity in the upper thoracic spine, either side or bilaterally.

● Duodenal pathology: any two adjacent segments of muscular paraspinal rigidity and tenderness, right side thoracic spine, levels 6, 7, and 8.

● Pancreatic dysfunction: any two adjacent segments of muscular paraspinal rigidity and tenderness, bilaterally, thoracic spine, segments 6, 7, 8, and 9.

● Liver and gall bladder: any two adjacent segments of muscular paraspinal rigidity and tenderness, right side thoracic spine, segments 8, 9, and 10.

● Chronic fatigue related to "adrenal exhaustion" or stress: any two adjacent segments of muscular paraspinal rigidity and tenderness in thoracic spine, segments 9, 10, 11, and 12.

● Renal disease: tenderness and pain on pressure, aggravated by percussion, thoracic spine segments 11, 12 and lumbar spine, segments 1, 2.

● Female and male reproductive organ problems: lumbosacral area tenderness or rigidity.

Notes

It is important to differentiate between segmental facilitation and spinal "splinting," which occurs as a result of underlying pathology, such as TB spine, vertebral metastasis (primary or secondary), and osteoporosis. In such cases splinting will usually be more widespread than just two adjacent segments.

CAUTION: No attempt should be made to reduce protective splinting.

How accurate is ARTT palpation?

A study compared Jones's (1981) palpation methods (see discussion of Jones's strain/counterstrain (SCS) later in this chapter) with standard osteopathic palpation procedures (i.e., ARTT). McPartland and Goodridge (1997) state that the study addressed five questions:

1. *What is the inter-examiner reliability of diagnostic tests used in strain–counterstrain technique?*

2. *How does this compare with the reliability of the traditional osteopathic examination (ARTT exam)?*

3. *How reliable are different aspects of the ARTT exam?*

4. *Do positive findings of Jones's points correlate with positive findings of spinal dysfunction?*

5. *Are osteopathic students more reliable with SCS diagnosis or ARTT tests?*

The examiners palpated for tender points which corresponded to those listed by Jones (1981) for the first three cervical segments. These points were located by means of their anatomical position, as described in Jones's original textbook, and were characterized as being areas of "tight" nodular myofascial tissue.

The ARTT exam comprised assessment for:

● tender paraspinal muscles

● asymmetry of joints

- restriction in ROM
- tissue texture abnormalities.

Of these, zygapophyseal joint tenderness and tissue texture changes were the most accurate.

In Jones's methodology the location of the tender point is meant to define the nature of the dysfunction. However, McPartland and Goodridge found that: "Few Jones points correlated well with the cervical articulations that they presumably represent." They did find, overall, that use of Jones's tender points (i.e., soft tissue tenderness) was a more accurate method of localizing dysfunction, in symptomatic patients, than use of joint tenderness evaluation as used in the ARTT exam, and that "students performed much better at SCS diagnosis than ARTT diagnosis."

Both methods are valuable, and have stood the test of time. It is for you to see which offers you the best way to identify dysfunction.

Exercise 5.1 *ARTT Palpation*

Time suggested **5–10 minutes**

If possible, examine a person with known visceral (cardiovascular, digestive, liver, etc.) disease.

- Targeting only spinal and paraspinal tissues (i.e., palpating no further away from the spine than the tips of the transverse processes), touch the skin (using the elements suggested in the previous chapter of scanning, skin-on-fascia pushes, skin stretches, and drag palpation) to evaluate the efficiency of these methods in identifying "suspicious areas" for further, deeper palpation.

- Now palpate the superficial and deeper musculature paraspinally (see layer palpation Exercises 3.17–3.24 in Chapter 3) in order to see whether a local segment (i.e., involving at least two adjacent vertebrae) can be identified that matches the description given by Magoun earlier in this chapter, i.e., *if involved in viscerosomatic adaptation the tissues will display homogeneous tension/hardness (and possibly fibrotic thickening), as well as hypersensitivity in both superficial and deeper layers.*

- There should therefore be superficial and deep contraction of tissues, on one or both sides of the spine, at an appropriate segmental level (described earlier in this chapter, as McFarlane Tilley's (1961) paraspinal sites relating to segmental facilitation).

- If possible, compare your palpation findings with those adjacent to a known structural (spinal) problem where only the deeper tissues should be contracted and sensitive.

- Also compare your findings with the feel of "normal" paraspinal tissues.

- Can you locate a segment in which asymmetrical evidence exists of tissue change and abnormal tenderness. (*Note*: Range of motion restriction is not included at this stage, as this topic is not covered until Chapter 8.)

- Record your findings in your journal.

Identifying segmental facilitation by palpation

Beal (1983) conducted a study in which over 100 patients with diagnosed cardiovascular disease were examined for patterns of spinal segment involvement. Approximately 90% had "segmental dysfunction in two or more adjacent vertebrae from T1 to T5, on the left side." More than half also had left side C2 dysfunction.

Beal reports that the estimation of the intensity of the spinal dysfunction correlated strongly with the degree of pathology noted (ranging from myocardial infarction, ischemic heart disease, and hypertensive cardiovascular disease to coronary artery disease). He further reported that the greatest intensity of the cardiac reflex occurred at T2 and T3, on the left.

Beal's description of the texture of the soft tissues, is of interest: "Skin and temperature changes were not apparent as consistent strong findings compared with the hypertonic state of the deep musculature." The major palpatory finding for muscle was of hypertonicity of the superficial and deep paraspinal muscles with fibrotic thickening. Tenderness was usually obvious, although this was not specifically assessed in this study. Superficial hypertonicity lessened when the patient was supine, making assessment of deeper tissue states easier in that position.

Beal's palpation method for identifying thoracic areas of segmental facilitation

With the patient supine, the thoracic spine is examined by the practitioner sliding the fingers under the transverse processes and applying an anterior (toward the ceiling) compressive force, assessing the status of the superficial and deep paraspinal tissues, as well as the response of the transverse process to an anterior, compressive, springing force (hence Beal's term of "compression test" for this method) (Fig. 5.1).

This compression is performed, one segment at a time, progressively down the spine, until control becomes difficult or tissues inaccessible. It is also possible to perform the test with the patient seated or side-lying, though neither is as effective as the supine position.

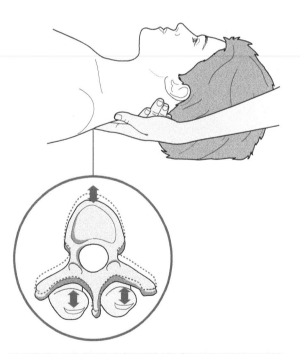

Figure 5.1
Beal's "springing" assessment for paraspinal facilitation rigidity associated with segmental facilitation.

Exercise 5.2 *Beal's Compression Palpation*

Time suggested **5–7 minutes**

As an exercise in developing this particular skill, you should take some time carefully springing the thoracic paraspinal tissues (and transverse processes), with a supine partner, *precisely as described by Beal in the previous paragraph.*

If possible, try to perform such palpation on people both with and without known cardiovascular (or other visceral) dysfunction, in order to develop a degree of discrimination between normal and abnormal tissue states.

- Your palpation model is supine and you are seated at the head of the table.

- Slide one hand under the spine of the patient, so that fingers are placed precisely as shown in Figure 5.1, at the level of T1–2.

- Using minimal force, ease the contact fingers toward the transverse processes, taking out available tissue slack.

- Spring the compressed tissues toward the ceiling to evaluate the degree of "give" or elasticity, as in Figure 5.1.

- Repeat the spring/compression evaluation until easy access is lost at around T6–7.

- Compare and record your findings with those you gathered when you performed Exercise 5.1.

Exercise 5.3 *Combined Viscerosomatic Reflex Palpation*

Time suggested **10–12 minutes**

- Use all the elements in Exercises 5.1 and 5.2, on the same patient, at the same time, and see which methods produce the most reliable evidence of viscerosomatic reflex activity.

- Apply words listed below (under the heading Descriptions of palpatory findings) to describe the sensations associated with these palpation methods.

Descriptions of palpatory findings

It may be useful to consider how practitioners performing similar palpations to those in Beal's exercise described what they actually felt. The five terms most commonly used to describe their palpatory findings in viscerosomatic conditions (Rosero et al. 1987) were selected from 16 descriptive terms provided for their use:

- "resistant" (firm, tense)
- "temperature/warm"
- "ropiness" (cord-like)
- "heavy musculature" (increased density)
- "edematous."

Of these, "resistant" and "temperature/warm" were the descriptions most commonly used.

Did you feel the "resistant and warm" tissues when doing Exercises 5.1, 5.2, and 5.3? If not, perhaps you should repeat the exercises.

Notes

It is suggested at this point that you revisit Special topic 1. In particular read up on Pick's advice on different levels for palpation – surface, "working," and rejection. Special topic Exercise 1.1 would offer an excellent way of enhancing skills before plunging into the exercises that follow in this chapter.

Muscles and facilitation

When considering paraspinal soft tissues we should not forget the very small intersegmental muscles that can be dramatically affected by facilitation. Korr (1976) reminds us:

Intersegmental mobility is very finely tuned by the small and easily forgotten muscles that run from segment to segment. Their critical role is not always appreciated in considerations of longstanding degenerative changes. We can see that the large muscles, for example the erector spinae group, initiate large movements, but which mediates the trans-lation of forces from one segment to the next? What concentrates the force of a particular motion at one particular locality, not once but a hundred thousand times in 20 years or so?

The intersegmental muscles are the conditioning agents and if their function is disturbed the result may be a change in the tracking characteristics at that particular junction, which in time will show impaired function.

Korr also reminds us that the more active a muscle is, in fine movement, the greater the number of muscle spindles there will be present (as in the hands). He continues:

Studies such as those involving the deep occipital muscles have indicated roughly the same ratio between spindles in the small and large muscles [as in the hand, i.e., 26:1.5]. **Although disturbances here are not apparent on routine examination they are detectable when the clinician has a well developed palpatory sense** *[my emphasis]. Locating these disorders, and modifying or removing them, insofar as possible, is a most logical and important element in preventive medicine.*

Discussion of palpatory progress involving Exercises 5.1–5.3

By applying the ARTT palpation sequence (albeit without range-of-motion evaluation at this stage), and by palpating for the changes described by Beal, and, most importantly, by understanding the mechanisms involved in facilitation and viscerosomatic influence, you will have begun to discriminate between primary biomechanical dysfunctions (such as overuse, strains) and reflexogenically induced changes.

ARTT palpation can, of course, be used to locate dysfunction of many types, including those of mechanical or overuse origin; however, combining the ARTT sequence with the compression method (Exercise 5.2), allows you to focus on the phenomena described by Beal and others.

Neuromuscular technique

Neuromuscular technique (NMT) evolved in Europe in the 1930s, as a blend of traditional Ayurvedic (Indian) techniques and methods derived from other sources. The person who created this method of combined diagnostic and therapeutic value was Stanley Lief ND DC. He and his son Peter (a graduate of the National College of Chiropractic, Chicago), and his cousin Boris Chaitow (also a National graduate) developed the techniques now known as NMT into an economical diagnostic (and therapeutic) tool.

In this text we will focus on the palpatory, assessment/diagnostic potential of NMT (rather than its therapeutic potential), for this is a modality that allows methodical, sequential, systematic, controlled combing of the major accessible (to palpating digits) sites of trigger points and other forms of localized soft tissue dysfunction (Chaitow 1991, 2002; Chaitow & Delany 2008).

Nimmo's contribution

Another assessment method, commonly used in seeking out trigger points, is receptor-tonus technique (Nimmo 1966). In the USA this has been incorporated into NMT methodology, where increasingly, the two versions of NMT (Lief's and Nimmo's) are blended (Chaitow & Delany 2008). Nimmo's contribution to the understanding of local myofascial dysfunction is outlined later in this chapter, with specific detail in Box 5.2.

Many "point" systems

Within shortened muscles, and within weakened ones as well, there is often an abundant crop of palpable, localized, discrete, sensitive areas of altered structure that may or may not be active trigger points, but which are all *potential* trigger points. One simple definition of a trigger point is that it is a palpable, sensitive, localized structure within the soft tissues that, when active, sends aberrant, noxious, neurological impulses to a distant site and on pressure, refers symptoms – usually involving pain, but with other symptoms possible – to that predictable target area.

Travell and Simons, authors of the major texts on myofascial trigger points to date (Simons et al. 1999; Travell & Simons 1992), offer a broader definition of trigger points, which is summarized later in this chapter.

All palpable sensitive tissue changes are of potential importance in palpatory analysis and by no means all such areas are trigger points. It is important to realize that even if painful (to pressure) "points" do not refer symptoms

(pain, numbness, etc.), they may still be of potential diagnostic value. They could, as examples, be points described in some other system, such as Chapman's neurolymphatic reflexes (described and illustrated in the previous chapter), Jones's strain/counterstrain "tender" points, or Lewit's periosteal pain points. These are discussed later in this chapter.

All such points are characterized by the overlying skin being less elastic than surrounding tissue (see Chapter 4), or by having a measurable degree of lowered electrical resistance (relating to altered hydrosis, and therefore palpable as "drag" – see Chapter 4).

Lief's methods

The major sites of these self-perpetuating troublemakers (trigger points) are often close to the origins and insertions of muscles, and this is where NMT probes for information more effectively than most other systems.

There are numerous ways of locating such localized areas of dysfunction, as witness the methods advocated by Travell, Pruden, and Nimmo described in this chapter, and others.

Lief advocated that the exact same sequence of contacts be followed on each occasion, whether assessing or treating, the difference between these modes being merely one of repetition of the strokes, with some degree of added pressure when treating. Lief's recommendation did not, however, mean that the same treatment was given each time, for the essence of NMT is that the pressure applied, both in diagnosis and in therapy, is variable and that this variability is determined by the tissues themselves.

Thus, while repetition of a diagnostic or therapeutic stroke might appear identical to its predecessor, it would differ depending upon the state of the tissues it was passing through. This concept will become clearer as we progress.

Palpating digit

- A light lubricant is always used in NMT, to avoid skin friction.

- The main contact is made with the tip of the thumb(s), more precisely the medial aspect of the tip, as a rule (Fig. 5.2).

- In some regions the tip of the index or middle finger is used instead (Fig. 5.3), as these allow easier insertion between the ribs for assessment (or treatment) of, for example, intercostal musculature.

- This "finger contact" is similar to that suggested in *bindegewebsmassage*, except that in the German system no lubricant is used.

Practitioner's body mechanics

The practitioner's posture and positioning are particularly important when applying NMT, as the correct application of forces dramatically reduces the energy expended, and the time taken to perform the assessment/treatment.

- The examination table should be at a height that allows the therapist to stand erect, legs separated for ease of weight transference, with the assessing arm straight at the elbow.

- This allows the practitioner's bodyweight to be transferred down the extended arm through the thumb, imparting any degree of force required, from extremely light to quite substantial, simply by leaning on the arm.

- This application of pressure presents a problem for a small number of practitioners whose thumbs are too flexible or unstable. A solution is for them to use only the finger contact described below.

- Weight transference, from the back to the leading leg, with knees slightly flexed, is an energy saving way of controlling accurately the degree of pressure application.

- It is important that the fingers of the assessing/treating hand act as a fulcrum, and that they lie ahead of the contact thumb, allowing the stroke being made by the thumb to run across the palm of the hand, in the direction of the ring or small finger, as the stroke progresses (see Fig. 5.2).

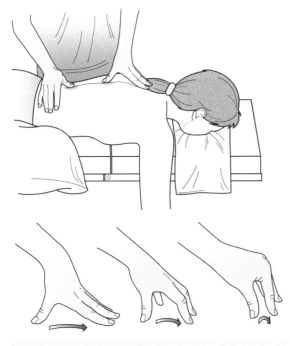

Figure 5.2
Neuromuscular thumb technique. The practitioner uses the medial tip (ideally) of the thumb to sequentially "meet and match" tissue density/tension and to insinuate the digit through the tissues seeking local dysfunction.

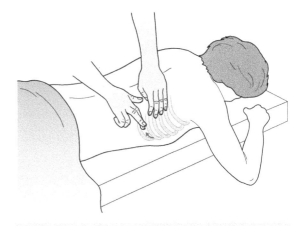

Figure 5.3
Neuromuscular finger technique. The practitioner utilizes index or middle finger, supported by a neighboring digit (or two), to palpate and assess the tissues between the ribs for local dysfunction. This contact is used instead of the thumb if it is unable to maintain the required pressure.

Chapter 5

Achieving control and delicacy of touch

The way the hand and body are used in NMT, as described above, produces numerous benefits, the most important being control. Were the thumb merely *pushed* along through the tissues, a lack of delicacy and fine control would result.

- For the thumb stroke, the finger/fulcrum (Fig. 5.2) remains stationary, as the thumb moves intelligently toward it, across the palm.

- This is quite different from a usual massage stroke, in which the whole hand moves.

- Here the hand is stationary and only the thumb moves.

- Each stroke, whether it be diagnostic or therapeutic, extends for approximately 4–5 cm before the thumb ceases its motion, at which time the fulcrum/fingers can be moved further ahead, in the direction that the thumb needs to travel.

- The thumb stroke then continues, feeling and searching through the tissues.

Variable pressure: the key to successful NMT palpation

- Another vital ingredient, indeed the very essence of the thumb contact, is its application of *variable pressure* (initial diagnostic pressure is measured in tens of grams, only) which allows it to "insinuate" and tease its way through whatever fibrous, indurated, or contracted structures it meets.

- The degree of resistance or obstruction presented by the palpated tissues determines the degree of effort required.

- Thus, in heavily tensed tissues, kilos of pressure may be needed for a subsequent diagnostic stroke.

- Tense, contracted, or fibrous tissues are never simply overcome by force, as this would irritate and add to dysfunction.

- Rather, the fibers are "worked through," using substantial pressure at times but in a constantly varying manner in which both angles of application of pressure and degrees of pressure are constantly altered to meet the particular demands of the tissues.

The intelligent thumb or fingertip

A degree of vibrational contact, as well as the variable pressure mentioned above, allows the stroke, and the contact, to have an "intelligent" feel that does not risk traumatizing or bruising tissues, even when heavy pressure is used.

It helps to try to see the thumb tip as an extension of the brain, so that an intelligent quality can be added to the mechanical nature of its search through tissue. The patient rapidly picks up on this quality, and senses that the approach is not just a mechanical process, but an intimate response to the addressing of pain or dysfunction.

- As in much palpation, it is usual to suggest that NMT be applied with eyes closed.

- A "nice hurt" is the most that should be complained of, even when pressure is fairly deep.

- It is helpful to try to use the medial tip of the thumb for precise contact and, as a rule, this is achieved after a little practice, unless there is hypermobility of the thumb joints preventing a stable contact of this sort.

Relax the working arm

Whether thumb or finger contact is used (see below for discussion on finger contact), energy conservation and ease of application of NMT is enhanced if the arm is relaxed and not tense. If the muscles of the forearm are unduly tense, or if the fingers that form the fulcrum towards which the thumbs move, are rigid:

- energy will be wasted

- the arm will tire rapidly

- control will diminish

- the "feel" to the patient will be harsh rather than gentle

- perception will be dulled in the process.

The finger-fulcrum should not grasp, or "dig into," the tissues on which it rests, but simply maintains contact, with minimal pressure, as the thumb travels towards it. Effort, if any is required, is achieved by shifting body-weight through the almost straight arm, *and not by using arm or hand strength.*

The finger stroke

(see Fig. 5.3)

When a finger contact is used instead of the thumb (which always travels away from the practitioner in a controlled manner), the hand is drawn towards the practitioner's body, with the treating finger slightly hooked, as in the methods of *bindegewebsmassage*. This allows for control of the hand and a different use of bodyweight to that applied during a thumb stroke.

- Unlike the thumb stroke, in which the hand apart from the thumb is stationary, during the finger stroke the whole hand (and sometimes the whole arm) moves.

- Another major area where finger contact is useful, apart from the intercostal structures, is the lateral pelvic region and lateral thigh.

- As the palpating hand is brought toward you, over a curved surface, its main usefulness will be perceived.

- By leaning backwards, transferring weight to the back leg, the hooked finger can be pulled through the tissues in a controlled manner.

- A moderate degree of counterweight, from the patient's inertia, can increase the depth of penetration with minimal effort from the practitioner.

Standing on the side opposite the one being treated, the hooked finger, supported by its neighboring digit if possible, can, as examples, be inserted deeply into the intercostal space (see Fig. 5.3), or the lateral pelvic musculature, above the trochanter.

As the practitioner leans back and allows the weight of the patient to apply pressure onto the fingers, these are slowly drawn through the tissues, allowing assessment of the nature of dysfunction. Alternatively cross-fiber friction, or sustained inhibitory contacts, are possible when finger contacts are used therapeutically rather than diagnostically.

Assessment palpation using NMT

The pattern of strokes that Lief and Chaitow suggest allows maximum access to potential dysfunction in the shortest time, and with least demand for altered position and wasted effort. These strokes are illustrated, together with the suggested practitioner foot positions, for each spinal region (see Figs 5.5–5.9).

- Assessment using NMT contacts usually involves one superficial and one moderately deep contact only.

- If treatment is decided then several more strokes, applied from varying angles, are applied to relax the structures, to stretch them, to inhibit contraction, or to deal with trigger points elicited in the examination phase.

- Trigger point treatment is possible using direct inhibitory pressure followed by stretching of the affected musculature (fully described in Chaitow 1991, 2002; Chaitow & Delany 2008).

NMT for particular areas

In assessing (or treating) joint dysfunction or problems involving the extremities, it is suggested that all the muscles associated with a joint receive NMT attention to origins and insertions, and that the bellies of the muscles be assessed for trigger points and other dysfunction. In this way, not only the apparently affected joint receives attention but, at the very least, the ones above and below it.

A full spinal NMT assessment should be accomplished in approximately 15 minutes, once the method is mastered. (Treatment of those areas demanding extra attention will add another 5–10 minutes.)

It is suggested that every patient receive full spinal and abdominal (including thoracic) neuromuscular assessment, at the outset of any treatment program, and that this should be repeated periodically to evaluate changes. It is seldom necessary to undertake a full assessment at each visit – with assessment/evaluation of a localized region being all that may be necessary.

By following a pattern that does not vary, involving the regions illustrated, and most importantly by recording whatever findings there are at each visit, a clear individual pattern of dysfunction and localized structural changes can be established for each patient, and progress – or lack of it – monitored. With effective use of NMT, not only should localized, discrete "points" be discovered, but also patterns of stress bands, altered soft tissue mechanics, contractions and shortenings. Beal's rigid paraspinal tissues (see Exercise 5.2) are readily identified, as are the changes resulting from viscerosomatic activity and localized dysfunction (see Magoun's views, earlier in this chapter).

NMT, in its therapeutic mode, has proved itself as an adjunct to manipulation, as well as often being able to obviate the need for other soft tissue or osseous approaches. Even if only the diagnostic approach is adopted, the patient will still have received potentially beneficial "treatment."

Is the term "neuromuscular technique" accurate?

Knowledge of the function of the neural "reporting" stations, such as the various components of the muscle spindle and Golgi tendon organs, helps explain how NMT may achieve its results.

When used near origins and insertions, the load detectors – the Golgi tendon organs – are clearly receiving mechanical input, especially if the direction of the stroke is towards the belly of the muscle.

- The effect of any degree of pressure away from the origin and insertion, towards the belly, would be initially to increase tone and, if sustained, would produce reflex relaxation of the muscle (Walther 1988) (Fig. 5.4).

- If pressure is away from the belly of the muscle, near both the origin and insertion simultaneously, there will be a tendency for muscle to lose tone. The muscle

spindles register length of muscle and rate of change of that length, and pressure via NMT would alter length locally as well as having an inhibitory effect on neural discharge (Fig. 5.5).

Pressure-induced inhibition of neural discharge is the main NMT contribution to trigger point treatment. The overall effect of NMT via neural mediation is one in which reduced tone is created in hypertonic structures, over and above the purely mechanical effects introduced by stretching, friction and drainage of fluids and toxic wastes.

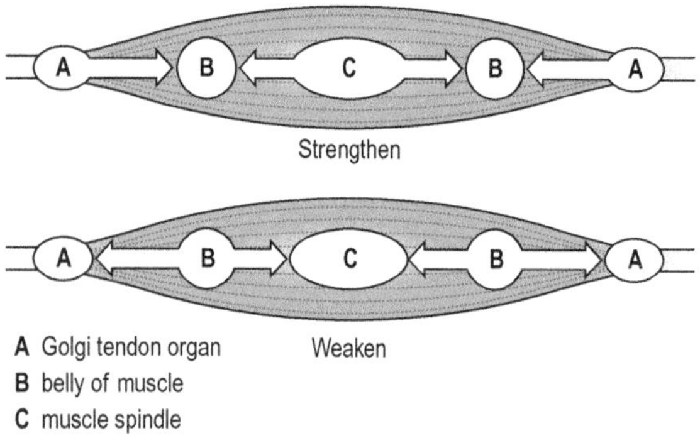

A Golgi tendon organ   Weaken
B belly of muscle
C muscle spindle

Strengthen

Figure 5.4
Proprioceptive manipulation of muscles.

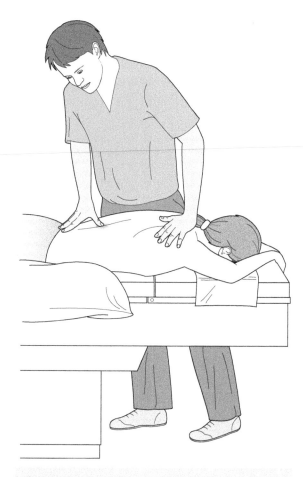

Figure 5.5
Practitioner using neuromuscular technique. Note position of feet; straight right arm; right hand position; thumb position.

Many hours of patient NMT work are required before achieving the degree of sensitivity that allows the smallest local area of dysfunction to be identified during palpation. Optimal palpatory literacy is the objective of those who utilize NMT.

Exercise 5.4 *Finger and Thumb NMT Strokes*

Time suggested **15 minutes**

Begin to practice NMT by concentrating on your body position.

- Make sure your treatment surface is of a height that allows you to stand as illustrated and described in Figure 5.5, without hunching.

- This position allows a straight arm position (when the thumb contact is being used as described below), as well as the ability to transfer weight, to increase pressure, without arm muscle strength being called for.

- After applying a light lubricant, position yourself and place your treating hand according to the illustration (Fig. 5.2) and description, with your fingers acting as a fulcrum, thumb (medial tip) feeling through the tissues, slowly and with variable pressure.

- Practice this, in no particular sequence of strokes, until the mechanics of the body-arm-hand-thumb positions are comfortable, and automatic.

- Pay attention to *varying the pressure*, so that it meets and matches tissue tone, and to using bodyweight, transferred through a straight arm, to increase pressure when needed.

- Also practice the use of the finger stroke, especially on curved areas, by drawing the slightly hooked and supported (by one of its neighboring digits) finger toward yourself in a slow, deliberate, searching manner (see Fig. 5.3).

Exercise 5.5 *Application of NMT in Assessment Mode*

Time suggested **10–15 minutes per segment**

- Choose any of the illustrated NMT sequences from Figures 5.6–5.11 (Fig. 5.8A or B would be an ideal uncomplicated starting sequence for practice; however, over time, practice all the sequences) and follow the stroke lines, as illustrated, as closely as possible.

Notes

> The direction of strokes need not always follow arrow directions, as illustrated, if the opposite direction is more comfortable

- The objective is to obtain information, without causing excessive discomfort to the patient and without stressing your palpating hands.

- NMT *in its treatment mode* involves greater pressure than during assessment, in order to modify dysfunctional tissues, but in these training sequences you are "information gathering" only, not treating.

- In time, with practice, treatment and assessment meld seamlessly together, with one feeding the other.

- Chart any findings you make, noting any particularly tender areas, stress bands, contracted fibers, edematous areas, nodular structures, hypertonic regions, trigger points, and so on.

- If trigger points are located, note their target area as well.

- In the sequence illustrated in Figure 5.8A and B, intercostal strokes are illustrated, and you should use the hooked finger contact to search these regions. For example, stand on the left side of the patient to assess right intercostals (see Fig 5.3).

- Record any findings.

Chapter 5

Exercise 5.5 *continued*

Work slowly and try to follow the descriptions given above, regarding the way the thumb insinuates its way through the tissues, never overwhelming them, and never gouging or pushing unfeelingly.

Time suggested for abdominal segment **20–30 minutes**

Allow your palpating contact to be your eyes. Try to work with your eyes closed so that sensory focus is heightened.

Record your feelings and findings in your journal, noting both your positive and negative feelings about this novel way of using your hands (which can take some weeks of regular use to become second nature).

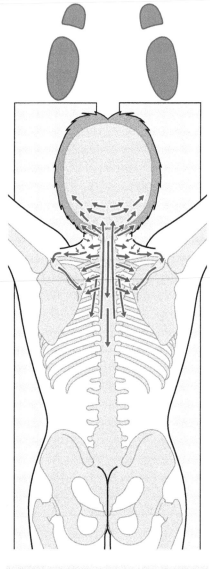

Figure 5.7
Neuromuscular technique working from head of patient to address upper trapezius and cervical region. Illustrating position of practitioner and lines of application.

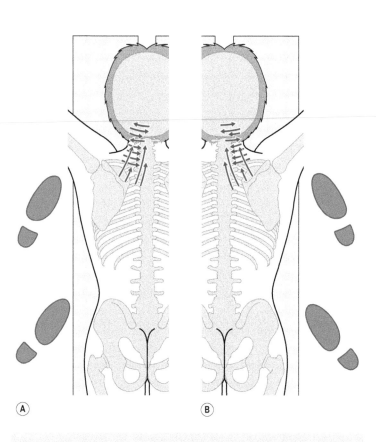

(A) (B)

Figure 5.6
(A, B) Neuromuscular technique for commencing upper thoracic and cervical region. Illustrating position of practitioner and lines of application.

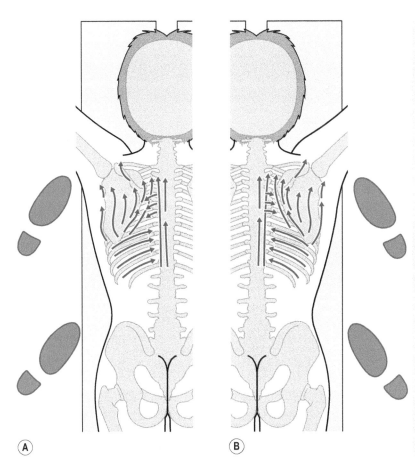

Figure 5.8
(A, B) Neuromuscular technique for the mid-thoracic region. Illustrating position of practitioner and lines of application.

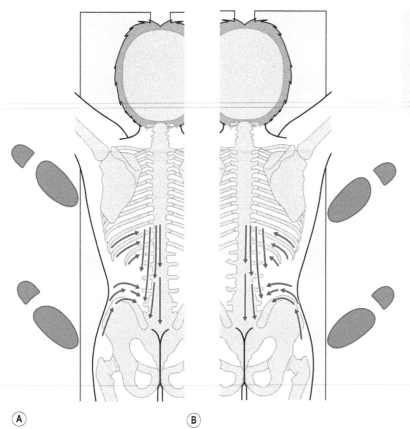

Figure 5.9
(A, B) Neuromuscular technique for lower thoracic and lumbar region. Illustrating position of practitioner and lines of application.

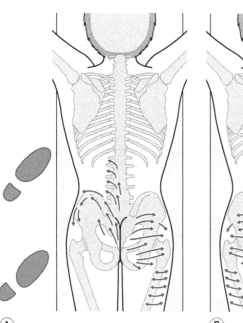

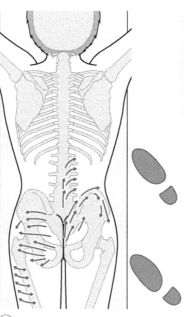

Figure 5.10
(A, B) Neuromuscular technique for gluteal and upper thigh region. Illustrating position of practitioner and lines of application.

Abdominal assessment using NMT

When assessing the abdominal area for soft tissue dysfunction, junctional tissues should receive particular attention (Simons et al. 1999). For example, you should be aware of the anatomical position and relationships of the following, by the time you start to assess the abdominal area.

- the central tendon
- the lateral aspect of the rectal muscle sheaths
- the insertion of the recti muscles and external oblique muscles into the ribs (Fig. 5.11)
- the xiphisternal ligament, as well as the lower insertions of the internal and external oblique muscles
- the intercostal areas from fifth to twelfth ribs
- below the costal margin for diaphragmatic attachments (Fig. 5.12).

It is also important to pay attention to scars from previous surgeries which may be the sites of formation of connective tissue trigger points (Simons et al. 1999). After sufficient healing has taken place, these incision sites can be examined by gently pinching, compressing, and rolling the scar tissue between the thumb and finger, to examine for evidence of trigger points (Chaitow & DeLany 2000).

Is the palpated pain in a muscle or in an organ?

When palpating the abdominal region there is no underlying osseous structure to allow easy compression of the musculature. A particular strategy is used that helps to decide whether palpated pain derives from superficial muscle tissues or from internal structures.

- When a local area of pain is noted using NMT or any other palpation method, it should be firmly compressed by the palpating digit, sufficient to produce pain/referred pain (if a trigger is involved) but not enough to cause distress.

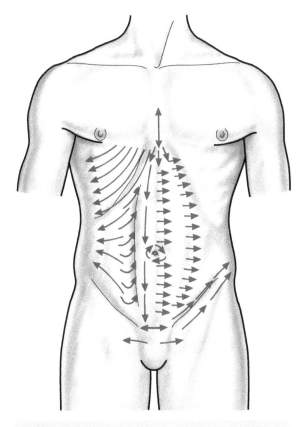

Figure 5.11
Neuromuscular general abdominal technique. Lines of application.

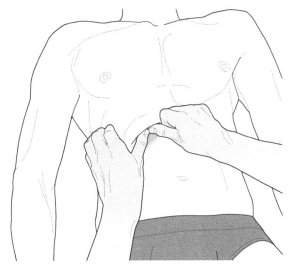

Figure 5.12
Palpation below costal margin to evaluate diaphragm attachment areas.

- The supine patient should then be asked to raise both (straight) legs from the table (heels must be raised several inches).

- As this happens there will be a contraction of the abdominal muscles, so that if pain *increases* at this time, the probability is that the pain site is muscular.

- If, however, pain *decreases* on the raising of the legs, the site of the pain probably lies beneath the muscle and probably involves a visceral problem (Thomson & Francis 1977).

- It is, of course, possible for there to be a problem in the viscera and also in the abdominal wall, in which case this test would not be able to differentiate the locality of the pain.

- The test described therefore gives a clue, but not an absolute finding, as to the locality of the problem causing the pain.

Exercise 5.6 *Anterior Thoracic and Abdominal NMT Palpation*

Time suggested 20–30 minutes initially, but aim to reduce this to 10 minutes with practice

Practice the abdominal/lower rib cage sequence as described in the text and illustrated in Figures 5.11 and 5.12.

- Remember to use lighter contacts than would have been appropriate for paraspinal musculature.

- See what soft tissue changes you can discover in these tissues, especially near origins and insertions, below the thoracic cage, near the pelvic and pubic insertions, in the lower intercostal structures.

- If there are scars, search diligently around these for sensitive and tight structures.

For greater guidance on this approach, and other NMT sequences, see *Modern Neuromuscular Techniques* (Chaitow 2002).

Anterior intercostal and abdominal palpation assessment

(see Figs 5.11 and 5.12)

The initial objective of the NMT strokes in this region is to evaluate for soft tissue changes (active or latent trigger points, tissue texture changes, asymmetry, tenderness, etc.) with a palpation contact that "meets and matches" tissue tension.

- You should be facing the supine patient at waist level, and be half-turned towards the head, with legs apart for an even distribution of weight, and with knees flexed to facilitate the transfer of pressure through the arms.

- Since many of the maneuvers in the intercostal area, and on the abdomen itself, involve finger and thumb movements of a light nature, the arms can be fairly relaxed during assessment.

- However, if deep pressure is called for, and especially when this is applied via the thumb (Fig. 5.12), the same criterion of weight transference, from the shoulder through the thumb, applies, for an economic and efficient use of energy.

- A series of strokes is applied with the tip of the thumb, along the course of the intercostal spaces, from the sternum laterally (see Fig. 5.11).

- It is important that the attachments of the internal and external muscles receive attention.

- The margins of the ribs, both inferior and superior aspects, should receive firm gliding pressure from the distal phalanx of the thumb or the middle or index finger.

- If there is too little space to allow such a degree of differentiated pressure, then a simple stroke along the available intercostal space has to suffice.

- If the thumb cannot be insinuated between the ribs a finger (side of finger) contact can be used, in which this is drawn towards the practitioner from the side contralateral to that being treated, toward the sternum.

- The intercostals, from the fifth rib to the costal margin below the 12th rib, should receive a series of two or three deep, slow-moving, gliding, sensitive strokes on each side, with special reference to points of particular congestion or sensitivity.

- It is useful to note the possible presence, in the intercostal spaces close to the sternum, of neurolymphatic (Chapman's) reflex points, which are discussed and illustrated in detail in the previous chapter (see Figs 4.7– 4.12).

- These points require only light circular pressure when being contacted in order to assess for their status.

- If a localized area of dysfunction is found that refers pain or other symptoms familiar to the patient, an active trigger point will have been located.

- Gentle probing on the sternum itself may elicit sensitivity in the rudimentary sternalis muscle, which has been found to house trigger points.

- It is not necessary to change sides during the assessment of the intercostals, unless it is found to be more comfortable to do so.

Having palpated and assessed the intercostal musculature and connective tissue, and having charted any trigger points you may have located, use either a deep thumb pressure or the pads of the fingertips to apply a series of short strokes in a combination of oblique lateral and inferior directions from the xiphoid process.

CAUTION: Pulsations

If, during palpation, any large pulsating mass is noted in the abdominal midline, between the xiphoid and the umbilicus, caution should be exercised. Kuchera (1997) notes:

A normal abdominal aorta in an adult should not be wider than an inch [2.5 cm]. Pulsations occurring anteriorly are normal, but lateral pulsations from the aorta suggest a weak vessel wall, or aneurysm. Palpate [also] the inguinal area for a good pulse and compare the right and left sides. If a decreased pulse is found on one or both sides, ask the patient about claudication and then palpate and evaluate the pulse at the popliteal, postero-tibial, and dorsal pedis arteries, in that leg, and compare [these] to pulses in the opposite leg.

Palpating the rectal sheath

Your thumbs or fingers may then be used to apply a series of deep, slow palpation strokes, along and under the costal margins (see Fig. 5.11). Whether diaphragmatic attachments can be located is questionable but sustained, firm (but not invasively aggressive) pressure allows gradual access to an area that can reveal trigger points of exquisite sensitivity, with often surprising areas of referral. Many seem to produce sensations internally, while others create sensations in the lower extremities, or in the throat, upper chest and shoulders.

- A series of short palpation strokes using fairly deep, but not painful, pressure is then applied by the thumb, from the midline up to the lateral rectal sheath. This series starts just inferior to the xiphoid and concludes at the pubic promontory. It may be repeated on each side several times, depending upon the degree of tension, congestion, and sensitivity noted.

- A similar pattern of assessment is followed (using the thumb if working ipsilaterally and fingers if working contralaterally), across the lateral border of the rectal sheath.

- A series of short, deep, slow-moving (usually thumb) palpation strokes should be applied from just beneath the costal margin of the rectal sheath until the inguinal ligament is reached. Both sides are assessed in this way.

- A series of similar strokes are then applied on the one side, and then the other laterally, from the lateral border of the rectal sheath (see Fig. 5.12). These strokes follow the contours of the trunk, so that the upper strokes travel in a slightly inferior curve whilst moving laterally (following the curve of the lower ribs), and the lower strokes have a superior inclination (following the curve of the crest of the pelvis), as the hand moves laterally. A total of five or six strokes should be adequate to complete these palpation movements, before performing the same strokes on the opposite side. You are seeking evidence of local soft tissue changes, as well as any underlying sense of tension or "drag" on supporting tissues.

- In palpating/assessing the side on which you are standing, it may be more comfortable to apply the stroke via the flexed fingertips, which are drawn towards you, or the usual thumb stroke may be used. In palpating/ assessing the opposite side, thumb pressure can more easily be applied, as in spinal technique, with the fingers acting as a fulcrum and the thumb gliding towards them in a series of 2 or 3 inch-long strokes. The sensing of contracted gangliform areas of dysfunction is more difficult in abdominal work and requires great sensitivity of touch and great concentration on your part.

Palpation of the symphysis pubis

The sheaths of the rectus abdominis muscles, from the costal margins downwards to the pubic bones, are evaluated by finger or thumb strokes. Attention should be paid to the soft tissue component of, as well as the insertions into, the iliac fossa, the pubic bones, and the symphysis pubis, including the inguinal ligaments (see Fig. 5.11).

● Commencing at the ASIS, palpation strokes should be made which attempt to evaluate the attachments of internal and external obliques and transversus abdominis.

● A deep but not painful stroke, employing the pad of the thumb, should be applied to the superior aspect of the pubic crest. This should start at the symphysis pubis and move laterally, first in one direction and, after repeating it once or twice, then the other.

● A similar series of palpation strokes, starting at the center and moving laterally, should then be applied over the anterior aspect of the pubic bone. Great care should be taken not to use undue pressure as the area is sensitive at the best of times and may be acutely so if there is dysfunction associated with the insertions into these structures.

● A series of deep slow movements should then be performed, with the thumb, along the superior and inferior aspects of the inguinal ligament, starting at the pubic bone and running up to and beyond the iliac crest.

Palpation of the lateral rectus sheath

Your thumbs or fingertips may then be insinuated beneath the lateral rectus border, at its lower margins, and deep pressure applied towards the midline. Your hand or thumb should then slowly move cephalad, in short stages, whilst maintaining this medial pressure. This lifts the connective tissue from its underlying attachments and helps to identify (and sometimes normalize) localized contractures and fibrous infiltrations.

Palpating in the region of the umbilicus

● A series of strokes should then be applied around the umbilicus. Using thumb or flexed fingertips, a number of stretching movements should be performed, in which the non-active hand stabilizes the tissue at the start of the palpation stroke, which first runs from approximately 1 inch (2.5 cm) superior and lateral to the umbilicus on the right side to the same level on the left side.

● The non-active hand then stabilizes the tissues at this end-point of the stroke and a further stretching and probing stroke is applied interiorly to a point about 1 inch (2.5 cm) inferior and lateral to the umbilicus, on the left side. This area is then stabilized and the stroke is applied to a similar point on the right.

● The circle is completed by a further stroke upwards, to end at the point at which the series began.

● Note that the superior mesenteric attachment, which supports the small intestine, is located 1 inch (2.5 cm) superior and 1 inch (2.5 cm) laterally to the left of the umbilicus (see Fig. 5.11). Additional strokes may be applied along the midline and the sheaths of the recti muscles from the costal margins downwards.

Notes

In all these strokes the intention should be to evaluate relative normality as compared with any undue imbalances, represented by tension, fibrous changes, areas of localized edema, etc.

Palpation of the linea alba

Additional strokes should be applied along the midline, on the linea alba itself, while searching for evidence of contractions, adhesions, fibrotic nodules, edema and sensitivity. Caution is always required to avoid deep pressure on the linea alba, especially if the patient has weakened this muscular interface via pregnancy, surgery or trauma. It should also be recalled that the linea alba is a place of attachment of the external obliques as well as transversus abdominis (Braggins 2000).

Exercise 5.7 *Comprehensive NMT Evaluation*

Time suggested **30–60 minutes**

Over a period of several weeks, work your way through the individually illustrated segments of the spinal NMT assessment, several times each (taking 20 minutes for each segment at first, reducing with practice to 8–10 minutes each, and then around 5–6 minutes each). Then put them all together, doing a full spinal assessment, charting everything you find. At first this will take up to an hour. With practice it can be effectively and thoroughly done in 20–30 minutes.

Always chart and record your findings.

Discussion regarding Exercises 5.4–5.7

Neuromuscular technique in its palpation mode (as opposed to treatment mode) is a delicate, efficient and, above all, proven (by over 70 years of use) method for assessment of soft tissue dysfunction. It is only by repetitious practice that skill can be achieved, and the exercises are designed to give you that opportunity.

Jones's strain/counterstrain palpation

Lawrence Jones (1981) described the evolution of his therapeutic methods, called strain/counterstrain (SCS), that partly depend upon the identification of "tender" points located in the soft tissues associated with joints that have been stretched, strained, or traumatized. These are identified, according to Dvorak and Dvorak (1984), as "swollen, flat regions in specific parts of the body."

The tender points are usually located in soft tissues that were shortened at the time of the strain or trauma (i.e., in the antagonists to those that were stretched during the process of injury – acute or chronic).

- For example, in spinal problems resulting from a forward-bending strain, in which back pain is complained of, the appropriate "tender" point would be found on the anterior surface of the body.

- The same process can take place in slow motion, so to speak, where chronic adaptation occurs rather than sudden strain.

- In such cases, once again, the tender points will be located in shortened structures, rather than in those which have lengthened.

- Tender points are usually exquisitely sensitive to pressure/palpation but painless otherwise.

- Once identified, such points are used as monitors (explained below) as the area, or the whole body, is repositioned ("fine-tuned" towards "ease") until the palpated pain disappears or reduces substantially.

- Tissue tension almost always eases at the same time as the easing of pain in the palpated point.

- If the "position of ease" is held for some 90 seconds, there is often a resolution of, or at least marked improvement in, the dysfunction which resulted from the trauma.

This method is fully explained in Jones's book (1981) and a modified version is described in *Positional Release Techniques* (Chaitow 2007).

The reason for inclusion of this topic in this survey of palpation is that awareness of its principles can help to account for unexplained and previously unreported sensitive areas, uncovered during palpation, whether or not Jones's methods of treatment are subsequently used.

Notes

Such points are similar to Ah Shi points (spontaneously tender points) as reported in Traditional Chinese Medicine (TCM) for several thousands of years. In TCM, however, they are not used in the manner described above, but are considered to be amenable to acupuncture or acupressure methods for as long as they remain sensitive. These points are sometimes also trigger points, in that they may refer pain to a distant target (Baldry 1993).

Exercise 5.8A *Jones's Tender Point Palpation: the "Box" Exercise*

Woolbright (1991) has devised a teaching tool that enables SCS skills to be acquired and polished. *This is not designed as a treatment protocol* but is an excellent means of acquiring a sense of the mechanisms involved.

Notes

As the individual's head and neck are passively positioned during this exercise (see Figs 5.13A, B and 5.14), no force should be used.

- Each position adopted is not the furthest the tissues can be taken in any given direction but rather it is where the first sign of resistance is noted.

- Thus, an instruction to take the palpation partner's head and neck into side-bending and rotation to the right would involve the very lightest of guidance towards that position, with no force and no effort, and no strain or pain being noted by the patient/model.

- As each position described below in this "box exercise" is achieved, three key elements require consideration:

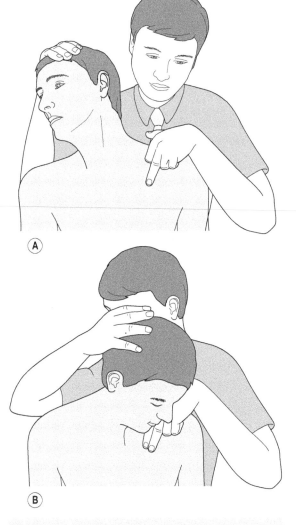

(A)

(B)

Figure 5.13
(A) Second head/neck position in the box exercise. (B) Fourth and final head/neck position of the box exercise.

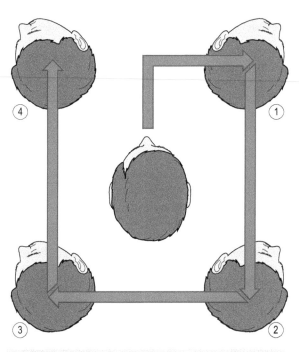

Figure 5.14
Box exercise. The head is taken into four positions, and as these are gently adopted, tenderness and tissue tension is palpated and monitored in tissues affected by the movements (in this exercise upper chest/intercostal muscles).

1. Is your palpation partner comfortable and unstressed by this position? If not, too much effort is being used, or they are not relaxed.

2. In this position, are the palpated tissues (in this exercise those on the upper left thoracic area) less sensitive to compression pressure than previously, as reported by your palpation partner?

3. In this position, are the palpated tissues reducing in tone, feeling more at "ease," with less evidence of "bind"?

Figure 5.13A shows the second head/neck position of the "box" exercise as pain and tissue tension is palpated and monitored (in this instance in the left upper pectoral area). Figure 5.13B illustrates the fourth and final head/neck position of the "box" exercise as pain and tissue tension is palpated and monitored.

Figure 5.14 summarizes the whole box exercise. The head is taken into four positions: flexion with side-bending and rotation right (1), extension with side-bending and rotation right (2), extension with side-bending and rotation left (3), flexion with side-bending and rotation left (4). As these positions are gently adopted, tenderness and/or tissue tension is monitored.

Method

As each position is reached you should pause to evaluate the tissue response to this new position, as well as enquiring of the patient/model what the "score" is for the pain/discomfort being produced by the palpating digit.

Try to be aware of changes in tone, as the head and neck move through the sequence of positions around the "box."

- Your palpation partner should be seated with you standing behind.

- Your right hand should rest very lightly on the crown of your palpation partner's head (palm on head, fingertips touching forehead, or the hand can be transversely placed on the head so that the heel of the hand is on one side and the fingertips on the other) while your left fingertips palpate an area of tenderness and tension a little below the left clavicle, in the pectoral muscles (see Fig. 5.13A and B).

- Sufficient pressure should be applied for a report to be made by your palpation partner of discomfort or pain.

- This is given a value of "10" and it is explained that whenever a request is made for the level of pain to be reported, a number (out of "10") should be given.

- The discomfort/pain will change as the head and neck alter their positions, and it is the primary objective of the exercise that you should be able to sense – by virtue of changes in the palpated tension in the tissues – whether the score is going to go up or down.

- As your palpation partner exhales, the head should be guided, *with minimal effort*, into flexion, after which it should be gently side-flexed and rotated to the right, to go to position 1 (see Fig. 5.13A).

- Pausing momentarily to assess changes in the palpated tissues and to obtain feedback regarding sensitivity (pain score), you should then take the head out of right rotation (while maintaining a slight right sidebend) and as the patient inhales, take it out of flexion and into slight extension.

- When the easy limit of extension is reached, rotation to the right should again be introduced taking it to position 2 (see Fig. 5.14).

- After a pause for evaluation of both tone and reported levels of pain/discomfort, and while maintaining slight extension, the head should then be moved towards side-bending left, rotation left, until an easy end-point is reached: position 3 (see Fig. 5.14).

- The head/neck should then, after a momentary pause to evaluate tissue tone and to obtain a pain score report, be eased out of left rotation and into flexion (during an exhalation) while left side-bending is maintained.

- Rotation to the left should once again be introduced as the head/neck comes to rest in flexion, in position 4 (see Fig. 5.13B).

- The head and neck should then be returned to the starting, neutral, position, before being moved around the box (as described above) a number of times, in order to assess for any additional relaxation (or increased bind) in the tissues under the palpating and monitoring hand.

- Note whether additional assistance to the process can be gained by having the patient/model, with eyes closed, "look" up or down or sideways – in the direction in which the head is being moved, as it moves.

- By experimenting with eye movements in this way, increased ease may be achieved, if the direction in which the eyes are looking is synchronized with the direction of movement (Lewit 1999).

- It is suggested that you may be able to make the process of moving the model/patient around the box more fluid by duplicating the movements of the palpation partner's eyes and breathing, as well as by leaning in the direction, and at the speed, of the movement of the head/neck.

- Repeat this exercise a number of times (with different people).

Exercise 5.8B *Jones's Tender Point Palpation: Using a Palpation Partner*

Time suggested 5–10 minutes per point

- Palpate the musculotendinous tissues, involving antagonists to those that were stretched during a joint or spinal trauma or strain.

- Tender points for this exercise should be located in areas *not complained of* as being painful.

- Any localized, extremely tender area in such tissue can be used as a *"Jones tender point"* and serve to monitor sensitivity as the tissues are fine-tuned towards an "ease" position.

- Apply enough pressure to such a point to cause mild to moderate discomfort.

- Inform your palpation partner (just as you would a patient if this was being performed clinically) that the discomfort being experienced should be ascribed a score of "10".

- Also inform your palpation partner that you will require regular feedback as to the score (out of 10) as you proceed with the exercise.

- Slowly position the joint, or area, in a way that removes the tenderness from the point or reduces it by at least 70% (from an initial score of "10" to "3" or less).

- Creating "ease" in the tissues housing the point usually involves producing some degree of increased slack in these tissues.

- Hold this position for 30 –90 seconds, then slowly return the tissues to a neutral position and repalpate.

- Has the tenderness reduced or vanished?

- Are the tissues more relaxed?

- Record your findings and continue to attempt to use this approach a number of times until the concept becomes imprinted.

Trigger point palpation

Travell and Simons (1992) and Simons et al. (1999), medical pioneers of our understanding of trigger points (TPs), describe specific characteristics which identify them from other myofascial changes.

1. A TP that is active causes pain to be referred to a predictable site, producing symptoms recognizable to the patient.

2. The trigger point itself is seldom located where the patient complains of pain.

3. There will be taut fibers (palpable bands) in the muscles which house TPs and pressure or tension applied to such a band (pressing or stretching the muscle, whether actively or passively) will usually refer pain to the target area.

4. There will be a palpable ropiness, or nodularity, in muscles which house TPs and the muscle will have a reduced range of motion.

5. A TP will be found at the site of the greatest sensitivity/tenderness in any taut band of muscle fibers.

6. If the tissue housing the TP is "rolled" briskly by fingers or thumb so that there is a sudden change of pressure on it, a "twitch" response may be observed.

7. Sustained digital pressure on the TP (or insertion into it of a needle) usually reproduces the referred pain pattern for which it is responsible.

8. Other autonomic phenomena may also be evoked, apart from pain.

Travell maintains that the high intensity of nerve impulses from an active trigger point can, by reflex, produce vasoconstriction, a reduction of the blood supply to specific areas of the brain, spinal cord, and nervous system, thus provoking a wide range of symptoms capable of affecting almost any part of the body. Among symptoms reported by Travell and others as a direct result of trigger point activity (as proved by their disappearance when the triggers were dealt with) are those listed in Box 5.1.

Box 5.1   Possible trigger point symptoms

- Pain
- Over- or undersecretion of glands
- Numbness
- Itching
- Localized coldness
- Oversensitivity to normal stimuli
- Paleness
- Redness of tissues
- Spasm
- Menopausal hot flashes
- Twitching
- Altered texture of skin (very oily, very dry)
- Weakness and trembling of muscles
- Increased sweat production
- In triggers found in the abdominal and thoracic muscles:
  - Halitosis (bad breath)
  - Heartburn
  - Vomiting
  - Distension
  - Nervous diarrhea and constipation
  - Disordered vision
  - Respiratory symptoms
  - Skin sensitivity

Trigger point compression guidelines

(Chaitow & DeLany 2000, 2002)

Central trigger points are usually palpable either with flat palpation (digital pressure against underlying structures using a thumb or finger) or with pincer compression (tissue held more precisely between thumb and fingers like a C-clamp, or held more broadly, with fingers extended like a clothes pin) (Fig. 5.15).

- Flat palpation into the tissues, using the thumb for example, should be slowly achieved, teasing and searching with the thumb tip, as tissues are slowly compressed toward underlying structures.

- Compressions may be applied wherever the tissue may be lifted without compressing neurovascular bundles.

- A more specific compression of individual fibers is possible by using the more precise pincer compression, applying the tips of the digits, or flat palpation, against underlying structures, both of which methods entrap specific bands of tissue.

- Compression between fingers and thumb has the advantage of offering information from two or more digits simultaneously, whereas flat palpation against

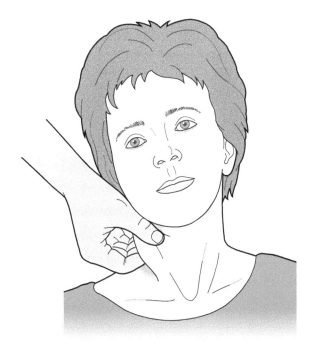

Figure 5.15
The sternocleidomastoid is examined with a flat pincer compression.

underlying tissues offers a more solid and stable background against which to assess the tissue.

- Once compressed by flat or pincer palpation, the patient/model is asked whether the pain is local, referring, radiating, and if radiating or referring, what the target area is, and whether the pain is familiar, a common symptom experience, in which case it is an active trigger.

- All other trigger points are "latent" and of less importance clinically.

- Additionally, the tissue can be rolled between fingers and thumb to assess quality, density, fluidity, and other characteristics that may offer information to the discerning touch.

Exercise 5.9 *Trigger Point Palpation*

Time suggested **15 minutes**

Locate – on yourself or on a suitable palpation partner – a number of trigger points, using NMT or other palpation method such as "skin drag" and the compression guidelines outlined above.

- A good place to start looking for a trigger point is in the upper trapezius, between the angle of the neck and the shoulder joint, where most adults have trigger points, although these are not always active.

- Establish precisely the "target" or reference area to which pain is being referred when each identified trigger point is compressed.

- If located in the sternomastoid, scalene, or upper trapezius muscles, the points should be lightly "compressed" rather than pressed by a single-digit contact (see Fig. 5.15).

- Go through the Simons/Travell guidelines to evaluate whether any of the other possible trigger point-related symptoms are present, as listed in Box 5.1.

- Record your findings.

Nimmo's perspective on trigger points

Nimmo (1966) developed a system he called "receptor tonus" that systematically uncovered trigger points and then "deactivated" them by inhibitory pressure, followed by stretching of the muscles involved if they were hypertonic, or strengthening if they were hypotonic.

Nimmo also applied himself to what he termed "noxious" points in ligaments. He diagnosed all noxious points by their degree of sensitivity, claiming that properly applied pressure would elicit painful points in all hypertonic and hypotonic muscles. He summarized his approach by saying: "We have three things to deal with: noxious or trigger points, ligament and tonus".

His method of identification of trigger or noxious points can be understood if we examine the following quote from his lecture notes (Nimmo 1966), which covers examination of the subscapular area for trigger points affecting the shoulder:

> Look about 2.5 inches [6.5 cm] to the left of spinous processes, on a level with the lower scapula border. Let the fingers glide along until a slight difference is found in the small muscles. If such a point is sensitive it should be treated.

After describing his method for dealing with the trigger (5 seconds sustained pressure, repeated if necessary) he continues:

> After holding pressure on a point, say on the level of the lower scapula border, move in a straight line upwards along the internal margin of the scapula about one inch [2.5 cm]. Here, usually, another point may be found. Treat it in the same manner and move upward about another inch [2.5 cm] and look for another point.

Nimmo stated that 90% of all patients have trigger points in one of these sites, and referred pain will be to the shoulder or head from these points on applied pressure. He continued by suggesting that practitioners search the body in the sites listed in Box 5.2, where the given percentages (Nimmo's figures) demonstrate active, sensitive, "noxious" points. Only sensitive points are treated, never non-painful ones.

Box 5.2   Nimmo's suggested search sites (and reported percentages) for sensitive points

1. Superior angle of scapula, on tendon of *levator scapulae*. This refers to head, face, neck, and shoulders. 90% incidence reported.

2. Between and on the ribs, between the transverse processes and around rib heads. Triggers here indicate an imbalance between *paraspinal musculature* due to Davis's law which states: "If hypertonus exists on one side, tonus is released on the other side." These triggers are said to affect most people.

3. Inferior angle of scapula, on inner insertions of *infraspinatus*. Also along inner border until spine of scapula is reached. 90% of patients have triggers here.

4. Press on internal aspect of *supraspinatus*, moving laterally towards its insertion. Triggers here are a common cause of "tired" shoulders. A 40% incidence is reported.

5. Search outer border of scapula for *teres major* points. Triggers are common if patient cannot raise arm behind back. 60% of patients were found by Nimmo to have triggers in these muscles.

6. *Upper trapezius* is searched by squeezing it between fingers and thumb, moving slowly from shoulder region towards spine until triggers are found. Pain refers to mastoid area or to forehead. Very common – 90%.

7. Pressure ("firm," says Nimmo) on superior border of sacrum, between iliac spine and sacral spinous process, produces pressure on SI ligament. Move contact superiorly and inferiorly searching for sensitivity. Triggers here are involved in all low back syndromes and 50% of all patients, according to Nimmo.

8. Press just superiorly to sacral base adjacent to spine, medial to PSIS. This is the *iliolumbar ligament*. Heavy pressure is required to find triggers which are involved in most low back problems. Search both sides. 90% incidence reported.

9. Hook thumb under *sacrosciatic* and *sacrotuberous ligaments* medial and inferior to ischial tuberosity, lifting and stretching laterally if painful. Nimmo reports a 30% incidence of triggers here.

Note: **Nimmo used a palm-held, rubber-tipped wooden T-bar, in order to apply pressure to areas requiring high poundage such as iliolumbar ligament.**

10. Medial pressure is applied by the thumb to lateral border of *quadratus lumborum* (QL), avoiding pressure on tips of transverse processes, starting below last rib down to pelvic rim. A "gummy" feel will be noted if contracture exists (plus sensitivity) in contrast to resilient, homogeneous feel of normal muscle. Often associated with low back problems. If *latissimus dorsi* is also involved, pain may radiate to shoulder or arm. 80% of patients show trigger activity in these muscles.

11. Search area below posterior aspect of ilia for noxious points associated with *gluteal muscles*.

12. Search central region of belly of *gluteus medius* for triggers which can produce sciatic-type pain. 90% incidence.

13. Search midway between trochanters and superior crest of ilium, in central portion of *gluteus minimus* where trigger affecting lateral aspect of leg or foot, or duplicating sciatic-type pain, is common. This also has a 90% incidence of triggers, as opposed to gluteus maximus, which produces active triggers in only 4% of patients.

14. The point of intersection, where imaginary lines drawn from the PSIS and the trochanter, and the ischium and the ASIS meet, is the access point for contact with the insertion of the *piriformis muscle*. If the line from the ASIS is taken to the coccyx, the intersection is over the belly of piriformis. These two points should be palpated; if sensitivity is noted, the muscle requires treatment. Sciatic-type pain distribution to the knee is a common referred symptom. A 40% incidence of triggers is reported by Nimmo.

15. *Hamstring* trigger points lie about a hand's width above the knee joint in about 20% of patients.

Box 5.2 *continued*

16. Trigger points in *abductor magnus muscle* lie close to its origins and insertions, notably near the tendinous insertion, and close to the ischium.

17. The area *posterior* to the *tibia* is a site for trigger points relating to calf pain. 90% of patients display triggers here.

18. Triggers abound in the region of the *external malleolus*, especially if recurrent ankle strains have occurred.

19. With patient side-lying and practitioner standing facing patient at chest level, reach across with cephalad hand to ease scapula into maximum abduction while thumb of the caudad hand is inserted under scapula to try to contact *serratus magnum* and *subscapularis muscles* (both have 90% incidence of triggers).

20. Search for triggers in the *upper cervical muscles* with patient face upwards and practitioner's thumb applying pressure against these muscles, medially and upwards (to ceiling) along length of lamina groove from occiput to base of neck. 90% of patients have triggers in these muscles.

21. Same position, right hand under and cupping lower neck, thumb anterior to *trapezius* fibers, rotate head to right allowing hand to slowly glide towards floor. The thumb can descend into a "pocket" created by the head position (Fig. 5.16A–C). When the thumb has reached as far as possible, pressure towards the opposite nipple allows contact to be made with insertion of splenius capitis muscle (around second thoracic vertebra). Referred pain to base of neck is a common symptom. Again, 90% of people have triggers here.

22. Standing at the head, place the right thumb just superior to clavicle, lateral to outer margin of *sternomastoid*; flex neck by raising head with other hand, allowing right thumb to enter area below clavicle over attachment of *anterior scalene muscle*. Patient's head is turned right, bringing *scalene* directly under thumb. Pressure laterally with thumb finds triggers located here, a common (90%) finding.

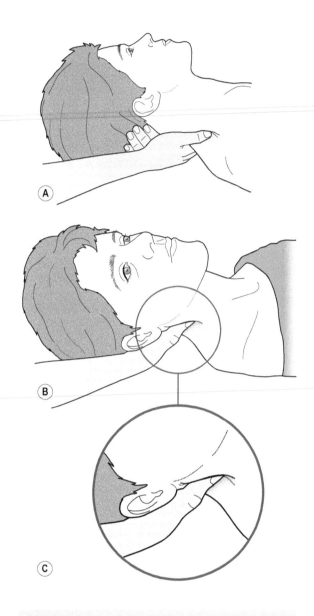

Figure 5.16
The thumb slides into a "pocket" formed anterior to the trapezius while remaining posterior to the transverse process to directly palpate a portion of lower splenii.

Box 5.2 *continued*

23. *Anterior cervical muscles* are palpated for changes and trigger points by facing seated patient and inserting thumbs under jawline to contact anterior surface of upper transverse processes. Gliding thumbs inferiorly allows contact with *longus capitis, colli*, and so on (70% trigger point incidence). Care is required as to degree of pressure and time spent in the region of carotid body.

24. *Sternomastoid* palpation is performed with patient face upwards, head turned towards side being assessed. Contact is by "squeezing" between finger(s) and thumb as direct pressure is avoided in this muscle (as in scalene, apart from its insertions).

25. Triggers lying in *masseter* and *external pterygoid muscles* are found with practitioner sitting at head of supine patient. Triggers here may relate to temporomandibular joint (TMJ) dysfunction, tinnitus, and salivary gland dysfunction.

26. Functional disturbances of the eyes may stem from active triggers in the *temporalis muscle*, which is palpated from same position as 25.

27. Standing to side of supine patient, grasp wrist with cephalad hand and abduct the arm; other hand contacts coracoid process and thumb contact glides towards sternum, assessing *subclavius muscle*. A similar stroke from coracoid process towards xiphoid assesses *pectoralis minor* (Nimmo reports a 90% incidence of triggers in both muscles, only 10% in *pectoralis major*).

28. Thumb pressure should be applied to the *biceps tendon* insertion for a distance of 2.5 cm or so below its insertion in search of a trigger which would relate to shoulder problems (90% incidence).

29. Trigger points are found on the sternum in the rudimentary *sternalis muscle* (40% incidence of triggers) as well as in *cartilaginous attachments* of ribs on sternum.

30. With patient supine, knees flexed, contact is flat of hand (fingers more than palm) with other hand on top of it, applying pressure from just inferior to rib margins, going under these as far as possible to approach triggers lying in *upper abdominal musculature* (90%). Finger pads are stroked in a series of movements from the most superior point reached under the ribs, towards the umbilicus. Tight bands will be felt, containing triggers.

31. *Serratus magnus* is searched with flat of hand stretching it towards its attachments (90% incidence).

32. Patient in the same position. Practitioner standing on side opposite that to be assessed and starting some 7.5 cm below umbilicus on a line from it to the ASIS, a firm flat hand contact is made; this is taken inferior and then medial, allowing contact to be made *anterior to fourth and fifth lumbar vertebrae* (site of hypogastric plexus and ganglionated cord). This is likely to be an area of referred sensitivity (upwards to chest) in 70% of patients. This contact could be avoided in the elderly, the obese, or patients with aneurysms or sclerotic aortas.

33. Patient in same position, practitioner standing on side to be examined. Place finger pads just superior to ASIS, pressing towards floor and then towards feet, allowing access under the pelvic crest to contact *iliacus muscle*. A gliding contact followed by flexing of the contact fingers allows searching of this area for triggers (90%).

34. Access to the *psoas muscle* is suggested from lateral margin of *rectus abdominis*, allowing finger contact to pass under the sigmoid on the left and under the caecum on the right. This accesses the belly of psoas in non-obese patients. Another access is directly towards the spine from the midline (patient with flexed knees) some 7.5 cm below umbilicus. On approaching the spine (denser feel), finger pad contact slides laterally over body of lumbar vertebrae (2, 3, or 4) to opposite side. This will contact origin of psoas, a common site for triggers (50–70%).

35. *Abductor longus* and *pectineus* can be contacted with patient in same position, as thumbs glide along abductor towards pubic attachment and then laterally to contact pectineus. 50% of patients have triggers in this muscle.

Box 5.2 continued

36. *Quadriceps* can be contacted and searched with thumbs, heel of hand or fingers, with patient supine. Triggers abound in both *rectus femoris* (90% incidence) and the *vasti* (70%).

37. *Tensor fascia lata* (TFL) is best contacted with patient side-lying, affected leg straight, supported by flexed other leg. Triggers here can produce sciatic-type pain (70%).

38. *Gracilis* attachment into the knee region (via its tendon) is a major trigger site (90%). The muscle itself should be assessed from tibial attachment to the pubis.

39. *Anterior tibialis muscle* may rarely contain triggers affecting feet or toes.

Exercise 5.10 *Palpation for Trigger Points Using Nimmo's Guidelines*

Time suggested **5–7 minutes per "Nimmo" site (Box 5.2)**

- Carefully read through the text of Box 5.2 and select particular aspects to use in this exercise.

- Or alternatively work steadily, in sequence, through Nimmo's suggested trigger point location protocols.

- For example, to start with, take description 1 or 2 (levator scapula attachment and posterior rib attachment areas), and see whether you can find active trigger points in these areas using Lief's NMT assessment method (thumb or finger contact), and/or one of the skin palpation methods described in Chapter 4 ("drag," elasticity, etc.), in order to evaluate the accuracy of these methods in locating triggers in the areas identified by Nimmo.

- See whether any of the triggers you locate are associated with joint and other restrictions as described by Lewit (see below).

- *Note*: This will be assisted by use of the joint palpation methods as described in later chapters.

- Over time, attempt to evaluate all of Nimmo's target sites.

- It is important to include in this search methods previously covered, notably skin evaluation, NMT and layer palpation.

- Record your findings in your palpation journal, and compare your results with those suggested as likely by Nimmo (based on his percentages).

Lewit's view of trigger point significance

Lewit (1992, 1999) suggests that, apart from their local significance in terms of pain and their influence on target areas, trigger points can have a clinical importance due to their links with certain pathologies. For example, triggers in:

- the thigh adductors may indicate hip pathology

- iliacus may indicate lesions of segments L5–S1 (coccyx)

- piriformis may indicate lesions of segment L4–5 (coccyx)

- rectus femoris may indicate lesions of L3–4 (hip)

- psoas may indicate lesions of thoracolumbar junction (T10–L1)

- erector spinae muscles may indicate lesions of corresponding spinal level

- rectus abdominis may indicate problems at xiphoid, pubis, or low back

- pectoralis may indicate problems of upper ribs or thoracic viscera

- subscapularis are common in "frozen shoulder"

- middle trapezius may indicate radicular syndrome of the upper extremity

- upper trapezius may indicate cervical lesion

- sternomastoid may indicate lesion of CO–1 and C2–3

- masticatory muscles relate to headache and facial pain.

Periosteal pain points

Lewit also interprets periosteal pain points (PPP) as relating to specific functional or structural problems.

As tonus increases and becomes chronic, leading to changes in the structure of the soft tissues, with increased fibrous tissue and decreased elastic content becoming palpably apparent, so do stresses build up on the tendons and their osseous insertions into the periosteum. Many are characteristic of certain dysfunctional patterns, making them useful as diagnostic aids.

The feel of periosteal pain points varies; however, a frequently palpated common feature is of a sensitive "soft bump" at the point of attachment of tendons and ligaments. This is often observed on spinous processes where one side is tender, relating to tension or spasm in the muscles on that side, something that also prevents easy rotation of the body of that vertebra.

Intervertebral joints can be palpated directly in some areas; for example, the cervical joints are accessible when the patient is supine. Greater pressure is required through paraspinal tissues with the patient prone for access to other spinal joints (for example, using NMT approaches as described above).

Many extremity joints are available for direct palpation:

- The hip attachments can be reached via the groin if care is taken.

- Acromioclavicular and sternoclavicular joints are easily accessed, as is the TMJ anterior to the tragus.

Table 5.1 describes the sites of some PPP, and the significance accorded to them by Lewit (1999).

Table 5.1

Some PPP and their significance according to Lewit (1999)	
PPP	Significance
Head of metatarsals	Metatarsalgia (flat foot)
Calcaneal spur (a classic PPP)	Tension in plantar aponeurosis
Tubercle of tibia	Tension in long adductors, possibly hip lesion
Attachments of collateral	Lesion of the corresponding meniscus knee ligaments
Fibula head	Tension in the biceps femoris or restriction of the head of the fibula
PSIS	Common, but no specific indication
Symphysis pubis (lateral)	Tension in the adductors, SI joint restriction or a hip lesion
Coccyx	Tension in the gluteus maximus, levator ani or piriformis
Iliac crest	Gluteus medius or quadratus lumborum tension or dysfunction at thoracolumbar junction
Greater trochanter	Tension in the abductors or a hip lesion
T5–6 spinous process	Lesion of the lower cervical spine
Spinous process of C2	Lesion at C1–2 or C2–3 or tension in levator scapulae
Xiphoid process	Tension in rectus abdominis or 6th, 7th or 8th rib dysfunction
Ribs in mammary or axillary line	Tension in pectoralis attachments or a visceral disorder

Table 5.1 *continued*

Some PPP and their significance according to Lewit (1999)	
PPP	**Significance**
Sternocostal junction of upper ribs	Tension in scalene muscles
Sternum, close to the clavicle	Tension in sternomastoid muscle
Transverse process of atlas	Lesion of the atlas/occiput segment or tension in either rectus capitis lateralis or sternomastoid
Styloid process of the radius	Elbow lesion
Epicondyles	Elbow lesion or tension in muscles attaching to epicondyles
Attachment of deltoid	Scapulohumeral joint lesion
Condyle of the mandible	TMJ lesion or tension in masticatory muscles

Exercise 5.11 *Palpation for Periosteal Pain Points (PPPs)*

Time suggested 3–5 minutes per PPP and associated muscle

- Palpate selected potential PPPs, as described in Table 5.1, and see how many are present as sensitive structures, in your palpation partner.

- Try to assess the soft tissues associated with tender PPPs, as indicated in the descriptions in Table 5.1.

- For example, do muscles indicated in the table display signs of altered tone, or is the general "feel" of these attaching muscles altered?

- This will become increasingly pertinent when you incorporate tests for shortness of muscles linked to PPPs, as outlined later in this chapter (Lewit 1992, 1999).

- Record your findings.

Discussion of palpatory progress involving Exercises 5.8–5.11

- Assessment using skills covered in earlier exercises/chapters allows the localization of trigger points, Jones's tender points and periosteal pain points.

- These differently named "points" may in the end all represent the same phenomena, viewed and labeled differently.

- It matters little what we call particular reflex areas, as long as we can find them, and evaluate their influence on the individual and the symptoms being complained of.

- The palpation skills that reveal something as being "different" or "not normal" relate to variations in texture, tone, fluid content, etc.

- By being aware of these different perspectives (Nimmo, Simons, Travell, Jones, Lewit, etc.) and practicing the identification – through touch – of the points/zones/areas they describe, your skills will advance.

Altered muscle function

The final segment of this section deals with exercises in which postural muscles may be assessed for relative shortness, as well as aspects of their function evaluated. Before this sequence, three "functional assessments" are outlined that examine the way in which muscles are firing when particular actions are performed by the patient/model.

Muscle-firing sequences offer evidence of normality or dysfunction and, depending on the region, can point to the probability of particular muscles being short or inhibited (Janda 1983). Janda demonstrated that postural muscles have a tendency to shorten, not only under pathological conditions, but often under circumstances of normal use. It has been asserted that most problems of the musculoskeletal system involve, as part of their etiology, dysfunction relating to muscle shortening (Janda 1978, 1983; Lewit 1999; Liebenson 2006).

Postural muscles are genetically older, and have different physiological and probably biochemical qualities compared with phasic muscles, which normally weaken and exhibit signs of inhibition in response to stress or pathology. Where weakness (lack of tone) is judged to be a major feature, it is common for antagonists to be shortened, reciprocally inhibiting their tone.

Before any effort is made to strengthen such apparently weak muscles, hypertonic antagonists should be stretched and released, after which spontaneous toning occurs in the previously hypotonic muscles. If tone remains reduced then, and only then, should exercise and/or isotonic muscle energy technique procedures be brought in (Chaitow 2001; Janda 1978).

Firing sequences and functional assessment

The following simple tests allow for a rapid gathering of information with a minimum of effort. The tests are based on the work of Janda (1983) and interpretations of this by Liebenson (1996, 2006). After a description of each test, a palpation exercise will be outlined.

Prone hip extension test

The patient lies prone and the practitioner stands at the patient's waist level, hands placed so that the cephalad one spans the lower erector spinae on both sides, and the caudad hand rests with the thenar eminence on gluteus maximus and the fingertips on the hamstrings (Fig. 5.17).

The patient is asked to raise the leg into extension of the hip.

The normal activation sequence involves gluteus maximus and hamstrings firing more or less simultaneously, followed by the erector spinae (contralateral then ipsilateral).

If the hamstrings and/or the erectors adopt the role of gluteus, as indicated by their firing first, they are working inappropriately, are therefore "stressed" and will by implication have shortened.

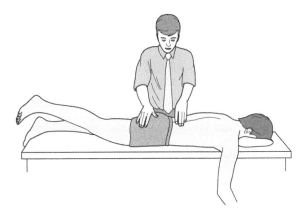

Figure 5.17
Hip extension test. The normal activation sequence is gluteus maximus, hamstrings, contralateral erector spinae, ipsilateral erector spinae.

Exercise 5.12 *Hip Extension Firing Sequence*

Time suggested **3 minutes**

- Your palpation partner should lie prone.

- You should stand at their waist level, with your cephalad hand spanning the low back so that the pads of your fingers touch one side of the erector spinae and the heel of your hand touches the other.

- Your caudad hand should be placed so that the heel is on gluteus maximus, and the finger pads are on the upper hamstrings.

- Ask your partner to raise the leg into extension.

- Note the firing sequence (i.e., which muscle fires first, which second, etc).

- Have your partner relax and perform the palpation test again several times.

1. Do the gluteal muscles fire first (they should)?

2. Do the hamstrings come in very fast, with gluteal muscles much later (they shouldn't)?

3. Most worryingly of all, do one or other of the erectors fire first?

- If the hamstrings or erectors fire early, then these are likely to have shortened and this will be demonstrable in the tests later in the chapter (Liebenson 2006).

Hip abduction test: observation and palpation

The patient is sidelying, with the lower leg flexed to provide support, and the upper leg straight, in line with the trunk. The practitioner stands in front of the patient at the level of the feet and observes (not touching) as the patient is asked to slowly abduct the leg:

- Normal – hip abduction to 45°.

- Abnormal – if hip flexion occurs (indicating TFL shortness) and/or leg externally rotates (indicating piriformis shortening), and/or "hiking" of the hip occurs at the outset of the movement (indicating quadratus lumbo-

rum overactivity, and therefore, by implication, shortness) (Fig. 5.18).

The test should be repeated with the practitioner standing behind the patient at their waist level, with a finger pad on the lateral margin of quadratus lumborum.

As the leg is abducted, if quadratus fires strongly, or before gluteus medius, a twitch or push will be felt by the palpating finger, indicating overactivity and probable shortness of quadratus lumborum (QL) (this would show visually as a "hip-hike," as mentioned above).

Exercise 5.13 *Hip Abduction Firing Sequence Test*

Time suggested **3–4 minutes**

- Your palpation partner should lie on his side, lower leg flexed, upper leg straight, in line with the trunk.

- You should stand in front, at the level of the feet and observe (no hands-on yet) as your partner is asked to abduct the leg slowly.

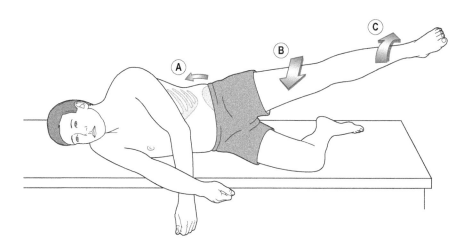

Figure 5.18

Hip abduction observation test. Normal firing sequence is gluteus medius or tensor fascia lata (TFL) first and second, followed by quadratus lumborum (QL). If QL fires first it is overactive and will be short (A). If TFL is short the leg will drift into flexion on abduction (B). If piriformis is short the leg and foot will externally rotate during abduction (C).

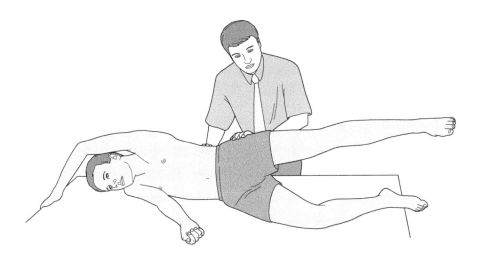

Figure 5.19
Palpation assessment for quadratus lumborum overactivity. The muscle is palpated, as is the gluteus medius and tensor fascia lata (TFL), during abduction of the leg. The correct firing sequence should be gluteus and TFL, followed at around 25° elevation by quadratus. If there is an immediate "hip-hike" (active contraction) of quadratus it indicates overactivity and therefore stress, and therefore shortness can be assumed.

- Observe the area just above the crest of the pelvis – does it "jump" at the outset of the abduction, or at least obviously activate before a 25° abduction has taken place? If so, QL is overactive and probably short.

- Have your partner relax completely and repeat the abduction.

- Does the leg drift anteriorly during abduction? If so, TFL is probably short.

- Do the leg and/or the foot, turn outward (externally rotate)? If so, piriformis is probably short (see Fig. 5.18).

- Now, standing behind your side-lying palpation partner, place one or two finger pads of your cephalad hand lightly on the tissues overlying QL, approximately 2 inches (5 cm) lateral to the spinous process of L3 (Fig. 5.19).

- Place your caudad hand so that the heel rests on gluteus medius and the finger pads on TFL. Assess the firing sequence during hip abduction. If QL fires early (you will feel a strong twitch or "jump" against your palpating fingers), it is overactive and short.

- The ideal firing sequence is TFL – gluteus medius – QL (but not before about 20–25° of abduction) (Liebenson 2006).

Scapulohumeral rhythm test

This important assessment offers information as to the status of the upper fixators of the shoulder.

The patient is seated with the arm at the side, elbow flexed and pointing forwards.

The practitioner stands behind, and observes as the patient abducts the arm towards the horizontal.

- Normal – elevation of shoulder occurs only after 60° of arm abduction.

- Abnormal – if elevation of the shoulder, or obvious "bunching" occurs between shoulder and neck, or winging of the scapulae, occurs within the first 60° of shoulder abduction (indicating levator scapulae and upper trapezius shortness, and lower and middle trapezius, as well as serratus anterior, weakness) (Fig. 5.20).

This pattern, of weak lower fixators and overworked and probably shortened upper fixators, is common in postural patterns involving a forward head carriage with round-shouldered stance.

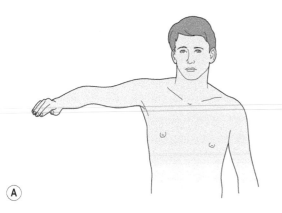

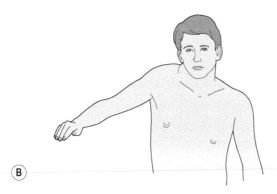

Figure 5.20
Scapulohumeral rhythm test. (A) Normal – elevation of the shoulder after 60° of abduction. (B) Abnormal – elevation of the shoulder before 60° of abduction.

Exercise 5.14 *Assessing Scapulohumeral Rhythm*

Time suggested 2 minutes

- Follow the description of the scapulohumeral rhythm test described above. This is a purely observational assessment, without touching.

- If the test is positive, seen as a bunching of upper trapezius before the abduction of the humerus has reached 60°, the implicated muscles (levator scapulae, upper

trapezius) should be tested for shortness (described later in this chapter).

Discussion of palpatory progress involving Exercises 5.12–5.14

- In these last few palpation and observation exercises the interface between structure and function has been reached, particularly with Janda's functional assessments.

- In those you were able to feel and observe inappropriate behavior and to link that to likely structural modification, in this instance shortness.

- These clues to structural change can then be confirmed by the sort of tests and assessments which form the remainder of this chapter.

- The palpation of neurolymphatic "points" was also a link between structure (the soft tissue changes) and function (the modified lymphatic flow). It is in this type of exercise that the clinical usefulness of such evaluations becomes obvious, as this impinges on the real world of people's problems, involving pain and restriction, and your role in trying to make sense of what has happened and what can be treated.

Assessing muscles for shortness

As part of a comprehensive palpation protocol, it is useful to learn to assess short, tight muscles in a standardized manner.

Janda (1983) suggests that to obtain a reliable evaluation of muscle shortness the following criteria should be observed:

- The starting position, method of fixation, and direction of movement, must be observed carefully.

- The prime mover must not be exposed to external pressure.

- If possible, the force exerted on the tested muscle must not work over two joints.

- The examiner should perform at an even speed a slow movement that brakes slowly at the end of the range.

- The examiner should keep the stretch even, avoiding jerking movements.

- Pressure or pull must always act in the required direction of movement.

- Muscle shortening can only be correctly evaluated if the joint range is not decreased, as might be the case with osseous limitation or joint blockage.

It is commonly in shortened muscle fibers, that reflex activity may be noted. This may take the form of local dysfunction, variously called trigger points, tender points, zones of irritability, hyperalgesic zones, neurovascular and neurolymphatic reflexes, etc. Localizing these is possible via normal palpatory methods (NMT, "drag," skin elasticity, etc.) or as part of neuromuscular diagnostic treatment.

Identification of tight muscles may also be systematically carried out as described below. Note that the assessment methods presented are not themselves diagnostic, but provide strong indications of probable shortness of the muscles being tested.

See Special topic 9, on "end-feel," for descriptions of different qualities of the end of range.

The following tests are derived from the work of Janda (1983), Kendall et al. (1952), Seffinger and Hruby (2008), and a variety of other sources.

Tests for postural muscle shortening

Ease and bind

Before starting a muscle-by-muscle sequence, in which postural muscles are tested for relative shortness, it is helpful to focus on acquiring the skill of being able to identify sensations of "bind" or resistance, as a muscle is moved towards its barrier of resistance.

Along with "bind"/resistance, being able to recognize the contrasting sensation of "ease" is also necessary. There can never be enough focus on these two characteristics that help soft tissues to reveal their current degree of comfort or distress.

Hoover (1969) describes "ease" as a state of equilibrium, or "neutral," that the practitioner senses by having at least one completely passive, "listening" contact, either the whole hand or a single or several digits, in touch with the tissues being assessed.

"Bind" is, of course, the opposite of "ease" and can most easily be recognized by lightly palpating the tissues surrounding a joint, as this is taken towards its resistance barrier, the end of range of movement.

In order to "read" hypertonicity, palpation skills need to be refined, and as a first step Goodridge (1981) suggests the following test, which examines medial hamstring and short abductor status, as a means of becoming comfortable with the reality of ease and bind, in a practical manner.

Exercise 5.15A *Palpating for the "Feather-Edge" Barrier in Muscle Shortness*

Time suggested **5 minutes**

This palpation exercise evaluates the concept of "ease and bind" during assessment of adductors of the thigh (Fig. 5.21A).

- Before starting, ensure that your palpation partner lies supine, so that the non-tested leg is abducted slightly, heel over the end of the table.

- The leg to be tested is close to the edge of the table.

- Ensure that the tested leg is in the anatomically correct position, knee in full extension and with no external rotation of the leg, which would negate the test.

- After grasping the supine patient's foot and ankle, in order to abduct the lower limb, close your eyes during the abduction and feel, in your own body, from the hand through the forearm into the upper arm, the *very beginning* of a sense of resistance.

- Stop when you feel it, open your eyes and note how many degrees in an arc the limb has travelled.

- In reality, by the time you sense resistance you will already have passed the tissue "barrier."

What you are trying to establish is that you learn to recognize the *very beginning of the end of range of free movement (the "feather-edge")*, where easy motion ceases and effort begins. This "barrier" is not a pathological one, but represents the first sign of resistance, the place at which tissues require some degree of passive effort in order to move them.

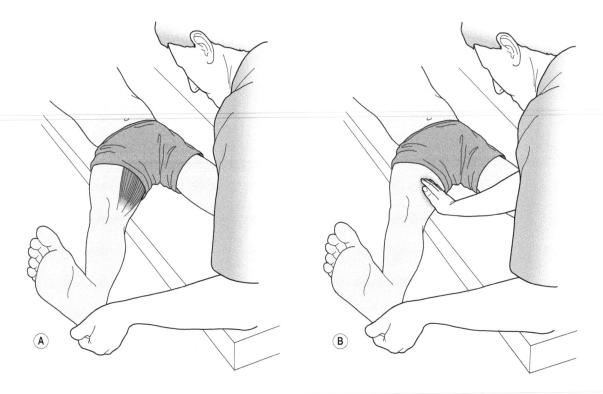

Figure 5.21

Assessment of "bind"/restriction barrier with the first sign of resistance in the adductors (medial hamstrings) of the right leg. (A) The practitioner's perception of the transition point, where easy movement alters to demand some degree of effort, is regarded as the barrier. (B) The barrier is identified when the palpating hand notes a sense of bind in tissues which were relaxed (at ease) up to that point.

This is also the position in which a sense of "bind" should be palpated, in the next part of this exercise.

It is suggested that the process be attempted several times, so that you get a sense of where resistance begins, before doing the next part of this exercise sequence. Then do the exercise again, but this time as described in Exercise 5.16B.

Exercise 5.15B *Goodridge's "Ease and Bind" Palpation (Fig. 5.21B)*

Time suggested **5 minutes**

- Stand between your palpation partner's partially abducted leg and the table, facing the head of the table, so that all control of the tested leg is achieved by using your lateral arm/hand, which holds and supports the leg at the ankle, while your table-side hand rests on the inner thigh, palpating the muscles which are being tested.

- This palpating hand (often called a "listening" hand) must be in touch with the skin, molded to the contours of the tissues being assessed, but should exert no pressure and should be completely relaxed.

- Abduction of the tested leg from its neutral resting position is introduced passively by the outside hand/arm, until the first sign of resistance is noted by the hand providing the motive force, i.e., the one holding the leg.

- As you approach this point of resistance (as noted in the previous exercise), can you sense a tightening of the tissues in the mid-inner thigh, which your table-side, listening hand is touching?

- This sensation is known as "bind."

- If this sensation is not clear, then take the leg back towards the table and out again, but this time go past the point where easy movement is lost and effort begins and towards its end of range. Here you will certainly sense bind.

- As you once more take the leg back towards the table you will note a softening, a relaxation, an "ease" in these same tissues.

Go through the same sequence with the other leg, becoming increasingly familiar with the sense of these two extremes (ease and bind), and try to note the very moment at which you can palpate the transition from one to the other, not to its extreme but where it begins, whether you are moving from ease to bind or the other way.

Normal excursion of the straight leg into abduction is around 45° and by testing both legs as described you can evaluate whether the two sets of adductors are both tight and short, or whether one is and the other is not.

Even if both are tight and short one may be more restricted than the other and this may be the one to treat first.

Suggestion

You should consider practicing palpation exercises, for ease and bind, on many other muscles than those described in Exercise 5.16A, while they are being both actively and passively moved, until you are comfortable with your skill in recognizing this change in tone.

The point at which you feel bind, or when a hand touching the tissues first senses that increased effort is required, is the resistance barrier, where an isometric contraction should start when muscle energy technique (MET) is applied to taut structures.

Record your experience, using the two methods of evaluating shortness in this muscle (Exercises 5.16A and B), and try wherever possible to use a directly palpating hand to assess bind as you perform the following exercises.

For each of the following exercises, involving assessment of individual muscle shortness, it is suggested that around 5 minutes be spent practicing each side, at first. This should, with practice, be reduced to around 2–3 minutes.

The muscles included here are representative ones (hamstrings, piriformis, erector spinae, upper trapezius). For a wider range of assessment and palpation methods see also:

Muscle Function Testing (Janda 1983)

Manipulative Therapy in Rehabilitation of the Locomotor System (Lewit 1999)

Muscle Energy Techniques (Chaitow 2006).

Evidence-Based Manual Medicine (Seffinger & Hruby 2008)

Orthopedic Assessment in Massage Therapy (Lowe 2006).

Exercise 5.16A *Palpation for Hamstring Shortness: Upper Fibers*

Time suggested **5 minutes**

In order to assess for shortened hamstrings (biceps femoris, semitendinosus, and semimembranosus), your palpation partner should lie supine with the leg to be tested outstretched, and the other leg flexed at knee and hip, to relax the low back (Fig. 5.22).

- In order to assess tightness in the left leg hamstrings (upper fibers), you should be standing at the side of the leg to be tested, facing the head of the table.

- The lower leg is supported by your caudad hand, keeping the knee of that leg in light extension and if possible resting the heel of that leg in the bend of the elbow to prevent lateral rotation.

- The cephalad hand can then rest on the hamstrings, around mid-thigh, to evaluate for bind as elevation takes place.

- The range of movement into hip flexion should (with a supple hamstring group) allow elevation of the tested leg to about 80° before bind is noted.

- Does the first sign of resistance, bind, occur before 80°?

- If so, hamstrings are shortened.

- Repeat the palpation exercise while your palpation partner lies with the head and neck turned fully away from

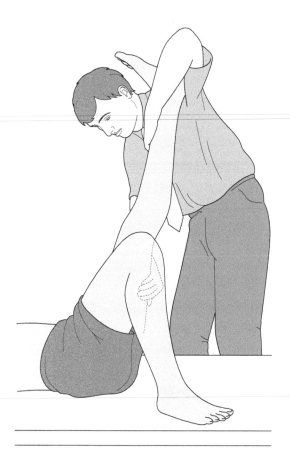

Figure 5.22
Assessment for shortness of hamstring, upper fibers, by palpation during leg raising.

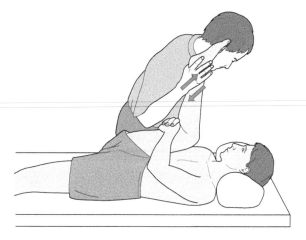

Figure 5.23
Assessment for shortness of hamstring, lower fibers, by palpation during leg straightening.

tested, they should test as tighter than previously (Murphy 2000). Was this apparent during the test?

Exercise 5.16B *Palpation for Hamstring Shortness: Lower Fibers*

Time suggested   3–5 minutes

● To make this assessment the tested leg is taken into full hip flexion (helped by the patient holding the upper thigh with both hands (Fig. 5.23)).

● You should place a hand onto the fibers just inferior to the popliteal space to assess for bind as the leg straightens.

● The knee is then passively straightened until resistance is felt or bind is noted by this palpation hand resting on the lower hamstrings.

● If the knee cannot easily straighten with the hip flexed, this indicates shortness in the lower hamstring fibers, and a degree of pull behind the knee and lower thigh will be reported during any attempt to straighten the leg.

● If the knee is capable of being straightened with the hip flexed, having previously not been capable of achieving an 80°, straight-leg raise, then the lower fibers are not

the side you are testing and then again fully turned toward the side you are testing.

● Was there any difference in the degree of elevation of the leg before bind was noticed when the neck was turned?

There may be a difference, due to the tonic neck reflex in which cervical rotation increases ipsilateral extensor tone and contralateral flexor tone while it decreases contralateral extensor and ipsilateral flexor tone.

Simply put, this means that when the neck is turned *away from the side being tested*, the hamstrings should be more relaxed. And when the neck is turned *toward the side being*

short, and it is the upper hamstring fibers that require attention.

Exercise 5.17 *Palpating for Shortness of Piriformis*

Time suggested **3–4 minutes**

When it is short, piriformis will cause the affected side leg of the supine individual to appear to be short and externally rotated.

- Have your palpation partner side-lying, tested side uppermost. You should stand in front of and facing the pelvis.

- In order to contact the insertion of piriformis, draw two imaginary lines: one runs from the ASIS to the ischial tuberosity and the other from the PSIS to the most prominent point of the trochanter (Fig. 5.24). Where these lines cross, just posterior to the trochanter, is the insertion of the muscle, and pressure here will produce marked discomfort if the structure is short or irritated.

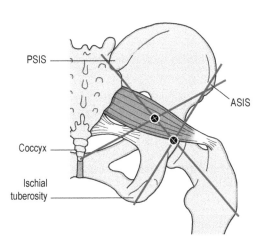

PSIS

ASIS

Coccyx

Ischial tuberosity

Figure 5.24

Landmarks are used as coordinates to locate the attachment of piriformis at the hip, and also the site of major trigger point activity in the belly of the muscle. ASIS, anterior superior iliac spine; PSIS, posterior superior iliac spine.

- In order to locate the most common trigger point site, in the belly of the muscle, the line from the ASIS should be taken to the tip of the coccyx rather than the ischial tuberosity. The other line, from the PSIS to the trochanter prominence, is the same.

- Pressure where one line crosses the other will access the mid-point of the belly of piriformis, where trigger points are common.

- Light compression here that produces a painful response is indicative of a stressed and probably shortened muscle.

Exercise 5.18 *Paravertebral Muscle Assessment (Fig. 5.25)*

Time suggested **3 minutes for observation, up to 15 minutes if additional palpation methods are introduced**

5.18A

- Your palpation partner should be seated on the treatment table, legs extended, pelvis vertical.

- Flexion is introduced in order to approximate the forehead to the knees, without strain.

- An even curve should be observed and a distance of about 4 inches (10 cm) from the knees achieved by the forehead.

- No knee flexion should occur and the movement should be a spinal one, not involving pelvic tilting.

5.18B

- Your palpation partner should be seated at the edge of the table, knees flexed and lower legs hanging over the edge, relaxing the hamstrings.

- Forward bending is introduced so that the forehead approximates the knees.

- If flexion of the trunk is greater in this position than in 5.19A, above, then there is probably tilting of the pelvis and shortened hamstring involvement.

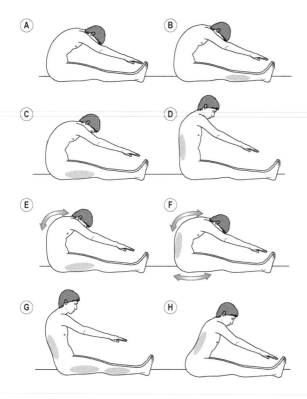

Figure 5.25
Tests for shortness of the erector spinae and associated postural muscles. (A) Normal length of erector spinae muscles and posterior thigh muscles. (B) Tight gastrocnemius and soleus; the inability to dorsiflex the feet indicates tightness of the plantarflexor group. (C) Tight hamstring muscles, which cause the pelvis to tilt posteriorly. (D) Tight low back erector spinae muscles. (E) Tight hamstring; slightly tight low back muscles and overstretched upper back muscles. (F) Slightly shortened lower back muscles, stretched upper back muscles and slightly stretched hamstrings. (G) Tight low back muscles, hamstrings, and gastrocnemius/soleus. (H) Very tight low back muscles, with lordosis maintained even in flexion.

Identifying and palpating areas of "spinal flatness" during Exercises 5.18A and 5.18B

During these assessments there should be a uniform degree of flexion throughout the spine, with a "C" curve apparent when looked at from the side. However, all too commonly areas of shortening in the spinal muscles may be observed, particularly as areas which are "flat" where little or no flexion is taking place.

In some instances lordosis may be maintained in the lumbar spine, even on full flexion, or flexion may be very limited, even without such lordosis. There may also be obvious overstretching of the upper back, as compensation for the relative tightness of the lower back.

Generally "flat" areas of the spine indicate involvement of local shortening of the erector spinae group.

- Can you observe "flat", tense areas of the spine during either or both of these flexion exercises?

- Identify one or two such areas and palpate them lightly as your partner moves into flexion.

- Compare the feel of the tissues as they tighten, bind, compared with those areas which are flexible, where the curve is normal.

- Also, if you identify flat areas, have your palpation partner lie prone and palpate lightly with your fingertips to assess the degree of hypertonicity and/or use skin palpation methods, discussed in Chapter 4, to evaluate other findings in the tense tissues (drag, for example, to locate trigger points) as compared with more normal ones.

- Evaluate whether these tight muscles alongside the spine are areas of facilitation, by using Exercises 5.1–5.3 again. Record your findings.

Notes

"Flat" areas in the thoracic spine, when the person is flexing, are particularly significant when considering breathing function, as there are likely to be associated rib restrictions and a limited ability for full and free inhalation/exhalation.

Exercise 5.19 *Palpating for Shortness of Upper Trapezius*

Time suggested **3 minutes**

5.19A

Your palpation partner should be seated as you stand behind, with one hand on the shoulder of the side to be tested, and the other hand on the ipsilateral side of the head.

- The neck is gently side-flexed, without allowing flexion, extension or rotation, to its "easy" barrier, i.e. no force at all, while the shoulder of the tested side is stabilised from above (Fig. 5.26).

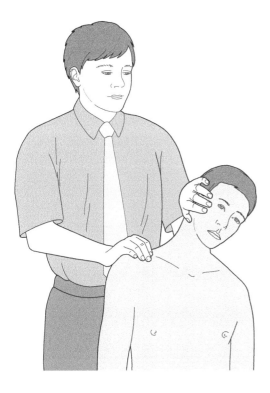

Figure 5.26
Assessment of relative shortness of right side upper trapezius. The right shoulder is stabilized while the neck is side-bent to its first sign of resistance ("bind") without force. One side is compared to the other. Normal range is thought to be approximately 45°.

- The range is compared on each side, and palpation (drag, for example) identifies the shortened fibers.

- The same procedure may be carried out in a supine position, with the ear being approximated to the shoulder during side-flexion.

5.19B

Time suggested **5–7 minutes**

- To test upper trapezius on the right side, your palpation partner should lie supine, initially with the neck fully (but not forcefully) rotated to the left.

- In order to evaluate the posterior fibers of upper trapezius, your left hand should support the upper neck/occipital area while your right hand, palm upward, rests so that the ulnar border lies against the right side of the neck.

- Your finger pads should be palpating the posterior fibers of upper trapezius, as you slowly side-flex it to the left, until you sense the *first sign of "bind"* with your finger pads or resistance with your hand which is supporting and transporting the head.

- You should now stabilize the head in this degree of side-flexion and rotation, with your right hand, and cross your left hand over to cup the shoulder (Fig. 5.27).

- Assess the ease with which the shoulder can be depressed (moved caudally), while the head and neck are held at their side-flexed and rotated barrier.

- There should be an easy "springiness" as you push the shoulder toward the feet, with a soft end-feel to the movement.

- Repeat this several times.

- If when "springing" the shoulder, there is a hard, wooden end-feel, those fibers of upper trapezius involved in the test are confirmed as shortened.

- This same evaluation should be performed with the head fully rotated away from the side being assessed (for upper trapezius posterior fibers), half turned away from the side being assessed (for upper trapezius medial fibers), and slightly turned toward the side being assessed (for upper trapezius anterior fibers), in order to respectively test for relative shortness, and functional efficiency, of the various subdivisions of the upper portion of trapezius.

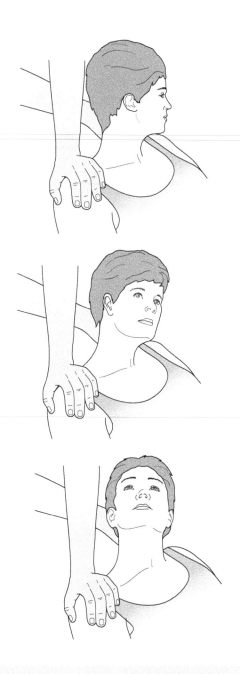

Figure 5.27
Assessment of shortness in upper trapezius. The three head positions relate to posterior fibers (head fully rotated and side flexed); middle fibers (head half rotated and side-flexed); anterior fibers, side-flexed and turned slightly toward side being assessed.

- When introducing side-flexion when assessing medial and anterior fibers, the respective parts of the muscle should be palpated in a similar way to that described above, palm up or down according to comfort.

Can you identify the barriers of resistance simultaneously, with the transporting hand, and the contacts feeling for bind?

Do the different assessments in this exercise confirm each other?

Which fibers are shortened based on these palpation tests?

Additional palpation exercises

Spend some time comparing the results of muscle tests, as described above, with the finding you made when searching for trigger points and other reflex activity.

- Are muscles that house such points consistently short on testing?

- Usually or only sometimes?

Begin the final exercises in this chapter with you and your partner repeating the assessments of postural muscles as described above, noting on a chart those found to be shortened. Results should then be compared with findings obtained after practicing basic spinal NMT (or abdominal NMT) assessment, in which there is charting of all areas, points, zones of soft tissue dysfunction (that palpate as abnormal, indurated, contracted, as well as sensitive).

Also practice Nimmo's assessment sequence as described in Box 5.2.

Greenman (1989) has described a pattern of palpation of muscle in the spinal region that is worth repeating, many times, until the tissues he asks you to feel for are indeed clearly identified. The following is a summary of part of his *"palpation prescription"* for this region, that commences with superficial palpation, similar to the palpation work described in Chapter 4.

Palpation skill status

In this chapter you have been exposed to a variety of approaches, all of which can be useful for uncovering evidence of functional integrity or dysfunctional adaptation, adding to the skills acquired in the previous chapter.

● If you have successfully completed the exercises in this chapter you should now be comfortably able to evaluate for muscle shortness in appropriate (postural) muscles, as well as being able to identify localized changes in these.

As has been established, structure and function are intertwined to a degree that makes them inseparable in reality. Just as we can use structural analysis and palpation to predict what functional changes are likely, so can we evaluate function to guide us towards what structural changes are probable. This was made clear in the functional assessments described in Exercises 5.13, 5.14, and 5.15.

In the next chapter, the methods used are no longer looking for structural change alone, but are concerned with altered function that accompanies altered structure.

Some of the methods described are subtle, others less so. All are of proven value if you have the patience to develop the sensitivity of touch needed to read the evidence waiting to be recognized.

Next

Refer back to Special topic 6 for a discussion on how to differentiate between muscular and a joint problems.

In Chapter 6, Tom Myers directs attention to palpation of fascia.

References

Ashina S, Bendtsen L and Ashina M (2005) Pathophysiology of tension-type headache. Current Pain and Headache Reports 9: 415–422.

Baldry P (1993) Acupuncture, trigger points and musculoskeletal pain. Edinburgh: Churchill Livingstone.

Beal M (1983) Palpatory testing for somatic dysfunction in patients with cardiovascular disease. Journal of the American Osteopathic Association 82: 822–831.

Becker R (1963) Diagnostic touch (part 1). Newark, OH: Yearbook of the Academy of Applied Osteopathy.

Becker R (1964) Diagnostic touch (part 2). Newark, OH: Yearbook of the Academy of Applied Osteopathy.

Becker R (1965) Diagnostic touch (part 3). Newark, OH: Yearbook of the Academy of Applied Osteopathy.

Braggins S (2000) Back care: A clinical approach. Edinburgh: Churchill Livingstone.

Chaitow L (1988) Soft tissue manipulation. Wellingborough: Thorsons.

Chaitow L (1991) Soft tissue manipulation. Rochester, MA: Inner Traditions.

Chaitow L (2001) Muscle energy techniques, 2nd edn. Edinburgh: Churchill Livingstone.

Chaitow L (2002) Modern neuromuscular techniques, 2nd edn. Edinburgh: Churchill Livingstone.

Chaitow L (2006) Muscle energy techniques, 3rd edn. Edinburgh: Churchill Livingstone.

Chaitow L (2007) Positional release techniques, 3rd edn. Edinburgh: Churchill Livingstone.

Chaitow L and DeLany J (2000) Clinical applications of neuromuscular technique (upper body). Edinburgh: Churchill Livingstone.

Chaitow L and DeLany J (2002) Clinical applications of neuromuscular technique (lower body). Edinburgh: Churchill Livingstone.

Chaitow L and DeLany J (2008) Clinical applications of neuromuscular technique (upper body), 2nd edn. Edinburgh: Churchill Livingstone.

Couppé C, Torelli P, Fuglsang-Frederiksen A et al. (2007) Myofascial trigger points are very prevalent in patients with chronic tension-type headache: A double-blinded controlled study. Clinical Journal of Pain 23: 23–27.

Chapter 5

Dvorak J and Dvorak V (1984) Manual medicine: Diagnostics. New York: Georg Thieme.

Frymann V (1963) Palpation – its study in the workshop. Newark, OH: Yearbook of the Academy of Applied Osteopathy, pp. 16–30.

Goodridge J (1981) MET, definition, explanation, methods of procedure. Journal of the American Osteopathic Association 81 (4): 249.

Greenman P (1989) Principles of manual medicine. Baltimore: Williams and Wilkins.

Higham T and Biewener A (2011) Functional and architectural complexity within and between muscles. Biological Sciences 366: 1477–1487.

Hoover H (1969) Method for teaching functional technique. Newark, OH: Yearbook of the Academy of Applied Osteopathy.

Janda V (1978) Muscles, central nervous motor regulation, and back problems, in Korr IM (ed) Neurobiologic Mechanisms in Manipulative Therapy. New York: Plenum.

Janda V (1983) Muscle function testing. London: Butterworths.

Jones L (1981) Strain/counterstrain. Colorado Springs: Academy of Applied Osteopathy.

Kendall H, Kendall F and Boynton D (1952) Posture and pain. Baltimore: Williams and Wilkins.

Kline CM (2011) Fascial manipulation, part I. Journal of the American Chiropractic Association 48 (3): 2–5.

Korr I (1976) Proprioceptors and somatic dysfunction. Newark, OH: Yearbook of the Academy of Applied Osteopathy.

Kuchera W (1997) Lumbar and abdominal region, in Ward R (ed) Foundations for osteopathic medicine. Baltimore: Williams and Wilkins.

Kuchera M, Bemben MG, Kuchera WF and Piper F (1990) Athletic functional demand and posture. Journal of the American Osteopathic Association 90 (9): 843–844.

Le Moal M (2007) Historical approach and evolution of the stress concept: A personal account. Psychoneuroendocrinology 32: S3–S9.

Lewit K (1992) Manipulative therapy in rehabilitation of the locomotor system, 2nd edn. London: Butterworths.

Lewit K (1999) Manipulative therapy in rehabilitation of the locomotor system, 3rd edn. London: Butterworths.

Lewit K (2009) Manipulative therapy: Musculoskeletal medicine. Edinburgh: Churchill Livingstone.

Liebenson C (1996) Rehabilitation of the spine. Baltimore: Williams and Wilkins.

Liebenson C (2006) Rehabilitation of the spine, 2nd edn. Baltimore: Williams and Wilkins.

Lowe W (2006) Orthopedic assessment in massage therapy. Sisters, OR: Daviau Scott.

McEwen B and Wingfield J (2010) What's in a name? Integrating homeostasis allostasis and stress. Hormones and Behavior 57 (2): 105.

McFarlane Tilley R (1961) Spinal stress palpation. Newark, OH: Yearbook of the Academy of Applied Osteopathy.

McPartland J and Goodridge J (1997) Osteopathic examination of the cervical spine. Journal of Bodywork and Movement Therapies 1 (3): 173–178.

Magoun H (1948) Osteopathic diagnosis and therapy for the general practitioner. Journal of the American Osteopathic Association December.

Masi A and Hannon J (2008) Human resting muscle tone (HRMT): Narrative introduction and modern concepts. Journal of Bodywork and Movement Therapies 12 (4): 320–332.

Mense S (2008) Muscle pain: Mechanisms and clinical significance. Deutsches Ärzteblatt International 105: 214–219.

Mense S and Simons D (2001) Muscle pain. Philadelphia: Lippincott, Williams and Wilkins.

Murphy D (2000) Conservative management of cervical spine syndromes. New York: McGraw-Hill.

Ng J, Richardson C, Kippers V et al. (1998) Relationship between muscle fibre composition and functional capacity of back muscles in healthy subjects and patients with back pain. Journal of Orthopaedic and Sports Physical Therapy 27: 389–402.

Nimmo R (1966) Workshop. London: British College of Naturopathy and Osteopathy.

Norris C (1998) Sports injuries, diagnosis and management, 2nd edn. London: Butterworths.

Pavan O, Stecco A, Stern R and Stecco C (2014) Painful connections: Densification versus fibrosis of fascia. Current Pain and Headache Reports 18: 441.

Rolf I (1962) Structural dynamics. Newark, OH: British Academy of Osteopathy Yearbook.

Rosero HO, Greene CH and DeBias DA (1987) Correlation of palpatory observations with the anatomic locus of acute myocardial infarction. Journal of the American Osteopathic Association 87: 118–122.

Seffinger M and Hruby R (2008) Evidence-based manual medicine. Philadelphia: Saunders.

Selye H (1984) The stress of life. New York: McGraw-Hill.

Simons DG (2008) New views of myofascial trigger points: Etiology and diagnosis. Archives of Physical Medicine and Rehabilitation 89 (1): 157–159.

Simons D and Mense S (1998) Understanding and measurement of muscle tone as related to clinical muscle pain. Pain 75: 1–17.

Simons D, Travell J and Simons L (1999) Myofascial pain and dysfunction: The trigger point manual, vol 1, upper half of body, 2nd edn. Baltimore: Williams and Wilkins.

Smith F (1986) Inner bridges: A guide to energy movement and body structure. New York: Humanics New Age.

Snider K, Schneider RP, Snider EJ et al. (2016) Correlation of somatic dysfunction with gastrointestinal endoscopic findings: An observational study. Journal of the American Osteopathic Association 116 (6): 358–369.

Thomson H and Francis D (1977) Abdominal wall tenderness: A useful sign in the acute abdomen. Lancet 1: 1053.

Travell J and Simons D (1992) Myofascial pain and dysfunction – the trigger point manual. Baltimore: Williams and Wilkins.

Upledger J (1987) Craniosacral therapy. Seattle: Eastland Press.

Walther D (1988) Applied kinesiology. Pueblo, CA: SDC Systems.

Ward R (ed) (1997) Foundations for osteopathic medicine. Baltimore: Williams and Wilkins.

Weppler CH and Magnusson SP (2010) Increasing muscle extensibility: A matter of increasing length or modifying sensation? Physical Therapy 90 (3): 438–449.

Woolbright J (1991) An alternative method of teaching strain/counterstrain manipulation. Journal of the American Osteopathic Association 91 (4): 370–376.

Some form of connective tissue matrix is everywhere within the body except the open lumens of the respiratory and digestive tubing, so we cannot palpate anywhere without contacting at least some corner of this unitary body-wide network (Myers 2014). The same is true of the neural, circulatory, and epithelial syncitia as well – every touch affects multiple types of tissue. With this caveat, that no tissue can be truly isolated or separated, this chapter points to some salient and prominent fascial or connective tissue features within this overall net. Our exploration here is limited to identifiable structures within the parietal myofasciae of the locomotor system – as opposed to the organic ligaments or meninges within the dorsal and ventral cavities. These structures are mapped here in terms of the myofasial meridians known as the *Anatomy Trains* (Myers 2014).

Before we begin this systematic process, a word about fascial layering. Although the fascial net takes its first form around the end of the second week of embryonic development as a single three-dimensional cobweb of fine reticular fibers and gels surrounding and investing the entire simple trilaminar embryo, the subsequent origami of embryonic development folds the original fascial netting into recognizable layers (Schultz 1996):

- In the mature phenotype (that would be us), picking up the skin anywhere in the body brings with it the first layer of fascial sheeting, the dermis, the backing for our carpet of skin, a layer so elastic it will move in any direction, and so tough that it resists entry to anything blunter than a sharpened blade.

- Although we note that each of these layers is incompletely separate from its neighbors as each layer is always connected to the next by variable fuzzy or gluey connections, the next identifiable layer is known as the areolar or adipose layer. This fascinating system (for it exists in most places in the body that must slide, and thus merits consideration as part of the articular system) is filled with a mixture of cells, including white blood cells and various types of fibroblasts, suspended in viscous proteoglycans that shift and change their connections easily in response to shifting forces,

including rotating acupuncture needles (Guimberteau and Armstrong 2015; Langevin et al. 2004, 2006).

- Below the areolar layer is the deep investing fascia, "fascia profundis," which forms a "unitard" around the musculoskeletal system. This very resilient fabric, given different regional names such as the crural fascia in the leg and the fascia lata in the thigh, etc., is again actually one systemic layer that holds our inner shape, and provides a leathery protection and orientation layer that neither the elastic dermis nor the soft areolar layer can provide.

- Around each muscle we can find a thin but tough epimysial layer, with smaller organizing perimysial and endomysial layers surrounding smaller bundles of muscles. In between groups of muscles, we find the tough but malleable intermuscular septa, which will feature in our palpations, since binding or shortening in these walls have definite structural and functional consequences. Continuous with these septa, but close to the bone under the deepest musculature, we find the periosteum as a cling wrap coating around the bone continuous with the joint-surrounding ligaments, and finally the bone, which is itself a connective tissue.

The arrangement of these layers, of course, differs from place to place, but the general order of the layers from superficial to deep applies. Since the front of your thigh is probably available to you just under this book, let us use that area as a place to palpate these layers (Fig. 6.1).

- Pick up the skin and roll it between your thumb and forefinger. You can feel the elastic layer on the back of the skin that holds the delicate skin cells together (see Chapter 4).

- Slide the skin back and forth to feel the easy gliding of the areolar layer on the layers underneath. No matter what direction you slide the skin, the areolar layer will allow a certain amount of sliding – a few centimeters – before the movement is checked. Move your exploring fingers down to the front of your tibia and try to lift the skin off this bone to see how limited the movement becomes when the areolar layer is very thin, as it is over this bone (see Chapter 4).

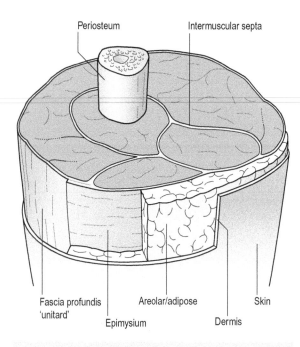

Periosteum   Intermuscular septa

Fascia profundis 'unitard'   Areolar/adipose   Skin

Epimysium   Dermis

Figure 6.1
Typical fascial layering, seen here in the thigh. Other areas contain more or fewer layers between skin and bone.

- Extend your knee to tighten the muscle under your fingers; the investing layer is like a thin but strong leotard between the loose, slippery superficial fascia and the muscle.

The density of the fascia within the muscle varies with your age, nutrition, genetics, and most of all with your training, but muscle cells themselves are very *gloopy* and surprisingly liquid when relaxed, as evidenced in dissection of untreated tissue, so it is the fascia (along with turgor and neurological tone) that is giving your leg its feeling of organized structure.

- Slide your fingers to the lateral part of your thigh to feel the iliotibial tract (ITT) as a distinct fascial sheet running down the outside of the thigh. Although this is not strictly an intermuscular septum (and we will be introducing others as we move through the body), it

will serve as an example of a similar heavy fascial sheet, albeit one that is easily accessible from the surface.

- You may also be able to feel the difference between the superficial muscle on the front of your thigh – the rectus femoris – and the denser, deeper muscle beneath it, the vastus intermedius. Between these two is another fascial plane, also an intermuscular septum, so that the "sausage" of the rectus femoris can be slid back and forth over the vasti.

The periosteum is very difficult to feel as a separate layer, as it is largely adjacent and often adherent to the bone, although you feel it very distinctly when you hit your shin on a stair, since the periosteum is very well innervated – and therefore more sharply painful when injured than either bone itself or muscle (see Chapter 5 for discussion of periosteal pain points).

- Palpation of the bone itself is most easily done, of course, where the bone emerges near the surface – at the patella or shin bone in your leg.

Under the presumption that muscles and bones are well-covered elsewhere in this volume (see Chapters 5 and 8), let us proceed to some of the salient connective tissue structures we can feel within the unity of the body's fascial system.

This series of explorations is arranged longitudinally, so that the front of the lower leg will be presented along with the front of the thigh and trunk, the side of the lower leg along with the rest of the side of the body, the calf with the hamstrings and the rest of the back, etc.

This will be frustrating to the reader who wants all the palpations for the lower leg gathered in one place, but this longitudinal approach has logic in terms of how these fascial structures relate to each other in real human functioning and stability. Labeling of each section will assist the reader who wants to quickly gather in the palpation guides for a given region.

Much more complete information on each of the myofascial meridians named below is given in the *Anatomy Trains* book (Myers 2014), supporting videos, and website: www.AnatomyTrains.com.

Exercise 6.1 *Palpation of the Superficial Front Line (Figure 6.2)*

Time suggested **20 minutes**

Foot and lower leg

- With your model supine, use one hand to hold the toes down into flexion while the model lifts them up and extends against your pressure.

- The other hand can explore the tendons of both the short and long toe extensors, which jump up through the thin skin of the dorsal surface of the foot as soon as the muscles are contracted.

- The short extensors angle off toward the lateral aspect of the foot; the long toe extensors pass under our first port of call, the extensor retinaculae.

- The most prominent tendon on the medial side is that of the tibialis anterior.

In anatomy atlases, the extensor retinaculae are distinct structures, looking like gauze bandages over the tendons. In reality, those sharp distinctions are made by the dissector's scalpel, while to the therapist's palpating hand, they are widely variable in both their thickness and their extent up the shin and down the foot.

- Keeping the muscles tight by having the model continue to extend her toes and dorsiflex against your resistance, pass your lightly touching fingers up those tendons where they cross the ankle to feel the retinaculae between these tendons and the skin.

- Depending on your model, they may be almost impossible to feel as distinct structures, or you may be able to feel the upper and lower sections as distinctly as they are often portrayed in the books.

- In any case, please note that the retinaculae are not really separate structures in themselves, but thickenings of the crural fascia that surrounds the whole lower leg like a support stocking.

Bony stations		Myofascial tracks
	15	Scalp fascia
Mastoid process	14	
	13	Sternocleidomastoid
Sternal manubrium	12	
	11	Sternalis/sternochondral fascia
Fifth rib	10	
	9	Rectus abdominis
Pubic tubercle	8	
Anterior inferior iliac spine	7	
	6	Rectus femoris/quadriceps
Patella	5	
	4	Subpatellar tendon
Tibial tuberosity	3	
	2	Short and long toe extensors, tibialis anterior, anterior crural compartment
Dorsal surfaces of toe phalanges	1	

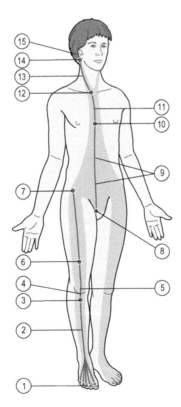

Figure 6.2
The Superficial Front Line.

149

Exercise 6.1 *continued*

- Move up onto the front of the shin and move the skin over the flat surface of the tibia. How much does it move over the bone?

- This can vary from model to model. Can you feel the distinct layer of deep investing fascia (crural fascia) between the easily moving skin and the immoveable bone?

- This investing layer can be "opened" or "moved" on the bone, and usually, in our experience, wants lifting cranially for best results.

Thigh

At the knee, you will find the subpatellar tendon just between the tibial tuberosity and the kneecap.

- Have your model extend her knee to bring this tendon (or ligament, depending on your preference) into sharp relief.

- This tendon on the sagittal midline is the strongest element within a complex "bridle" that attaches the patella to the knee joint and the tibial plateau.

- Have your model keep her knee extended while you explore the area below and on either side of the patella; see if you can feel some of the restraining bands within this "bridle."

- Again, they vary widely in their thickness and arrangement depending on use, but the practicing athlete will usually show palpable lines of thickening within this complex.

- Have the model relax the knee extension to feel the connections of the four quadriceps into the superior side of the patella. These strong fascial connections are obviously extensions of the muscles.

To the lateral side, one can sometimes feel the anterior edge of the iliotibial tract (ITT) covering the vastus lateralis, but we will take this structure up when we palpate the Lateral Line. On the medial side, the sartorius covers the medial intermuscular septum we will take up when we palpate the Deep Front Line.

- At the top of the thigh, find the anterior superior iliac spine (ASIS).

- Four distal structures come from below into this nexus of forces: the tensor fasciae latae (TFL), the rectus femoris, the sartorius, and the inguinal ligament.

- The TFL attachment is palpable just lateral and inferior to the ASIS if you have your model strongly medially rotate her leg.

- The sartorius attachment is palpable just medial and inferior to the ASIS, most easily palpable when the model laterally rotates her leg and lifts against the resistance you supply with your other hand.

- The rectus femoris is listed as going to the anterior inferior iliac spine (AIIS), so in between the two muscles discussed above, you will find the rectus femoris tendon, often in a little "pocket" between sartorius and TFL, diving into the body toward the AIIS.

In a certain percentage of people, though, there will be a fascial extension of the rectus femoris up to the ASIS, known affectionately in our school as the "Morrison ligament," after its discoverer.

- The inguinal ligament (which is misnamed – it is really the free but rolled up end of the layers of abdominal fasciae and not really a ligament) runs in a straight line from the pubic tubercle on the side of the pubic bone up to the ASIS.

- It can be palpated as a string you can gently strum about 1 cm (1/2 inch) above the fold between the leg and the trunk.

- Take care not to press hard on the neurovascular bundle that passes under this ligament between the pectineus and the iliopsoas.

The abdomen

The intrepid palpator can find the round lower attachments of the rectus abdominis on the superior side of the pubic bone.

- As this is generally a touchy area for your model, it is suggested that you have your supine model flex her knees fully, and then gently drop your fingers into the belly of your model halfway between the pubic bone and the navel, pushing past any accumulated fat well into the abdominal cavity.

- This should not be painful, and is contraindicated if it is.

Exercise 6.1 *continued*

- Then turn your fingertips down toward the pubic bone and resting there, let the model bring the pubic bone to your fingertips, by pushing on her feet and rolling the pelvis into a posterior tilt, rather than you pressing down toward the pubic bone with your own power.

- A model with a full bladder is a definite disadvantage in this palpation, and be sure to let the model bring their pubic bone to you, rather than pushing your way to the bone.

- Do not palpate heavily on the lateral side of the pubic tubercles, as there is a weakness in the fascial walls here, especially for the male of the species, and over-working here could predispose toward an inguinal hernia.

Once found, these lower attachments of the rectus are surprisingly round and spaced a couple of centimeters apart. In between lies the small but important adjustor of the pyramidalis muscle. Just lateral to the rectus is the lateral edge of the rectus sheath.

The rectus abdominis arranges itself as a series of muscles, separated by tendinous inscriptions readily felt in the athlete, or Pilates devotee, as the familiar element in "six-pack abs."

More importantly, the rectus is wrapped in a sheath of fascia that is continuous with the other abdominal sheets of muscle. Where the rectus sheath meets these other muscles, just lateral to the muscle, is a very important fascial raphe for abdominal tone and stability.

- To feel this fascial structure, explore along the edge of the rectus abdominis, which widens as it rises toward the ribs.

- The fascial raphe (or semilunar line) is just between the medial edge of the obliques and transversus and the lateral edge of the rectus, and extends from the pubic bone all the way up and out to the subcostal arch.

- This fascial "crossroads" among the four abdominal muscles has connections into the diaphragm, as well as onto the ribs, and constitutes part of the Front Functional Line, as well as this Superficial Front Line.

The anterior rib cage

Above the costal arch at the level of the 5th rib, you can feel a distinct horizontal fascial band between the top of the rectus and the lower edge of the pectoralis major, essentially along the "bra line." This "strap," which has no name in the atlases but is commonly called the "Schultz band" after its describer, the late Dr Louis Schultz, is very important when too short or bound, in restricting breathing, upward movement of the chest, and free movement of the arms.

- Despite its power to limit movement, this band is fairly superficial, and can usually be moved up and down over the underlying sternum and ribs.

- It invites widening and lifting to loosen its grip on the model's movement.

- The sternal fascia – actually a portion of the deep investing "leotard" of pectoral fascia – can be moved on the sternum, and additional fascial build-up can often be felt on the raised structures of the knuckle-like sternochondral joints on either side of the sternal "valley" at the midline.

The neck

The sternocleidomastoid (SCM) will be familiar to most palpators, easily seen and palpated by having the model turn her head to the side and lift it ceilingward against your resistance.

- The fascial element of this palpation comes at the superior end of the muscle.

- The muscle tissue itself ends at the mastoid process, but its fascial extension can be felt another inch or two (3–5 cm) up toward the asterion (where the parietal, temporal, and occipital bones meet, and a strong attachment point for the tentorium cerebelli on the inside). The asterion itself can be felt as a fingertip-sized dimple in the flesh approximately 3 cm behind the upper attachment point of the ear.

- Have your model turn her head to the side, place your fingers on and above the mastoid, and have her lift her head to feel this fascia tighten. The clinical point here is that the sternocleidomastoid (and by extension the upper part of the Superficial Front Line) can pull down on and affect the movement of the dural meninges – the tentorium cerebelli in particular.

Exercise 6.2 *Palpation of the Superficial Back Line (Figure 6.3)*

Time suggested **20 minutes**

Foot and lower leg

The front line is complemented by a line running up the back of the body.

- The first and familiar fascial feature within this line is the plantar aponeurosis, readily palpable when it is tightened by extending the toes.

- As wide as all five toes at the ball of the foot, its edges are readily palpable (and sometimes tender) passing back along the sole, narrowing as it goes to the width of only 3/4 inch (2 cm) as it blends into the periosteum at the front of the heel.

- A branch of this fascia, the lateral band, can be felt between the outer, lower edge of the calcaneus and the prominent base of the 5th metatarsal bone.

- This fascia is a major stabilizer of the lateral arch, and is recommended for treatment in both pronated and supinated feet.

The plantar fascia blends into a "bridle" of fascial fabric around the heel that continues into the Achilles tendon. These are not usually shown as joined, but we have dissected this connection many times.

- Follow this tendon up the calf to feel how thin it becomes as it spreads wide over the posterior surface of the soleus.

- At the popliteal fossa of the knee, there is a fascial connection between the heads of the gastrocnemius and the hamstring tendons linking around them.

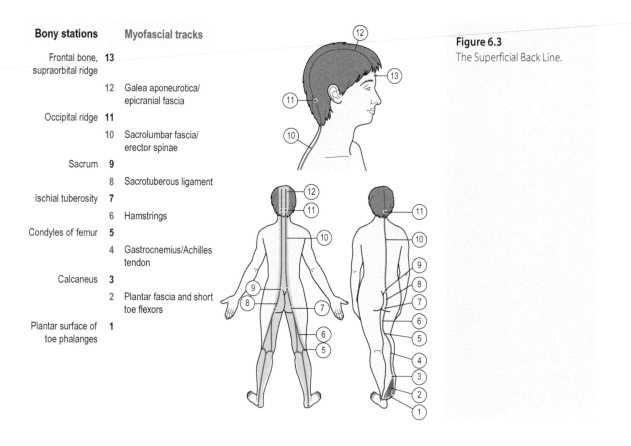

Bony stations	Myofascial tracks
Frontal bone, **13** supraorbital ridge	
	12 Galea aponeurotica/ epicranial fascia
Occipital ridge **11**	
	10 Sacrolumbar fascia/ erector spinae
Sacrum **9**	
	8 Sacrotuberous ligament
Ischial tuberosity **7**	
	6 Hamstrings
Condyles of femur **5**	
	4 Gastrocnemius/Achilles tendon
Calcaneus **3**	
	2 Plantar fascia and short toe flexors
Plantar surface of **1** toe phalanges	

Figure 6.3
The Superficial Back Line.

Exercise 6.2 *continued*

Thigh

At their distal end, the division between the medial and lateral hamstrings is clear.

● Palpate superiorly from here and see how far up toward the ischial tuberosity the hamstrings can be easily separated.

● In runners, the medial and lateral hamstrings can be bound fascially together so that they cannot be separated more than a few inches above the knee.

● This limits the differential movement between these two, which is required in football, say, or skiing.

● With your model prone and knee flexed to 90°, put your fingertips in this septum between the hamstrings, and have them rotate the lower leg strongly medially and laterally – you will feel the inner "semis" and the lateral biceps working alternately as the lower leg rotates, making it easy to find the fascial "valley" in between.

● How easily can you sink toward the femur and how far superior can the separation between medial and lateral hamstrings be detected?

● At their proximal end, notice how the hamstrings are attached to the posterior (not the inferior) surface of the ischial tuberosity, "touching down" on the back of the bone as the fascia continues into the sacrotuberous ligament.

Pelvis

● At the upper end of the hamstrings, you can track the fascial continuity onto the sacrotuberous ligament, a tough, almost bony-feeling strip between the ischial tuberosity along the medial edge of the gluteus maximus to the lower edge of the sacrum.

● The sacral and thoracolumbar fascia (TLF) is a vast expanse of many fascial layers laid over the sacrum and lumbars in a diamond shape. Palpation with a skeleton nearby will impress the reader with how much soft-tissue (largely collagenous, but including the sacral multifidus) lies between the skin and the sacrum. The TLF includes the aponeurosis of the latissimus dorsi and abdominal muscles, but for the Superficial Back Line provides the "sausage casing" for the entire erector spine group.

Back

The erector spinae fill in the space between the spinous processes and the angle of the ribs.

● Between the lower ribs and the posterior iliac crest, on the outer edge of the iliocostalis lumborum, you can find the lateral raphe, a fascial band that complements the band running along the outside of the rectus abdominis in front.

● This thick fascial structure lies at the confluence of the erector fascia, the posterior limit of the abdominal fascia, and near the outer edge of the quadratus lumborum, for which it is often mistaken.

Head

Though the erector spinae are quite densely fascial, as muscles go, the next directly fascial structure on the Superficial Back Line is the epicranial fascia that traverses the head from the nuchal line to the brow ridge.

● If the person carries a head-forward posture, the epicranial fascia thickens over the occipital and occasionally even the parietal bones in response to the changing angle of pull from the erectors.

● The back of the skull is relatively smooth.

● If you can feel bumps, waves, or furrows as you palpate beneath the hair on the back of the head, this is the thickening and extra fibrous tissue in the epicranial fascia.

● Part of setting the head back up on top of the body is to ease this fascia out and down, until the skull feels smooth once again.

Exercise 6.3 *Palpation of the Lateral Line (Figure 6.4)*

Time suggested **20 minutes**

Foot and lower leg

Turning to the fascial continuity running up the side of the body, we can palpate the tendons of fibularis longus and brevis (peroneals) just inferior to the fibular malleolus. The fibularii run up the side of the lower leg to the lateral side of the fibula.

● If you have your model point her toes (strongly plantarflex), these dense muscles will be readily palpable between the bulge of the soleus and the tibialis anterior.

Exercise 6.3 *continued*

On either side of these muscles are intermuscular septa that divide this lateral compartment from its neighbors. These compartment walls are well connected to the crural fascia that surrounds the lower leg, and are often shortened and tight in compartment syndrome. Relief of compartment syndrome symptoms will often result from deep release work on the crural fascia over the fibularii, as well as work into these intercompartmental septa.

- The anterior septum, between the tibialis anterior and the peroneals, can be found by palpating up from the fibular malleolus, tracking the small "valley" between these muscles, ending just in front of the fibular head. Having your model dorsiflex and plantarflex contracts these two muscles sequentially, making the palpation of the wall between them easier.

- The posterior septum can be tracked by starting in the space between the Achilles tendon and the back of

the ankle, running in front of the soleus up the posterior edge of the fibula and ending just behind the fibular head.

- In the ideal, these "valleys" should be easily accessed down to the fibula; in many cases, however, they are so bound that differential movement or any valley at all is difficult to feel.

- This is an indication for spreading work to open the valleys.

Thigh and pelvis

The iliotibial tract is a well-known fascial structure of the thigh, comprising a strong band of vertical fibers that interweave with the fascia lata that surrounds the thigh (continuous with the crural fascia below via the anterior ligament of the head of the fibula at the anterior superior aspect of the head of the fibula).

The iliotibial tract runs from a strong, rounded, tendon-like structure easily felt just above the knee on the lateral side, which widens as it passes up the thigh and over

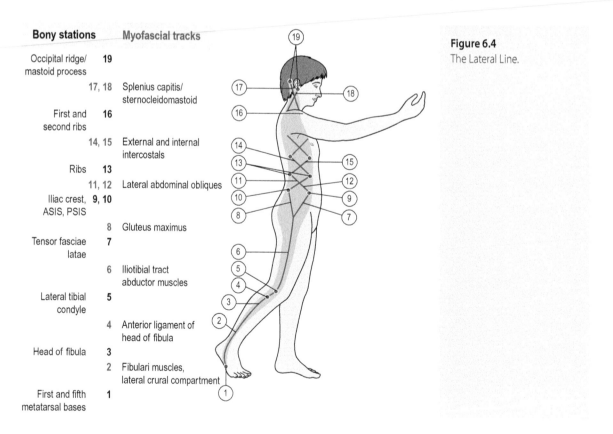

Bony stations		Myofascial tracks
Occipital ridge/ mastoid process	**19**	
	17, 18	Splenius capitis/ sternocleidomastoid
First and second ribs	**16**	
	14, 15	External and internal intercostals
Ribs	**13**	
	11, 12	Lateral abdominal obliques
Iliac crest, ASIS, PSIS	**9, 10**	
	8	Gluteus maximus
Tensor fasciae latae	**7**	
	6	Iliotibial tract abductor muscles
Lateral tibial condyle	**5**	
	4	Anterior ligament of head of fibula
Head of fibula	**3**	
	2	Fibulari muscles, lateral crural compartment
First and fifth metatarsal bases	**1**	

Figure 6.4
The Lateral Line.

Exercise 6.3 *continued*

the greater trochanter to join with the gluteus maximus, medius, and tensor fasciae latae muscles. Between the tensor and the medius, a heavy fascial extension of the iliotibial tract can be felt running up to the coronal midpoint of the iliac crest.

This structure should be strong and tight, as it is an essential support for transfer of weight from the pelvis to the femur, although excess tightness can restrict ab- and adduction movements at the hip. The tract fades into the fascia lata anteriorly, but thickens posteriorly to create the lateral intermuscular septum between the vastus lateralis and the biceps femoris.

- To palpate and assess the iliotibial tract, lay your hand along the thigh of your side-lying model, fingers pointing down the thigh to the knee.

- Where is the iliotibial band the tightest – in the front, in the middle, or on the posterior edge?

- In most people, the back edge feels thicker and tighter, but with practice, you can assess whether the anterior or middle part of the band is carrying an excess of tension by comparison.

- Shortness in the anterior part of the band often accompanies an anterior tilt of the pelvis, while excess shortness in the posterior part accompanies a posterior tilt or an anterior shift.

- Once assessed, you can adjust your work to emphasize the part most in need of attention.

Trunk

The Lateral Line passes up the trunk in a series of muscular "X"s formed by the lateral abdominal obliques and intercostal muscles. Palpation of these is covered in Chapter 5. A deeper structure with more fascial volume is the fascia running parallel to the outer edge of the quadratus lumborum, the lateral raphe.

- To find this fascia, which runs from the lateral iliac crest to the outer end of the 12th rib, hook your finger onto the inside edge of the iliac crest of your side-lying model.

- "Walk" your fingers back along the inside of the iliac crest from the ASIS toward the back. At the lateral midline or

just posterior, you will find a sharpish edge of a fascial band that sweeps up and medial toward the 12th rib (which is quite variable in length).

- This fascia is frequently short in lordotic or compressed lumbar patterns, and its release is a central part of relieving such patterns.

Neck

Although the sternocleidomastoid (SCM) and splenius muscles form the neck portion of the Lateral Line, and are readily palpable when your side-lying model lifts her head and rotates it, a deeper and more fascial part of this line is the underlying "skirt" of the scalenes.

- Readily palpable as a hard group behind the trailing edge of the SCM, these muscles act as a "quadratus lumborum of the neck" in controlling side-to-side movement of the head on the trunk.

- They are also secondary breathing muscles, supporting the ribs and lungs from above.

- Unfortunately, they can also serve to pull the lower cervicals into flexion, "turtling" the neck into the torso.

An unusual but effective access to the scalene fascia can be made via the axilla.

- With your model side-lying, with no pillow, and with you standing behind her shoulders, pick up her head and sidebend it toward you (away from the table).

- Lay your other hand comfortably in her axilla, fingers pointing toward her head.

- Slide your fingers into the axillary space, parallel to the ribs, letting her shoulder fall upward toward the head to allow you access to the highest ribs possible without discomfort. Her ear and shoulder are by now close or touching.

- Press your fingerpads gently but firmly down toward the ribs, and then slowly lower her head down toward the table. Have her lift her head off your hands to feel the fascial sheet that is the extension of the scalenes come into sharp relief.

- You will feel the extension of the scalene fascia pulling along under your fingers.

- Repeat with more pressure to turn this palpation into a treatment for shortened scalene fascia.

Palpation of the Spiral Line (Figure 6.5)

The double helix of the Spiral Line winds in and out of all the lines previously and subsequently described. All the fascial features of the Spiral Line are covered elsewhere in this chapter.

Exercise 6.4 *Palpation of the Shoulder and Arm Lines (Figure 6.6)*

Time suggested 10 minutes

Many of the muscles of the shoulders and arms are covered elsewhere in this book, so we will confine ourselves here to a few salient fascial features of the arms.

The Superficial Front Arm Line

The palmar aponeurosis covers the palm of the hand much as the plantar aponeurosis covers the sole of the foot.

It is tightened by the palmaris longus, whose tendon can be palpated and often seen above the flexor retinaculum when the wrist is strongly flexed. Since this muscle is anomalous, it cannot always be found.

When the fingers are extended, the palmar aponeurosis can be felt tightening like the head of a drum. The middle of this aponeurosis can be shortened in the pathology of *Dupuytren's contracture.*

- The flexor retinaculum can be felt just distal to the radiocarpal joint, running from the base of the thenar muscles of the thumb to the base of the hypothenar muscles of the little finger.

- This strong fascial band covers the carpal tunnel, whose flexor tendons can be felt sliding under the skin just proximal to the wrist if you "play piano" with your fingers.

- In those with carpal tunnel syndrome, the retinaculum often presents as too short, creating an excessive "arch" that crowds the carpal tunnel.

- The common flexor tendon can be felt just distal to the medial humeral epicondyle on the inside of the elbow. Just proximal to the epicondyle you can feel the medial intermuscular septum, sometimes presenting as a "bass string" when it is overly tight.

- This septum, which divides the upper arm flexors from extensors and encloses the neuromuscular bundle, runs

up toward the glenohumeral joint with the attachments of the latissimus dorsi and pectoralis major muscles on the medial side of the proximal humerus.

Exercise 6.5 *Palpation of the Superficial Back Arm Line*

Time suggested 5 minutes

- The extensor tendons can be easily felt along the back of the hand.

- The extensor retinaculum is much "lighter" than its counterpart on the flexors, but can nonetheless be detected by sensitive fingers on the back of the wrist.

At the proximal end of the forearm, the common extensor tendon lies just distal to the lateral humeral epicondyle, where it frequently presents with tender spots. Just proximal to the epicondyle is the lateral intermuscular septum, which is a bit thinner and less easily felt than its medial counterpart. This small septum runs between the brachialis and the triceps to the distal end of the deltoid, running deep to a small part of the brachialis that lies over it.

- Within the deltoid, you can feel the multipennate tendons, the largest of these running over the front of the humeral head.

Exercise 6.6 *Palpation of the Deep Front Arm Line*

Time suggested 10 minutes

- The radial collateral ligaments can be felt between the styloid process of the radius and the carpals at the base of the thumb.

- Near the proximal end of the radius, you can find both tendons of the biceps brachii.

- To feel the radial tendon, hold your arm against your belly with your elbow flexed, and put your index finger into the flesh just above the cubital fossa.

- The biceps tendon is an obvious large cord.

- Follow this cord down into the fossa, pronating and supinating the forearm to feel the tendon move around the radius.

Bony stations		Myofascial tracks
Occipital ridge/mastoid process atlas/axis TPs	1	
	2	Splenius capitis
Lower cervical/ upper thoracic SPs	3	
	4	Rhomboids major and minor
Medial border of scapula	5	
	6	Serratus anterior
Lateral ribs	7	
	8	External oblique
	9	Abdominal aponeurosis, linea alba
	10	Internal oblique
Iliac crest/ASIS	11	
	12	Tensor fasciae latae, iliotibial tract
Lateral tibial condyle	13	
	14	Tibialis anterior
First metatarsal	15	
	16	Fibularis longus
Head of fibula	17	
	18	Biceps femoris
Ischial tuberosity	19	

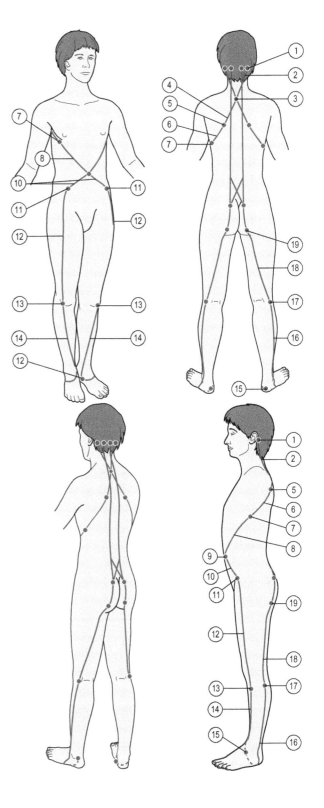

Figure 6.5
The Spiral Line.

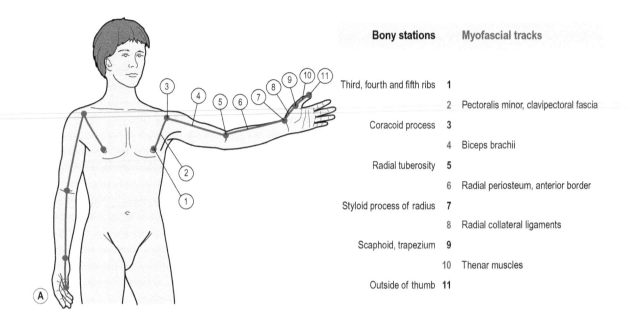

Bony stations		Myofascial tracks
Third, fourth and fifth ribs	1	
	2	Pectoralis minor, clavipectoral fascia
Coracoid process	3	
	4	Biceps brachii
Radial tuberosity	5	
	6	Radial periosteum, anterior border
Styloid process of radius	7	
	8	Radial collateral ligaments
Scaphoid, trapezium	9	
	10	Thenar muscles
Outside of thumb	11	

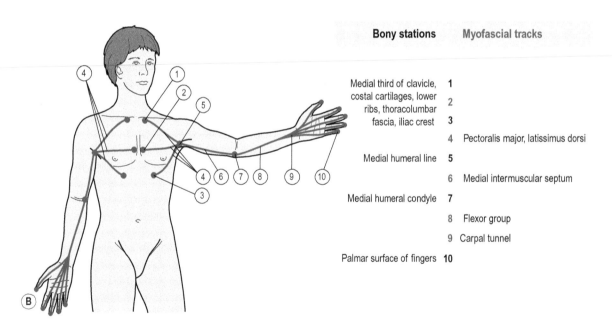

Bony stations		Myofascial tracks
Medial third of clavicle, costal cartilages, lower ribs, thoracolumbar fascia, iliac crest	1	
	2	
	3	
	4	Pectoralis major, latissimus dorsi
Medial humeral line	5	
	6	Medial intermuscular septum
Medial humeral condyle	7	
	8	Flexor group
	9	Carpal tunnel
Palmar surface of fingers	10	

Figure 6.6
The Arm Lines.

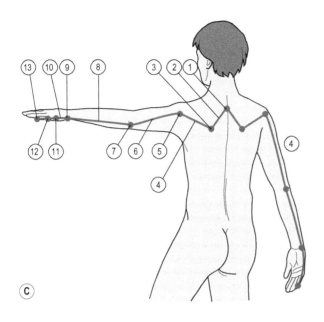

Bony stations		Myofascial tracks
Spinous process of lower cervicals and upper thoracic, C1–C4 TPs	1	
	2	Rhomboids and levator scapulae
Medial border of scapula	3	
	4	Rotator cuff muscles
Head of humerus	5	
	6	Triceps brachii
Olecranon of ulna	7	
	8	Fascia along ulnar periosteum
Styloid process of ulna	9	
	10	Ulnar collateral ligaments
Triquetrum, hamate	11	
	12	Hypothenar muscles
Outside of little finger	13	

C

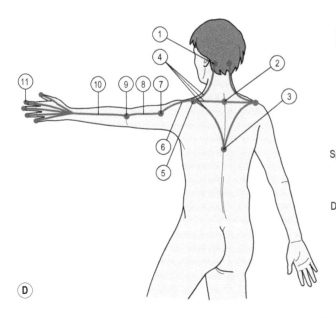

Bony stations		Myofascial tracks
Occipital ridge, nuchal ligament, thoracic spinous processes	1, 2, 3	
	4	Trapezius
Spine of scapula, acromion, lateral third of clavicle	5	
	6	Deltoid
Deltoid tubercle of humerus	7	
	8	Lateral intermuscular septum
Lateral epicondyle of humerus	9	
	10	Extensor group
Dorsal surface of fingers	11	

D

Figure 6.6 (continued)
The Arm Lines.

Exercise 6.6 *continued*

- To find the other lower attachment of the biceps – the bicipital aponeurosis or tendon of Lacertus – laterally rotate the upper arm so your hand is away from your body, but with the elbow still adducted and flexed.

- Run your fingers down the near (medial) side of the tendon to feel the fascia spread and gradually disappear, blending into the myofascia of the flexor group. This is the bicipital aponeurosis, or tendon of Lacertus.

This is a clear example of a "muscle attaching to a muscle," and is used to reduce strain on the elbow when carrying a heavy load.

The short head of the biceps attaches to the coracoid process, which is the distal attachment of the important pectoralis minor. The pectoralis minor lies within a fascial sheet – the clavipectoral fascia – which lies deep to, and is almost as large as, the pectoralis major.

The clavipectoral fascia runs from the clavicle on the superior side to the inner border of the anterior axilla on its inferior edge. It is bilaminar, and includes the subclavius muscle within its layers, as well as the pectoralis minor.

- It can be felt by entering the axilla under the pectoralis major.

- The fascia may present as a tight sheet, or be loose enough so that the pectoralis minor is all that can be distinguished of this fascia.

The subclavius, found on the infraclavicular surface, is a very fascial muscle, acting as an adjustable ligament for the sternoclavicular joint. Just inferior to the subclavius, between it and the shortest head of the pectoralis minor, is a thickening of the clavipectoral fascia named the costocoracoid ligament.

- This band, running from the 2nd rib to the coracoid process, can often be palpated through the overlying pectoralis major as a tougher band of fascia, which can feel like a slip of the pectoralis minor, but if followed, will lead to the coracoid process.

- Each and all of these fasciae can restrict full shoulder movement from the front.

Exercise 6.7 *Palpation of the Deep Back Arm Line*

Time suggested 10 minutes

The ulnar collateral ligaments can be felt between the styloid process of the ulna and the carpals at the base of the little finger.

The fascia running over the ulna connects these ligaments to the olecranon, where the fascial tendon of the triceps can be palpated just proximal to the point of the elbow.

- The tendons of the rotator cuff can be palpated on the back of the humeral head by following the long head of the triceps to the teres minor on the lateral edge of the posterior scapula.

- Walk your fingers out the teres minor (about the size of your little finger and frequently tender) to the posterior aspect of the humeral head.

- Rotating the humerus will reveal where the teres and infraspinatus tendons blend with the glenohumeral joint capsule.

- The tendon of the subscapularis can be palpated by putting the fingers into the axilla with the finger pads facing posteriorly, passing over the latissimus tendon and teres major to the multipennate subscapularis. The tendon can be felt as one slides distally toward the humeral head. Sliding proximally into the so-called "scapulothoracic joint," one can feel the technically "loose areolar" but factually often quite dense cottony layer of fascia between the subscapularis and the serratus anterior, often the cause of disturbed scapulohumeral rhythm.

On the proximal side of the scapula, this line is completed by the rhomboid muscles and the levator scapulae leading to the rectus capitis lateralis. Of fascial interest here is the septum between the rhomboid major and minor, running superiorly and medially from the medial end of the scapular spine, and the ubiquitously sore attachment of the levator scapulae, which, when under eccentric postural strain, can manifest extra attachment fibers to the apex of the scapula.

Exercise 6.8 *Palpation of the Functional Lines (Figure 6.7)*

Time suggested **5 minutes**

The rest of the Arm Line structures, and the myofasciae of the Functional Lines, are covered elsewhere in this chapter or in this book. We note only that in the front, the intrepid palpator can track the fascial connection from the adductor longus tendon on one side, through the pubic symphysis to the fascia on the outside of the rectus abominis on the other – the semilunar fascia already covered in the Superficial Front Line section. This passes into the strong band of fascia on the inferior edge of the pectoralis major.

In the back, the more superficial laminae of the dense and easily palpated diamond of lumbar fascia carry the force from the latissimus dorsi on one side across the sacrolumbar junction to the inferior gluteus maximus on the other. This line carries on from the lower distal end of the gluteus into the vastus lateralis in the thigh, passing diagonally under the vertical iliotibial tract discussed in the section on the Lateral Line.

The Ipsilateral Functional Line presents two additional points of interest: note the strong attachment of the latissimus dorsi to the end of the 10th, 11th, and 12th ribs. The muscle commonly rolls over these attachments, keeping them out of sight and out of mind. These attachments are fascially continuous with the corresponding slips of the external oblique, which lead over the iliac crest and ASIS to the sartorius, which terminates in the fascial complex known as the pes anserinus. Find the pes on the medial side of the upper tibial shift and condyle, adduct and laterally rotate against gravity to feel the confluence of the sartorius, gracilis, and hamstring tendons stabilizing the inside of the knee and reinforcing the medial collateral ligament.

Exercise 6.9 *Palpation of the Deep Front Line (Figure 6.8)*

Time suggested **40 minutes**

The Deep Front Line (or "core" line) runs through the more obscure parts of our anatomy, which makes some of its fascial features difficult to palpate, for biomechanical, client safety (endangerment sites), and social acceptability reasons. The following palpations come with appropriate precautions,

but the general caveat for the less experienced practitioner/ student is to explore these dynamic and important but both literally and figuratively "profound" structures with precision, at a slow and sensitive pace, and in clear communication with your model (and where possible, try them on yourself first).

The lower leg

One can find the distal end of the three tendons that comprise the lower end of this line on the medial side of the ankle.

- When the big toe is actively or passively extended, the flexor hallucis longus tendon can be palpated on the bottom of the foot running parallel to the inner edge of the plantar aponeurosis.

- At the ankle, this tendon can be felt by putting one's thumb or fingertip in the medial space just in front of the Achilles tendon and behind the medial malleolus.

- Be careful of the tibial nerve, but one can feel, when the model flexes and extends the big toe, the tendon moving on the back of the bone where it supports the talus in the medial arch.

- The strong tendon of the tibialis posterior can be felt by putting your fingertip just below the tip of the your model's medial malleolus, and then having her point her toes and invert her foot.

- A substantial tendon will push out at your finger.

- The tendon continues under the foot to many other bones but is too deep to be palpable there.

- The flexor digitorum longus muscle tendon is about 1 cm posterior to the tibialis posterior, but the tendon is small and sometimes hard to find.

The three muscles are palpable only a few inches above the medial side of the ankle before they disappear beneath the bulky soleus. The deep transverse septum, however, that runs behind them, separating these deep muscles of the Deep Front Line from the triceps surae of the Superficial Back Line, can be palpated – at least its outer edges.

- Place your model supine with one knee flexed, and the foot flat on the surface.

- Sitting by the foot, put your thumbs on the front of the shin, about midway up, and insinuate the fingers of the your inside hand tightly behind the posterior edge of the tibia.

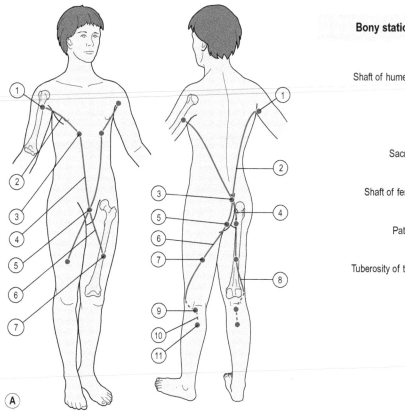

Bony stations		Myofascial tracks
Shaft of humerus	1	
	2	Latissimus dorsi
	3	Lumbodorsal fascia
	4	Sacral fascia
Sacrum	5	
	6	Gluteus maximus
Shaft of femur	7	
	8	Vastus lateralis
Patella	9	
	10	Subpatellar tendon
Tuberosity of tibia	11	

Figure 6.7
The Functional Lines.

Exercise 6.9 *continued*

- Do the same with the outer hand, going around the fibularii (peroneal) muscles, to come through behind them to the posterior edge of the fibula.

- Once your hands are "pinching" the deep transverse septum in this way, have the model lift and lower her heel, and then forefoot, to feel the muscles of the deep posterior compartment moving past this septum.

- This approach is a better assessment tool than trying to read these muscles by palpating directly through the bulk of the soleus and gastrocnemius.

Though not strictly part of this line, the pes anserinus on the inside of the knee presents itself here for palpation; the three tendons of the sartorius, gracilis, and semimembranosus can be palpated near their inferior end on the medial side of the femoral condyle just above the tibia.

The thigh

- Just above the pes, on the medial side, one can locate the edge of the medial femoral epicondyle, and the accompanying heavy distal tendon of the adductor magnus.

- Take care not to palpate heavily just superior to this epicondylar attachment, as this is where the neurovascular bundle passes through the adductor hiatus.

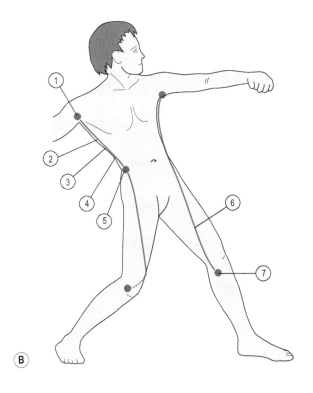

Bony stations		Myofascial tracks
Front Functional Line		
Shaft of humerus	1	
	2	Lower edge of pectoralis major
Fifth and sixth rib cartilage	3	
	4	Lateral sheath of rectus abdominis
Pubic tubercle and symphysis	5	
	6	Adductor longus
Shaft of femur	7	
Ipsilateral Functional Line		
Shaft of humerus	1	
	2	Latissimus dorsi, outer edge
End of ribs 10–12	3	
	4	External oblique
Anterior superior iliac spine	5	
	6	Sartorius
Pes anserinus, medial tibial condyle	7	

Figure 6.7 (continued)
The Functional Lines.

Exercise 6.9 *continued*

From the adductor magnus tendon, two heavy bilaminar septa traverse the inside of the thigh – one between the adductor group and the hamstrings posteriorly, and one between the adductors and the quadriceps anteriorly. The anterior wall, known as the medial intermuscular septum, is "capped" at the surface for most of its run by the sartorius muscle.

- To find and assess the posterior septum, lie your model on her side with the superior hip and knee flexed out of the way (and supported on bolsters) so that the medial aspect of the leg that lies on the table is presented to you.

- The lower end of this septum is easily found just above the knee between the adductor magnus attachment to the medial femoral epicondyle and the medial hamstring tendons – a space 2 cm wide on most people.

- Follow this "valley" upward toward the ischial tuberosity.

- If you can easily palpate the valley as you go up, this septum is appropriately allowing movement between these muscle groups.

- Often, however, the valley will fill in and disappear, becoming instead a tight wall, indicating a common but less then ideal binding of the hamstring and adductor compartments.

The upper end of the intercompartmental wall is thus hard to find in these people, but can be located with a simple test:

- Put three fingers on the posterior-inferior aspect of the ischial tuberosity, one fingertip on the posterior aspect, one fingertip on the inferomedial "corner," and one fingertip on the inferior aspect of the tuberosity.

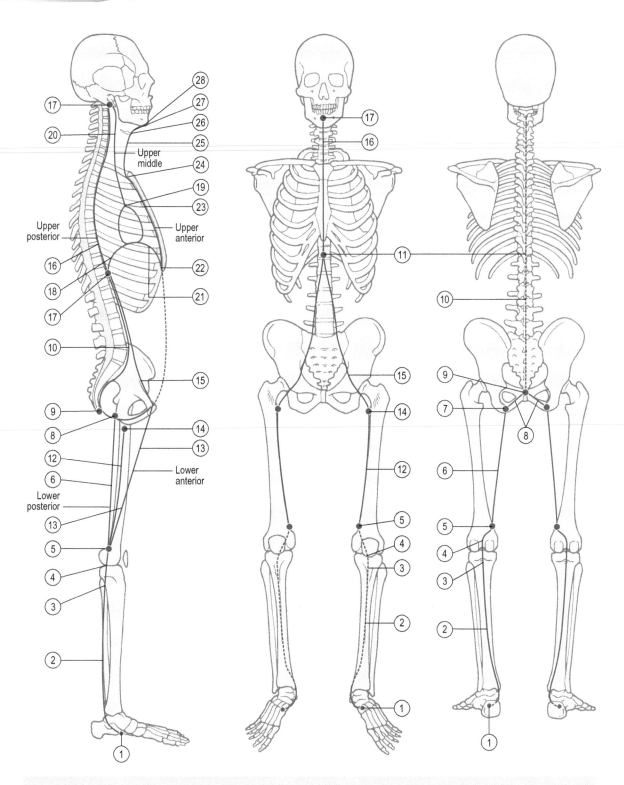

Upper middle

Upper posterior

Upper anterior

Lower anterior

Lower posterior

Figure 6.8
The Deep Front Line.

Bony stations		Myofascial tracks	Bony stations		Myofascial tracks
Lowest common			**Upper middle**		
Plantar tarsal bones, plantar surface of toes	1		Lumbar vertebral bodies	11	
	2	Tibialis superior, long toe flexors		18	Posterior diaphragm, crura of diaphragm, central tendon
Superior/posterior tibia/fibula	3			19	Pericardium, mediastinum, parietal plura
	4	Fascia of politeus, knee capsule		20	Fascia prevertebralis, pharyngeal raphe, scalene muscles, medial scalene fascia
Medial femoral epicondyle	5				
			Basilar portion of occiput, cervical TPs	17	
Lower posterior					
Medial femoral epicondyle	5				
	6	Posterior intermuscular septum, adductor magnus and minimus	**Upper anterior**		
Ischial ramus	7		Lumbar vertebral bodies	11	
	8	Pelvic floor fascia, levator ani, obturator internus fascia		21	Anterior diaphragm
Coccyx	9		Posterior surface of subcostal cartilages, xiphoid process	22	
	10	Anterior sacral fascia and anterior longitudinal ligament			
Lumbar vertebral bodies	11			23	Fascia endothoracica, transversus pretrachialis
			Posterior manubrium	24	
Lower anterior				25	Infrahyoid muscles, fascia petrachialis
Medial femoral epicondyle	5				
Linea aspera of femur	12		Hyoid bone	26	
	13	Medial intermuscular septum, adductor brevis/longus		27	Suprahyoid muscles
Lesser trochanter of femur	14		Mandible	28	
	15	Psoas, iliacus, pectineus, femoral triangle			
Lumbar vertebral bodies and TPs	11				
Upper posterior					
Lumbar vertebral bodies	11				
	16	Anterior longitudinal ligament, longus colli/capitis			
Linea aspera of femur	17				

Figure 6.8 (continued)
The Deep Front Line.

Exercise 6.9 *continued*

- Have your model lift her knee to the ceiling.

- This will contract the adductor magnus and should "pop" your finger on the inferior aspect.

- Have the model lower her leg, and then flex her knee against resistance (which your thigh can provide) – this should contract the hamstrings and "pop" your fingertip behind the ischium.

- The superior end of the septum will thus lie with your finger lying between the two at the corner of the ischial tuberosity.

- Just anterior to the adductor magnus tendon and behind the gracilis is often a small "window" in the fascia where one can palpate (if tolerated by the model) the psoas and iliacus tendon, at their distal attachment to the "fingertip" of bone you can sometimes feel – the lesser trochanter. This is not the easiest of palpations for the model, but as the lowest attachment of the major "guy-wire" to the spine, it is a rewarding place to be able to reach.

Above the ischial tuberosity is the sacrotuberous ligament, running from the hamstrings up the medial edge of the gluteus maximus to the lower base of the sacrum. Just medial to this is the ischiorectal fossa, which allows access to the posterior triangle of the pelvic floor fascia.

- Place your model supine or side-lying, and put three fingertips on the medial side of the ischial tuberosity, with your index finger along the edge of the sacrotuberous ligament, using it as a "guide."

- Move your fingertips in the direction of the model's umbilicus, sliding into the open space between the anal verge and the ischium, the ischiorectal fossa.

- Your fingerpads will pass the hardness of the ischium and onto the softer area of the obturator internus until your fingertips reach the fascia of the inferior side of the pelvic floor.

- Have your model contract and relax the pelvic floor; with practice, you can assess both the muscular as well as the fascial tone of the pelvic floor, as well as its relative position in the superior/inferior dimension.

The anterior (medial intermuscular) septum is more easily found:

- Look for a palpable "valley" just behind the sartorius muscle, heading from the medial lower thigh around toward the anterior upper thigh.

- This valley is usually easily found at the surface of the thigh, but its journey to the bone is a curved one, so to really assess the condition of the septum, one must curl one's fingers around the quadriceps, toward the linea aspera on the posterior side of the femur.

- With your model supine, stand beside the thigh facing in, and search out the surface valley behind and beneath the sartorius.

- Carefully and sensitively follow the valley into the thigh with your fingertips; it will follow a curved path into the thigh toward the posterior edge of the femur.

- With a little practice, you can again assess whether the septum is free all the way into the thigh, or (as is common) free at the surface but bound deeper in the thigh.

At the upper end, this septum opens into the femoral triangle, bounded by the sartorius laterally, adductor longus tendon medially, and the inguinal ligament superiorly.

- The adductor longus tendon originates from the pubis, and the intrepid palpator can follow the tendon to the bone to find the round attachment near the pubic tubercle.

- Just lateral and deep to this attachment is the attachment of the pectineus on the iliopectineal ridge.

- Posterior to this tendon, one can palpate the tendinous attachment of gracilis running along the ischiopubic ramus posteriorly to the adductor magnus superior attachment detailed above.

The abdomen

Above the inguinal ligament, one can find the iliac fascia between the iliacus and psoas major muscles. If fibrotic, this fascia can inhibit gliding between the two muscles (which are separate almost from the inferior attachment – "iliopsoas" is a misnomer); if it is short, it can pull the psoas laterally toward the iliacus, and imbalance the pull on the lumbar spine.

- Place your model supine with both knees up.

- Find the ASIS, and go in and posterior just medial and superior to the ASIS.

Exercise 6.9 *continued*

- The iliacus muscle is immediately available under your fingerpads.

- If you slide posteromedially on this muscle, as if skiing down a slope, your fingertips will run into the psoas eventually, which you can confirm by feeling it tense as they lift that foot from the table.

- If the iliac fascia is too short or unusually dense, you will have trouble skiing down the slope, the journey will end in a tough and "muddy" fascia, and the separation between the two parts of the iliopsoas will not be clear. When this fascia is loose, the "valley" between the iliacus and psoas is readily palpable, especially when the psoas is contracted by lifting the leg off the table.

The umbilicus is like a "grommet" that pins together all the layers of the abdomen into one from the skin all the way down to the peritoneum.

- Putting your thumbs on one side of the rectus and your fingertips on the other, pick up the umbilicus on your supine model, usually with, or if necessary without, the rectus abdominis, and bring it anteriorly (ceilingward).

- This is a strange sensation for the model, but with a little practice they can learn to tolerate it, as it is not really painful but feels quite strange to the neophyte.

- With even a mild lifting, you can "weigh" the abdominal contents, and feel the connections of the peritoneum around the body wall.

- With practice, this palpation can be used to assess adhesions in the peritoneal attachments and ligaments all the way around to the kidneys.

The anterior longitudinal ligament (ALL) is a primary soft-tissue structure in the body, running up the front of the original notocord, or in our case, up the front of the intervertebral discs. As such, its very bottom, at the coccyx, would only be accessible by entering the lower body cavity, which is beyond the scope of practice of most readers. You can access the ALL at the sacral promontory on some willing clients. Although we are describing palpations here, not techniques, lifting the ALL here and in the neck (see below) can have profound effects.

Make sure your model has an empty bladder, and preferably is not swollen (e.g., pre-menstrually) before you attempt this palpation.

Pain is an immediate contraindication.

- Have her lie supine with her knees up to soften the abdomen.

- Drop your fingertips gently into the abdomen below the navel, but above the line of the pubic hair, headed straight posteriorly.

- Let your fingers "swim" through the tissue – force will not work.

- If you come across the pulse of the aorta, you are too high; come out and go in more caudally.

- About halfway through the body, you will find the front of the spine.

- The sacral promontory is an edge of bone, where the spine turns from nearly horizontal (along the front of the sacrum) to vertical (along the front of L3 or so).

- The ALL is the tough fabric running over the sacrum, the L5–S1 disc (which is softer to the touch), and onto the L5 body (which is slightly scalloped, so that the ALL can be felt here distinct from the bone itself.

- Usually, trying to go any higher up the spine than this is frustrated by the joining of the common iliac arteries into the aorta with its characteristic pulse. Do not challenge its authority.

The thorax

The structures of the Deep Front Line – the mediastinum, pleura, and endothoracic fascial layers – lie entirely within the embrace of the ribcage, and are only palpable by indirect methods.

Chronic shortness in the mediastinum, pericardium, and central tendon of the diaphragm can be seen and inferred, even if it is not palpable, when a hollow is seen at the level of the xiphoid process, or indeed if the sternum seems to be pulled into the body. At its most extreme, this causes the condition known as "pectus excavatum." But nothing has been excavated or pushed; instead the sternum is kept close to the thoracic spine by restricting fascia while the ribs grow around the restriction.

The neck

The scalene muscles are more fascial than most, forming a strong skirt around the cervical spine that supports the neck on the upper ribs, as well as supporting both the upper ribs and the pleura of the lungs as well. These muscles form a fascial complex with the envelope for the brachial plexus, as well as being the secondary muscles of breathing, readily palpable during the latter part of inhalation.

- You can palpate the fascial extension of the scalene complex down the outside of the ribcage.

- With your model side-lying, put one hand in the axilla, palm down and fingertips as far up into the axillary space as is comfortable.

- With your other hand, lift the model's head toward you (side-bending their neck away from the table).

- At the same time slide your hand into the axilla, allowing the shoulder to drop up toward her ear.

- Slowly lower your model's head back toward the table to feel the extension of the scalene fascia move out from under your fingers on the surface of the ribs.

- Have your model lift her head toward you again to feel the fascia tense as a sheet.

Coupled with these muscles are the two muscular reinforcements for the ALL in the neck, the longus colli and longus capitis muscles.

- With your model supine and you sitting at the head of the treatment table, lean in to place your hands palm down with your fingertips of both hands facing each other just at the trailing (posterior) edge of the sternocleidomastoid muscle (SCM).

- Lift the SCM slightly forward with the fingernail side of your fingertips, and slip in behind the SCM, but in front of the hard cylinder of muscle surrounding the neck, including the scalenes.

- With a little practice, it becomes easy and comfortable to slip between the motor cylinder and visceral cylinder of the neck.

- This puts you behind the alar fascia (and thus behind the visceral endangerment sites), but in front of the prevertebral fascia and the ALL.

- The anterior scalene will be readily palpable under the cleidal head of the SCM as a 1/2 inch (1.25 cm) band that gets taut during or at the top of the breath.

- A bit further medial, and the "bumps" of the anterior tubercles of the transverse processes can be felt.

- Still further medial, if your model can tolerate it and you can keep your fingers soft and exploratory, you will find the longus colli or capitis muscles (depending on where you are superiorly or inferiorly in the neck). Have your model lift their head slightly to feel these muscles fire up. Do they also fire when the model flattens the back of her neck to the table? This would indicate a good balance between these neck flexors and the very strong upper cervical extensors of the Superficial Front and Superficial Back Lines.

- These muscles often need to be strengthened to reinforce the ALL in those with a hyperextended cervical spine, or eased in those with a reduced curve (military neck).

This concludes our tour of some of the more prominent and available larger features in the fascial network of the myofascia, organized in terms of the continuous myofascial meridians, which we hope you have enjoyed and valued. In closing, we would like to re-emphasize the idea that the structures we have identified are not separate entities, but simply palpable geography within a body-wide net that is increasingly identified as dynamic, responsive, and highly communicative over its whole length and breadth.

With practice, the skilled palpator can assess the state of any one part of that net from a station at any other part, through coupling client movement with a refined sense of "end-feel."

References

Guimberteau J-C and Armstrong C (2015) Architecture of human living fascia. Edinburgh: Handspring.

Langevin HM, Konofagou EE, Badger GJ, Churchill DL, Fox JR, Ophir J and Garra BS (2004) Tissue displacements during acupuncture using ultrasound elastography techniques. Ultrasound in Medicine and Biology 30: 1173–1183.

Langevin HM, Bouffard NA, Badger GJ, Churchill DL and Howe AK (2006) Subcutaneous tissue fibroblast cytoskeletal remodeling induced by acupuncture: evidence for a mechanotransduction-based mechanism. Journal of Cellular Physiology 207 (3): 767–774.

Myers T (2014) Anatomy trains, 3rd edn. Edinburgh: Churchill Livingstone.

Schultz L (1996) The endless web. Berkeley: North Atlantic Books.

Leon Chaitow

In this chapter we will be examining some useful assessment techniques relating to what has been described as "abnormal tension in the neural structures." Before doing so it is necessary to look at some of the potential implications, other than pain, which such "abnormal tensions" can lead to. We need therefore to briefly examine one physiological component which may be involved: *the trophic function of nerves.*

Neural transportation

Irvin Korr, the primary researcher into the neurological and pathophysiological processes involved in osteopathic medicine, studied the phenomenon of the transport and exchange of macromolecular materials along neural pathways.

- Among his pertinent (to our study) findings are that the influence of nerves on target organs and muscles depends largely upon the delivery to them of specific neuronal proteins.

There is also evidence of a return pathway by means of which messenger substances are transferred back from target organs, to the central nervous system, and brain, along neural structures.

In one of Korr's examples (Korr 1981) it is shown that red and white muscles, which differ morphologically, functionally, and chemically (and as we have seen in Chapter 5, differently in response to stress), can have all these differences reversed if their innervation is "crossed," so that red muscles receive white muscle innervation and vice versa. "This means, that the nerve instructs the muscle what kind of muscle to be, and is an expression of a neurally mediated genetic influence," says Korr.

In other words, it is the nerve that determines which genes in a muscle will be suppressed, and which expressed, and this information is carried in the material being transported along the axons.

When a muscle loses contact with its nerve (as in anterior poliomyelitis, for example) atrophy occurs, not as a result of disuse, but because of the loss of the integrity of the connection between nerve cells and muscle cells at the myoneural junction, where nutrient exchange occurs irrespective of whether or not impulses are being transmitted.

These and other functions depend upon the flow of axonally transported proteins, phospholipids, glycoproteins, neurotransmitters and their precursors, enzymes, mitochondria and other organelles. Korr's words can help us to appreciate this phenomenon further.

- *The rate of transport of such substances varies from 1mm/day to several hundred mm/day, with "different cargoes being carried at different rates".*

- *"The motor powers (for the waves of transportation) are provided by the axon itself."*

- *"Retrograde transportation" seems to be a fundamental means of communication between neurons and between neurons and non-neuronal cells.*

Korr showed this process to have an important role in maintenance of "the plasticity of the nervous system, serving to keep motor-neurons and muscle cells, or two synapsing neurons, mutually adapted to each other and responsive to each other's changing circumstances."

Implications

What are the clinical implications of this knowledge and, more specifically, how is this related to our study of palpation?

Awareness of the trophic influence of nerves on the structural and functional characteristics of the soft tissues they supply, should alert us to situations that may disrupt the two-way flow along these nutrient highways. Korr explains:

Any factor that causes derangement of transport mechanisms in the axon, or that chronically alters the quality or quantity of the axonally transported substances, can cause the trophic influences to become detrimental. This alteration in turn would produce aberrations of structure, function, and metabolism, contributing to dysfunction and disease.

Among the negative influences frequently operating on these transport mechanisms, Korr informs us, are: "deformations of nerves and roots, such as compression, stretching, angulation and torsion". These stresses occur all too often in humans, says Korr, and are particularly likely where neural structures are most vulnerable: "In their passage over highly mobile joints, through bony canals, intervertebral foramina, fascial layers, and tonically contracted muscles (for example, posterior rami of spinal nerves and spinal extensor muscles)."

Korr further amplifies his concern over negative influences on neural trophic function when he discusses "sustained hyperactive peripheral neurons (sensory, motor and autonomic)." For when there is a high rate of discharge from neural structures (facilitated segments and trigger points, for example) the metabolism of neurons are affected "and almost certainly their synthesis and turnover of proteins and other macromolecules."

These thoughts (and others of Korr's, given below) relating to the vital trophic role of the nervous system, over and above its conduction of impulses, should be borne in mind as we examine methods of assessing adverse mechanical tension in the nervous system. For, as Che et al. have observed (2016): "The bidirectional transport of cargos along the thin axon is fundamental for the structure, function and survival of neurons. Defective axonal transport has been linked to the mechanism of neurodegenerative diseases."

Assessment of adverse mechanical tension in the nervous system

Testing for, and treating, "tensions" in neural structures offer us an alternative method for dealing with some forms of pain and dysfunction, since such adverse mechanical tension (AMT) is often a major component cause of musculoskeletal dysfunction as well as more widespread pathology (bear Korr's research in mind).

Maitland (1986) suggests that we consider this form of assessment and treatment to involve "mobilization" of the neural structures, rather than simply stretching them. He and others recommended that these methods be reserved

for conditions which fail to respond adequately to normal mobilization of soft and osseous structures (muscles, joints and so on). Maitland and Butler (Butler & Gifford 1989) have, over the years, discussed those mechanical restrictions which impinge on neural structures in the vertebral canals and elsewhere.

There is no general agreement as to the terminology which should be used in describing such biomechanical changes in the neural environment. Maitland et al. (2001), for example, suggest that "abnormal neural movement" is a more accurate description than "neural tension." Whatever we term the dysfunctional pattern, Butler and Gifford's focus on those "adverse mechanical" changes that negatively influence neural function, and cause a multitude of symptoms, including pain, has been a singular contribution to our understanding of some aspects of pain and dysfunction.

Many of the concepts and methods advocated by Maitland, Butler and others in regard to management of adverse neural tension have subsequently been validated and refined (Efstathiou et al. 2015; Saurab Sharma et al. 2016).

Base tests

Butler and Gifford (1989) have outlined a series of "base tests" that can be used to discover precise mechanical restrictions relating to the nervous system. Five of the "base (tension) tests" that will be described are useful not only for diagnosis but for passive mobilization of the structures involved. The tissues involved in "mechanical tension" often include the nerve itself, as well as its surrounding muscle, connective tissue, circulatory structures, dura and so on.

The five tension test methods described below are:

- straight leg raising (SLR)
- prone knee bending (PKB)
- passive neck flexion (PNF)
- a combination of these called "slump" position and variations of this
- upper limb tension tests (ULTT).

These tests are often performed in conjunction with each other (for example, "slump" together with PKB). Despite some of these tests being familiar in other settings, if reliable results are wanted it is vital that the methodology for their use, as described in this particular context, is followed closely.

Butler and Gifford report that studies have shown that changes in tension in lumbar nerve roots have been demonstrated during stretching maneuvers and that there is often an instant alteration in neck and arm (and sometimes head) pain via the addition of ankle dorsiflexion during SLR. Additional stretches, such as ankle dorsiflexion performed during SLR, are described in this work as "sensitizing" maneuvers.

Adding tension to neural structures can be alternated in practice by adding glide/slide as described and illustrated below (see Fig. 7.3A, B) (Beltran-Alacreu et al. 2015).

Correct positioning important

Butler and Gifford (1989) noted that careful positioning of the region being tested is vital as changes in pain are assessed as well as the use of passive stretches (or glides) as a means of inducing release of restrictions when they are discovered. The developers of tension tests for adverse mechanical tension in the nervous system point out that body movements (and therefore these tests) not only produce an increase in tension within the nerve but also move (slide/glide) the nerve in relation to surrounding tissues.

Meet the mechanical interface

The tissues that surround neural structures have been called the mechanical interface (MI). These adjacent tissues are those that can move independently of the nervous system (e.g., supinator muscle is the MI to the radial nerve, as it passes through the radial tunnel).

- Any pathology in the MI can produce abnormalities in nerve movement, resulting in tension on neural structures with unpredictable ramifications.

- Good examples of MI pathology are nerve impingement by disc protrusion or osteophyte contact and carpal tunnel constriction.

These problems would be regarded as mechanical in origin as far as the nerve restriction is concerned. Any symptoms resulting from mechanical impingement on neural structures will be more readily provoked in tests that involve movement, rather than pure (passive) tension.

Chemical or inflammatory causes of neural tension also occur, resulting in, for example, "interneural fibrosis" that leads to reduced elasticity and increased "tension", which would become obvious with tension testing of these structures. (See Chapter 5, discussion of progression from acute to chronic in soft tissue dysfunction under the heading "Local adaptation syndrome.")

Pathophysiological changes resulting from inflammation, or from chemical damage (i.e., toxic), are noted as commonly leading to internal mechanical restrictions of neural structures in a different manner to mechanical causes, such as those imposed by a disc lesion, for example.

Adverse mechanical tension changes (or "abnormal neural movement") do not necessarily and automatically affect nerve conduction, according to Butler and Gifford. However, Korr's research shows it to be likely that axonal transport would be affected by such changes. Current neuroscience research has validated much of Korr's work (Che et al. 2016).

Adverse mechanical tension and pain sites not necessarily the same

When a tension test is positive (i.e., pain is produced by one or another element of the test – initial position alone or with "sensitizing" additions), it indicates only that there exists AMT somewhere in the nervous system – and not that this is necessarily at the site of reported pain.

Butler and Gifford (1991) report research indicating that 70% of 115 patients with either carpal tunnel syndrome or lesions of the ulnar nerve at the elbow showed clear electrophysiological and clinical evidence of neural lesions in the neck. This is, they maintain, because of a "double crush" phenomenon in which a primary and often long-standing disorder, perhaps in the spine, results in secondary or "remote" dysfunction at the periphery.

This phenomenon can also work in reverse, for example where wrist entrapment of the ulnar nerve leads ultimately to nerve entrapment at the elbow (they term this "reversed double crush").

Tension points and test descriptions

Butler and Gifford (1991) note that certain anatomical areas, where the nervous system moves only a small amount relative to the surrounding interface during motion, or where the system is relatively fixed, are the most likely regions for AMT to develop. This is often where nerves branch or enter a muscle. Such areas are called "tension points" and these are referred to in the test descriptions.

1. A positive tension test is one in which the patient's symptoms are reproduced by the test procedure and where these symptoms can be altered by variations in what are termed "sensitizing maneuvers," which are used to "add weight to" and confirm the initial diagnosis of AMT. Adding dorsiflexion during SLR is an example of a sensitizing maneuver.

2. Precise symptom reproduction may not be possible, but the test is still possibly relevant if other abnormal symptoms are produced during the test and its accompanying sensitizing procedures. Comparison with the test findings on an opposite limb, for example, may indicate an abnormality, worth exploring.

3. Altered range of movement is another indicator of abnormality, whether this is noted during the initial test position or during sensitizing additions.

Variations of passive motion of the nervous system during examination and treatment

1. An increase in tension can be produced in the *interneural component*, where tension is being applied from both ends, so to speak, as in the "slump" test.

2. Increased tension can be produced in the *extraneural component*, which then produces the maximum movement of the nerve in relation to its mechanical interface (such as in SLR) with the likelihood of restrictions showing up at "tension points."

3. Movement of *extraneural tissues* in another plane can be engineered.

Before beginning the exercises below, look at Box 7.1, which gives some general precautions and contraindications for their use.

Box 7.1 General precautions and contraindications for Exercises 7.1–7.6

1. Take care of the spine during the "slump test" if disc problems are involved or if the neck is sensitive (or the patient is prone to dizziness).

2. Take care not to be excessive in side bending of the neck during ULTT.

3. If any area is sensitive, take care not to aggravate existing conditions during performance of tests (arm is more likely than leg to be "stirred up").

4. If obvious neurological problems exist, take special care not to exacerbate by vigorous or strong stretching.

5. Similar precautions apply to patients with diabetes, multiple sclerosis, or who have recently had surgey, or where the area being tested is much affected by circulatory deficit.

6. Do not use the tests if there has been recent onset or worsening of neurological signs or if there is any cauda equina or cord lesion.

Implications of adverse mechanical tensions

Bearing in mind the evidence as to the many ways in which soft tissue (and osseous) dysfunction can impinge on neural structures, it is logical that maximum relaxation of any muscle involved in interface tissue should be achieved, by normal methods, before such tests (or subsequent treatment based on such tests) are considered.

It is not within the scope of this text to describe methods for releasing abnormal tensions except to suggest that, as in (most of) the examples of tests for shortened postural muscles given in Chapter 5, the treatment positions are a replication of the test positions.

Butler suggests that, in treating adverse mechanical tensions in the nervous system in this way, initial stretching should commence well away from the site of pain in sensitive individuals and conditions. Re-testing regularly during treatment is also wise, in order to see whether gains in range of motion or lessening of pain provocation during testing are being achieved.

CAUTION: It is critical that any sensitivity provoked by treatment should subside immediately. If it does not, the technique/test should be stopped or irritation could be caused to the neural tissues involved.

Exercise 7.1 *Straight Leg Raising (SLR) Test*

Time suggested **3–4 minutes for each "sensitizing" addition**

See also the text relating to hamstring test (for shortness) in Chapter 5 (Exercise 5.16A) and its accompanying figure (5.22).

The leg is raised in the sagittal plane, with the knee extended, until a barrier or resistance is noted or symptoms are reported.

Sensitizing additions might include:

- ankle dorsiflexion (this loads the tibial component of the sciatic nerve)
- ankle plantarflexion plus inversion (this loads the common peroneal nerve, which may be useful with anterior shin and dorsal foot symptoms)
- passive neck flexion
- increased medial hip rotation
- increased hip adduction
- altered spinal position (the example is given of left SLR being "sensitized" by lateral flexion to the right of the spine).

Perform the SLR test and incorporate each sensitizing addition, in order to assess changes in symptoms, new symptoms, restrictions, etc.

Can the leg be raised as far as it should normally go (approximately 80°), and as easily, without force and without symptoms (new or old) appearing, when the sensitizing additions are incorporated?

Notes on SLR test

On SLR there is caudad gliding movement of the lumbosacral nerve roots in relation to interfacing tissue (which is why there is a "positive" indication – pain and limitation of leg-raising potential – from SLR if a prolapsed intervertebral disc exists).

Less well known is the fact that the tibial nerve, proximal to the knee, moves caudad (in relation to the mechanical interface) during SLR, whereas distal to the knee it moves cranially. There is no movement of the tibial nerve behind the knee itself, which is therefore known as a "tension point".

The common peroneal nerve is attached firmly to the head of the fibula (another "tension point").

Exercise 7.2 *Prone Knee Bend (PKB) Test*

Time suggested **3–4 minutes for each "sensitizing" addition in each position (1 and 2)**

Method 1

Your palpation partner should be prone.

You flex the knee, taking the heel towards the buttock, in order to assess reproduction of existing symptoms or other abnormal symptoms or altered range of movement (heel should approximate buttock relatively easily).

During the test the knee is flexed, while the hip and thigh are stabilized, and this moves the nerves and roots from L2, 3, 4 and, particularly, the femoral nerve and its branches.

Method 2

If, however, the test is conducted with the person side-lying, the hip should be maintained in extension during the test (this alternative position is thought more appropriate for identifying entrapped lateral femoral cutaneous nerve problems).

The PKB test stretches rectus femoris and rotates the pelvis anteriorly, thus extending the lumbar spine, which can confuse interpretation of nerve impingement symptoms.

Reliance on sensitizing maneuvers helps with such interpretation. These include (in either prone or side-lying use of the test) the addition of:

- cervical flexion
- adopting the "slump" position (Exercise 7.3) – but only in the side-lying variation of the test
- variations of hip abduction, adduction, rotation.

Can the knee easily be fully flexed, without force and without symptoms (new or old) appearing, when the sensitizing additions are incorporated?

Exercise 7.3 *The "Slump Test"*

Time suggested 3–4 minutes for each "sensitizing" addition

This is regarded by Butler as the most important test in this series. It links neural and connective tissue components from the pons to the feet and requires care in performance and interpretation (Fig. 7.1).

This test is suggested for use in all spinal disorders, most lower limb disorders, and some upper limb disorders (especially those which seem to involve the nervous system).

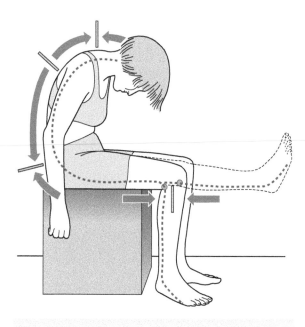

Figure 7.1
The slump test position stretches the entire neural network from pons to feet. Note the direction of stretch of the dura mater and nerve roots. As the leg straightens, the movement of the tibial nerve in relation to the tibia and femur is indicated by arrows. No neural movement occurs behind the knee or at levels C6, T6, or L4 (these are the "tension" points).

The test involves your palpation partner introducing the following sequence of movements:

- thoracic and then lumbar flexion, followed by
- cervical flexion
- knee extension
- ankle dorsiflexion
- sometimes also with hip flexion (produced by either bringing the trunk forwards on the hips or by increasing SLR).

Sensitizing maneuvers during slump testing are achieved, as a rule, by changes in the terminal positions of joints. Butler gives examples:

- Should the "slump position" reproduce (for example) lumbar and radiating thigh pain, a change in head position – say away from full neck flexion – could result in total relief of these symptoms.
- A change in ankle and knee positions could significantly change cervical, thoracic or head pain.
- In both instances this would confirm that AMT was operating, although the site would remain unknown.

Additional sensitizing movements with the person in the slump position might involve the addition of trunk side bending and rotation – or even extension, hip adduction, abduction, or rotation – and varying neck positions.

The "slump test" involves *tension* on the nervous system rather than *motion*.

Notes on "slump" position

Cadaver studies demonstrate that neuromeningeal movement occurs in various directions, with C6, T6, and L4 intervertebral levels being regions of constant state (i.e., no movement, therefore "tension points").

Butler reports that many restrictions, identified during the "slump" test, may only be corrected by appropriate spinal manipulation and that SLR is more likely to pick up neural tension in the lumbosacral region.

It is possible for SLR to be positive (e.g., symptoms are reproduced) and "slump" negative (no symptom reproduction) and vice versa, so both tests should always be performed.

The following findings have been reported in research using the slump test:

Exercise 7.3 *continued*

1. Mid-thoracic to T9 are painful on trunk and neck flexion in 50% of "normal" individuals.

2. The following are considered normal if they are symmetrical:

- hamstring and posterior knee pain, occurring with trunk and neck flexion, when the knees are extended and increasing with ankle dorsiflexion

- restrictions in ankle dorsiflexion during trunk/neck flexion, while the knee is in extension

- there is a common decrease in pain and an increase in range of knee extension or ankle dorsiflexion on release of neck flexion.

If the patient's symptoms are reproduced by the slump position, and can be relieved by sensitizing maneuvers, you have a positive test. This is further emphasized if, as well as symptom reproduction, there is a symmetrical decrease in the range of motion which does not happen when tension is absent. For example, bilateral ankle dorsiflexion is restricted during slump, but disappears when the neck is not flexed.

In some instances, anomalous reactions are observed in which, for example, pain increases when the neck is taken out of flexion or when trunk on hip flexion decreases symptoms. Mechanical interface (MI) pathology may account for this.

Notes

A variation on the slump test – turning it into "gliding" exercise – is described in Exercise 7.6, below.

Exercise 7.4 *Passive Neck Flexion (PNF) Test*

Time suggested   1–2 minutes for each variation

As with SLR, this test takes up slack from one end only. It allows movement of neuromeningeal tissues in relation to the spinal canal, which is its mechanical interface (MI).

In an industrial survey 22% of patients with back pain were found to have a positive PNF test.

- The head and neck are supported by your hands as you take the chin toward the chest.

- In a normal neck the chin should approximate the sternum without force or symptoms.

- Variations such as neck extension, lateral flexion and PNF, in combination with other tests, should be used for screening purposes for AMT.

Exercise 7.5 *Upper Limb Tension Tests (ULTT 1 and 2)*

Time suggested   3–4 minutes for each "sensitizing" addition to each version of the test

ULTT 1

- Your palpation partner should be supine.

- Place the tested arm into abduction, extension, and lateral rotation of the glenohumeral joint. Once these positions are established, supination of the forearm is introduced together with elbow extension.

- This is followed by addition of passive wrist and finger extension.

- If pain is experienced at any stage during placement of the person into the test position or during addition of sensitization maneuvers (below), particularly reproduction of neck, shoulder, or arm symptoms previously reported, the test is positive and confirms a degree of mechanical interference affecting neural structures.

Additional sensitization is performed by:

- adding cervical lateral flexion away from the side being tested

- introduction of ULTT 1 on the other arm simultaneously

- the simultaneous use of straight leg raising, bi- or unilaterally

- introduction of pronation rather than supination of the wrist.

Exercise 7.5 *continued*

Notes on ULTT 1

A great deal of nerve movement occurs during this test. In cadavers, up to 2 cm (0.8 inches) movement of the median nerve in relation to its mechanical interface has been observed during neck and wrist movement. "Tension points" in the upper limb are found at the shoulder and elbow.

ULTT 2

Butler developed this test and finds it more sensitive than ULTT 1. He maintains that it replicates the working posture involved in many instances of upper limb repetition disorders ("overuse syndrome").

In using ULTT 2, comparison is always made with the other arm.

Example of right-side ULTT 2

- For a right-side test the person lies close to the right side of the table, so that the scapula is free of the surface.

- The trunk and legs are angled towards the left foot of the bed so that the patient feels secure.

- The practitioner stands to the side of the person's head, facing the feet with the practitioner's left thigh depressing the shoulder girdle (Fig. 7.2).

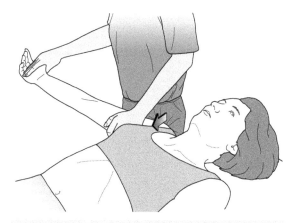

Figure 7.2
Upper limb tension test (2). Note the practitioner's thigh depresses the shoulder as sensitizing maneuvers are carried out.

- The person's fully flexed right arm is supported at both elbow and wrist, by the practitioner's hands.

- Slight variations in the degree and angle of shoulder depression ("lifted" towards ceiling, held towards floor) may be used, by alteration of thigh contact.

Holding the shoulder depressed, the practitioner's right hand grasps the patient's right wrist while the upper arm is held by the practitioner's left hand.

With these contacts sensitization maneuvers can be introduced to the tested arm – see below:

- shoulder internal or external rotation

- elbow flexion or extension

- forearm supination or pronation.

The practitioner then slides his right hand down onto the open hand and introduces supination or pronation or stretching of fingers/thumb or radial and ulnar deviations.

Further sensitization may involve:

- neck movement (side bend away from tested side, for example), or

- altered shoulder position, such as increased abduction or extension.

A combination of shoulder internal rotation, elbow extension and forearm pronation (with shoulder constantly depressed) is considered to offer the most sensitive test position.

> ### Notes
>
> Cervical lateral flexion away from the tested side causes increased arm symptoms in 93% of people and cervical lateral flexion towards the tested side increases symptoms in 70% of cases (Butler & Gifford 1991).

Butler and Gifford report that ULTT mobilizes the cervical dural theca in a transverse direction, whereas the "slump" mobilizes the dural theca in an anteroposterior direction as well as longitudinally.

Exercise 7.6 *Neurodynamic Stretching and Slider Exercises*

Note that Beltran-Alacreu et al. (2015) found that these exercises in neuromobilization had an immediate, widespread, hypoalgesic effect.

7.6A: neurodynamic stretching

The process of inducing a neural stretch effect requires repetitive and constant movement of the patient/model from a starting to a final position – and back again (Fig. 7.3).

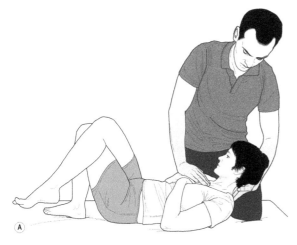

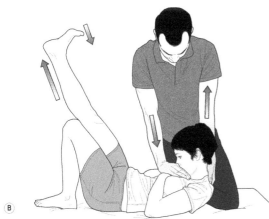

Figure 7.3
The starting (A) and finishing (B) positions employed in neurodynamic stretching.

The speed of application of the repetitions can vary, depending on the physical status of the subject, who must be kept in constant motion.

- To start, the subject is supine with knees flexed – and with the right leg resting on the left, supported at the popliteal area.

- A cushion/soft wedge may optionally be placed under the buttocks and the lower thoracic area, to increase thoracic flexion.

- Both the subject's hands should be crossed over the chest.

- You stand on the subject's right side, with one hand/arm supporting the upper thoracic, cervical, and occipital areas.

- The other hand is placed over the crossed hands of the subject (Fig. 7.3A).

- To achieve the final position you should flex the patient's thoracic and cervical spines – at the same time as applying steady pressure to the subject's crossed hands that are resting on her chest – so increasing thoracic kyphosis.

- *At the same time*, the subject is asked to extend the right knee as she raises the lower leg – while maintaining the contact between the popliteal area and the leg on which it rests – while also inducing maximal dorsiflexion of the ankle, and a maximum knee extension (Fig. 7.3B).

- The start position is then returned to, and the process repeated.

- This technique results in a neural stretch.

7.6B: neurodynamic sliding

The process of inducing a neural glide effect requires repetitive and constant movement of the patient/model from a starting (Fig. 7.4A) to a final (Fig. 7.4B) position – and back again. The speed of the repetitions depends on the objectives and the physical status of the subject, who must be constantly moving.

- To treat/test the right side, the subject sits with the right lower limb extended and the left lower limb flexed; both hands holding the left knee.

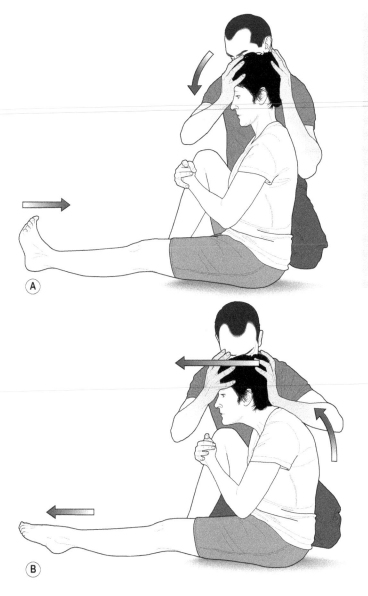

Figure 7.4
The starting (A) and finishing (B) positions employed in neurodynamic sliding.

Exercise 7.6 *continued*

- You should be on the side of the flexed limb, with your knee against the lower back, to prevent lumbar kyphosis.

- Using both hands you engage the subject's head (occiput and frontal) before introducing craniocervical flexion, while at the same time the subject performs dorsiflexion of the right ankle (Fig. 7.4A). This is the first position.

- To reach the final position, the subject increases thoracic kyphosis at the same time as performing plantarflexion in the right ankle, while you introduce craniocervical extension in the subject (Fig. 7.4B).

Exercise 7.6 *continued*

- The starting position is then resumed, and the process repeated.

- In application of the technique, the nerves glide because in the *initial movement* there is a stretch of the cervical spinal cord and shortening of the dorsal spinal cord, combined with stretch of the nerves in the posterior leg.

- In the *final movement*, the cervical cord shortens and the dorsal spine cord stretches, at the same time as slackening of the nerves in the posterior leg.

Discussion regarding Exercises 7.1–7.6

The inclusion of these tests, in a text primarily aimed at enhanced palpatory literacy, may be questioned. What have they to do with palpation?

I consider that the tests previously described (Chapter 5), evaluating muscle length, as well as those for joint play (Chapter 8 and Special topic 9 on joint play) and those in this chapter, which evaluate possible AMT in neural structures, are all logical extensions of palpation of the skin (and indeed of the region just below the skin) as well as of muscles and fascia.

The concepts of "end-feel," range of motion, and restrictive barriers are discussed elsewhere and assessment of such barriers and restrictions, as well as normal "end-feel," requires the delicacy of touch that is a major element of palpatory literacy. These skills are likely to be enhanced if the tests described in this chapter are performed with delicacy and care.

Awareness of what Butler calls *"tension" points* can be added to the knowledge we hold in mind as we palpate and test in other ways than those described above.

As we use the methods developed by Lief, Nimmo, Lewit, Beal, Smith or Becker (or any other method of palpation) such knowledge is potentially very useful indeed. If, for example, on NMT palpation, or application of Becker's palpation methods, soft tissue changes are palpated in "tension" point areas, as described by Butler, the possibility of neurological entrapment would be clear only if the concepts of AMT were understood.

Use of one or all of the tests described above might then either confirm or deny this possibility.

Use of additional tests to assess for shortened muscle structures (Chapter 5) and joint restrictions (Chapter 8) would also be appropriate, as such changes could easily be the cause of adverse tension in the nervous system.

The inclusion of these tests is intended to encourage a different way of evaluating somatic dysfunction, using some familiar procedures (such as straight leg raising) as well as the enhancement of the palpation skills required in the performance of some quite complex manual procedures (ULTT 2, for example).

Clinical use of the tests involved in, as well as the underlying concepts of, AMT in neural structures, requires adequate professional training in these methods.

If you have succeeded in performing these tests, and their sensitizing additions, and have acquired useful feedback and information which points towards AMT in the nervous systems of the model(s) you have worked with, then you may feel inspired towards further training in this subject, which has emerged out of physiotherapy methodology in recent years.

Chapter 7

References

Beltran-Alacreu H, Jiménez-Sanz L, Fernández Carnero J and La Touche R (2015) Comparison of hypoalgesic effects of neural stretching vs neural gliding. Journal of Manipulative and Physiological Therapeutics 38 (9): 644–652.

Butler D and Gifford L (1989) Adverse mechanical tensions in the nervous system. Physiotherapy 75: 622–629.

Butler D and Gifford L (1991) Mobilisation of the nervous system. Edinburgh: Churchill Livingstone.

Che DL, Chowdary PD and Cui B (2016) A close look at axonal transport: Cargos slow down when crossing stationary organelles. Neuroscience Letters 610: 110–116.

Efstathiou M, Stefanakis M, Savva C and Giakas G (2015) Effectiveness of neural mobilization in patients with spinal radiculopathy: A critical review. Journal of Bodywork and Movement Therapies 19: 205–212.

Korr I (1981) Axonal transport and neurotrophic function in relation to somatic dysfunction, in Korr I (ed) Spinal Cord as Organizer of Disease Processes, part 4. Newark, OH: Academy of Applied Osteopathy, pp 451–458.

Maitland G (1986) Vertebral manipulation. London: Butterworths.

Maitland G, Hengeveld E, Banks K and English K (2001) Maitland's vertebral manipulation, 6th edn. London: Butterworth Heinemann.

Saurab Sharma S, Balthillaya G, Rao R and Mani R (2016) Short term effectiveness of neural sliders and neural tensioners as an adjunct to static stretching of hamstrings on knee extension angle in healthy individuals: A randomized controlled trial. Physical Therapy in Sport 17: 30–37.

Special topic 7

Red, white, and black reaction
Leon Chaitow

Many researchers and clinicians from various thera-peutic backgrounds – osteopathy, chiropractic, and naturopathy – have described an assortment of responses in the form of "lines," variously colored from red to white and even blue-black, after appli-cation of manual, or tool-assisted, frictional pressure.

In the early days of osteopathy in the 19th century, the phenomenon was already in use. McConnell (1899) reported:

> I begin at the first dorsal and examine the spinal column down to the sacrum by placing my middle fingers over the spinous processes and standing directly back of the patient draw the flat surfaces of these two fingers over the spinous processes from the upper dorsal to the sacrum in such a manner that the spines of the vertebrae pass tightly between the two fingers; thus leaving a red streak where the cutaneous vessels press upon the spines of the vertebrae. In this manner slight deviations of the vertebrae laterally can be told with the great-est accuracy by observing the red line. When a vertebra or section of vertebrae are too posterior a heavy red streak is noticed and when a vertebra or section of vertebrae are too anterior the streak is not so noticeable.

Many decades later, Marshall Hoag (1969) wrote as follows regarding examination of the spinal area using skin friction.

> With firm but moderate pressure the pads of the fingers are repeatedly rubbed over the surface of the skin, preferably with extensive longitudinal strokes along the paraspinal area. The blunt end of an instrument or of a pen may be used to apply friction, since the purpose is simply to detect colour change, but care must be taken to avoid abrading the skin. The appearance of less intense and rapidly fading colour in certain areas as compared with the general reaction is ascribed to increased vaso-constriction in that area, indicating a disturbance in autonomic reflex activity. The significance of this red reaction and other evidence of altered reflex activity in relation to (osteopathic) lesions has been examined in research. Others give significance to an increased degree of erythema or a prolonged lingering of the red line response.

On the same theme, Upledger and Vredevoogd (1983) described this phenomenon thus:

> Skin texture changes produced by a facilitated seg-ment [localized areas of hyperirritability in the soft tissues involving neural sensitization to long-term stress] are palpable as you lightly drag your fingers over the nearby paravertebral area of the back. I usually do skin drag evaluation moving from the top of the neck to the sacral area in one motion. Where your fingertips drag on the skin you will probably find a facilitated segment. After several repetitions, with increased force, the affected area will appear redder than nearby areas. This is the "red reflex." Muscles and connective tissues at this level will:
>
> 1. Have a "shotty" feel (like buckshot under the skin);
>
> 2. Be more tender to palpation;
>
> 3. Be tight, and tend to restrict vertebral motion; and
>
> 4. Exhibit tenderness of the spinous processes when tapped by fingers or a rubber hammer.

De Jarnette (1934), the developer of chiropractic sacro-occipital technique (SOT), wrote extensively on the subject of the "red reaction," with some complex interpretations suggested in his classic text *Reflex Pain*.

De Jarnette initially made assessments of patients (partly based on blood pressure readings) into various categories, during which process he had them treated in order to alter the relative oxygenation levels which he believed to be the basis of these categories. None of these methods are pertinent to this survey of skin reactions, but are a necessary preamble to his descriptions, which would be confusing otherwise.

In his "Type 1" SOT patient – who had received the appropriate preliminary attention as outlined ("carbon dioxide elimination technic") – he suggested the following:

Sit or stand immediately behind the patient facing the patient's back. Have the patient bend slightly forward. Be sure the light is even on the patient's back to avoid shadows. Place the index and middle fingers of your right hand upon the 7th cervical vertebra, having the two fingers about an inch [2.5 cm] lateral from the spine of the 7th cervical vertebra. Keep the fingers evenly spaced as you go down the spine, so each line is as straight as possible. For the "Type 1" patient (normal BP after appropriate techniques) use a light touch. To produce an even pressure of both fingers on the back they may be fortified by placing the fingers of the left hand over them. As you go down the spine, your pressure will be just hard enough to cause the fingers to dent the skin.

Now draw your fingers down the spine very quickly ending at the coccyx. Step back and watch the reaction. A red line will usually appear all the way down the spine. This soon starts to fade and the fading is what you must watch. The area that appears reddest as this fading starts, is the major [lesion] for this patient and should be marked with a skin pencil. You will often notice on this type of patient that the major area is much wider than any other area of your lines down the back. This is caused by tissue infiltration.

The "Type 2" category SOT patient will have slightly high blood pressure after De Jarnette's preliminary treatment. After adopting the same starting position he suggests:

Making a firm pressure, draw fingers down the spine, with a fairly slow motion. You should be able to count to 15 while drawing the fingers from the 7th cervical to the coccyx, by counting steadily. With a good light on the back, the results should show a line which becomes red, some portions brighter and some very faintly coloured. Now watch the lines fade. The area which shows the whitest is marked as the major [lesion] for this is the most anaemic spinal muscle area. It will be paler than any portion of skin on the patient's body.

Moving next to the final SOT category (patients with high blood pressure), De Jarnette asks that you adopt the same start position and then:

Making heavy pressure, come down the spine slowly, counting 20 as you go from 7th cervical to coccyx. Now watch the reaction. The line that shows the whitest is the major [lesion]. In this type the blood pressure is over 180 (systolic), the whitest area shows a waxy, pale colour and may persist for several minutes.

Korr (1970) described how the red reflex phenomenon corresponded well with areas of lowered electrical resistance, which themselves correspond accurately to regions of lowered pain threshold, and areas of cutaneous and deep tenderness (termed "segmentally related sympatheticotonia"). Korr was able to detect areas of intense vasoconstriction which corresponded well with dysfunction elicited by manual clinical examination. He cautioned:

You must not look for perfect correspondence between the skin resistance (or the red reflex) and the distribution of deeper pathologic disturbance, because an area of skin which is segmentally related to a particular muscle does not necessarily over-

lie that muscle. With the latissimus dorsi, for example, the myofascial disturbance might be over the hip but the reflex manifestations would be in much higher dermatomes because this muscle has its innervation from the cervical part of the cord.

By use of a mechanical instrument which quantified the pressure applied at a constant speed, followed by measurement of the duration of the redness resulting from the action of the frictional stimulator on the skin, Korr could detect areas of intense vasoconstriction which corresponded well with dysfunction elicited by manual clinical examination.

It could be said that the opportunity to "feel" the tissues was being ignored during all these "strokes" and "drawing" of the fingers down the spinal musculature and this thought was not lost on Morrison (1969), who described his views of what he termed "induration" technique as follows.

Run your fingers longitudinally down alongside the dorsal and lumbar vertebrae (anywhere from the spinous processes extending laterally up to two inches [5 cm]) and stop at any spot of tissue which seems "harder" or different from normal tissue. These thickened areas, stringy ligaments, bunched muscle bands, all represent indurated tissue; they are usually protective and indicate irritation and dysfunction. Once these indurated areas are palpated press down and almost always they will be sensitive, indicating a need for treatment.

Morrison used methods for easing such contractions similar to those described by Lawrence Jones, in his Strain/Counterstrain system (Jones 1981).

Osteopathic researchers Cox et al. (1983) wrote regarding their work on identification of palpable musculoskeletal findings in coronary artery disease (see notes on facilitated segments in Chapter 5) and describe their use of the red reflex as part of their examination procedures (other methods included range of motion testing of spinal segments and ribs, assessment of local pain on palpation and altered soft tissue texture). In their work the most sensitive parameters, which were found to be significant predictors for coronary stenosis, were limitation in range of motion and altered soft tissue texture:

"Red reflex" cutaneous stimulation was applied digitally in both paraspinal areas [T4 and T9–11] simultaneously briskly stroking the skin in a caudad direction.

Patients were divided arbitrarily into three groups.

Grade 1 – erythema of the spinal tissues lasting less than 15 seconds after cutaneous stimulation.

Grade 2 – erythema persisting for 15 to 30 seconds after stimulation.

Grade 3 – erythema persisting longer than 30 seconds after stimulation.

In this context the Grade 3 – maintained erythema – is seen to represent the most dysfunctional response.

Roger Newman Turner (1984) describes the research of another osteopath/naturopath, Keith Lamont, who first described the "black line" phenomenon:

It is a common observation of osteopaths who use a spinal meter, to detect the most active lesions, that pressure on either side of the spine with a hemispherical probe of approximately 0.5 cm diameter, will, in some patients, elicit a dark blue or black line. The pressure of the probe is usually very light since it is intended to register variations in skin resistance (to electricity), but it has a pinching-off effect on the arterioles and venules of the capillary network beneath the skin. Local engorgement of the capillary bed with deoxygenated venous blood causes the appearance of the line which slowly fades as the circulation returns.

This is considered by some to relate to a nutrient deficit in those patients in whom this sign is seen. Newman Turner suggests that Lamont, who first drew attention to the black line phenomenon, found that administration of vitamin E, bioflavonoid complex, and homoeopathic ferrum phosphate corrected this deficiency.

Hruby et al. (1997) describe the thinking regarding this phenomenon.

> *Perform the red reflex test by firmly, but with light pressure, stroking two fingers on the skin over the paraspinal tissues in a cephalad to a caudad direction. The stroked areas briefly become erythematous and almost immediately return to their usual color.*

> *If the skin remains erythematous longer than a few seconds, it may indicate an acute somatic dysfunction in the area. As the dysfunction acquires chronic tissue changes, the tissues blanch rapidly after stroking and are dry and cool to palpation.*

You are reminded that Hilton's law confirms simultaneous innervation to the skin covering the articular insertion of the muscles, not necessarily the entire muscle. Hilton's law states that the nerve supplying a joint also supplies the muscles which move the joint and the skin covering the articular insertion of those muscles.

Making sense of the red reaction

Clearly there is a good deal to learn from and about the simple procedure of stroking the paraspinal muscles. Whether or not De Jarnette's preliminary methods are validated does not alter the possible wisdom of his subsequent observations, employing variable pressures and looking at the fading of redness, rather than the initial red reaction itself, for evidence of altered function.

Similarly, Lamont's nutritional observations would need verification, something which does not alter the fact that some patients demonstrate this unusual "black streak." As with so much in palpation, there is little question over whether "something" is being felt or observed. It is the interpretation of what the "something" means that excites debate.

The observations of Upledger, Korr, Hoag, Hruby, Morrison and McConnell (and their co-workers) are readily applicable and should be tested against known dysfunction to assess the usefulness of these methods during assessment.

The research of Cox et al. indicates that one musculoskeletal assessment method alone is probably not sufficiently reliable to be diagnostic; however, when, for example, tissue texture, changes in range of motion, pain and the "red reaction" are all used, the presence of several of these is a good indication of underlying dysfunction which may involve the process of facilitation. This supports the thoughts expressed in Chapter 1.

A simpler use for the reaction

A less complex use of the red reaction is to go back more than a century to McConnell's method, in order to highlight spinal deviations. By creating erythema paraspinally you can stand back and visualize the general contours of the spine as well as any local deviations in the pattern created by application of your firm digital strokes.

Question

How do you know whether your palpating fingers or thumbs are applying equal pressure bilaterally during such assessments, or when palpating elsewhere bilaterally? A useful guide to the uniformity of pressure can be obtained by comparing the relative blanching of your nailbeds: are they equally white, pink, red?

Special topic exercise 7.1 **Red Reflex Assessment**

Time suggested: 20 minutes

- Perform the various "strokes," as described above.
- Run your fingers or probes firmly down the tissues close to, and parallel to, the spine.

- Observe the "red reaction" as well as how it fades.

- Look for areas which become more irritated and those that become less irritated when compared with surrounding tissues.

Having marked the ones that respond most dramatically, and those that fade fastest, repalpate the tissues using some or all of the methods discussed in Chapters 4, 5, 6 and 8, in order to evaluate what it is you sense as being different about the tissues.

- Do tissues which seem hypertonic respond to brisk stroking of this sort differently to normal or more flaccid tissues?

- Do you note increased sensitivity in areas which redden or blanch when stroked in this way or is there little difference?

- How does the degree of skin "tightness" vary over these different areas?

- What is the degree of skin adherence to underlying connective tissue (when skin rolling or lifting) in the different areas?

- If you scan from off the body, can you sense differences in temperature in these contrasting areas?

- Is eliciting of the "red reflex" likely to be of any clinical value to you?

References

Cox J, Gorbis S, Dick L and Rogers J (1983) Palpable musculoskeletal findings in coronary artery disease (double blind study). Journal of the American Osteopathic Association 82 (11): 832.

De Jarnette B (1934) Reflex pain. Nebraska City, NB: privately published.

Hoag M (1969) Osteopathic medicine. New York: McGraw-Hill.

Hruby R, Goodridge J and Jones J (1997) Thoracic region and rib cage, in Ward R (ed) Foundations for osteopathic medicine. Baltimore: Williams and Wilkins.

Jones L (1981) Strain/counterstrain. Colorado Springs, CO: Academy of Applied Osteopathy.

Korr I (1970) The physiological basis of osteopathic medicine. New York: Postgraduate Institute of Osteopathic Medicine and Surgery.

McConnell C (1899) The practice of osteopathy. Kirksville, MO: Journal Printing Company.

Morrison M (1969) Lecture notes. Presentation/seminar, Research Society for Naturopathy, British College of Osteopathic Medicine, London.

Newman Turner R 1984 Naturopathic medicine. Wellingborough: Thorsons.

Upledger J and Vredevoogd W (1983) Craniosacral therapy. Seattle: Eastland Press.

Special topic 8

Percussion palpation and treatment
Leon Chaitow

There are a variety of percussion approaches, some of which are discussed below (Miller-Keane and O'Toole 2006):

- *Auscultatory percussion*: auscultation of the sound (dull resonance) produced by percussion against a *pleximeter* (layer of material such as plastic on the body surface, or the examiner's finger of the other hand (*plexor*)). This process is also known as *mediate or indirect percussion*.

- The *pleximeter* is usually the middle finger of the examiner's left hand (if right hand dominant) which is firmly applied to the area being assessed (chest wall, liver area, etc.) so as to displace any air between it and the body. The pleximeter is moved in order to evaluate different areas, for example lower border of the liver.

- The distal phalanx is struck repetitively (not on the nail), with the plexor effort deriving from a wrist motion rather than the whole forearm.

- *Immediate or direct percussion*: in which the percussion is against the body surface rather than a pleximeter. This is also used therapeutically in *spondylotherapy* and *percussive trigger point* treatment, as described below.

- *Palpatory percussion* is a combination of palpation and percussion offering tactile, rather than a purely auditory effect.

How valid is this method?

With modern technology (ultrasound imaging, for example) it may be thought that "old fashioned" methods such as this have been consigned to history. The following examples demonstrate that this is not the case.

Skrainka and colleagues (1986) reported:

- *In 75 hospital patients an estimation of liver span was made independently by students, fellows, and consultants. These bedside estimates were made three times at full inspiration in a right parasagittal line one third of the sternal length from the midline by palpation, direct, and indirect percussion. These bedside estimates were compared to each other and to ultrasound in full inspiration in the supine position and to scintiscan in quiet respiration.*

- *We found that bedside estimate of liver span by direct percussion was as accurate as ultrasound, but that indirect percussion estimate of liver span was inaccurate. Scintiscanning during quiet respiration over-estimates the liver span in comparison to ultrasound. Previous suggestions that clinical estimates of liver span should be abandoned may be in error.*

Gilbert (1996) has reported:

- The comparative value of palpation, light percussion, and auscultatory percussion for detecting the liver below the costal margin was studied in 45 normal subjects and 20 patients.

- The presence of the liver 2 cm or more below the costal margin was considered abnormal, since this organ was found no more than 1 cm below in a few normal subjects *only by auscultatory percussion*.

- In the patient group, auscultatory percussion detected the liver of 12; four livers and one case of gallbladder-hydrops were detected only by this method.

- Also, auscultation behind the right flank during percussion identified one hydronephrotic kidney.

- The liver was detected by palpation in 12 patients and was found only by this method in 6 of them.

- Light percussion detected the liver in only 6 patients, but was useful in 2 for determining that the liver dome had been depressed in the rib cage. Results of liver function tests were abnormal in 15.

- These findings suggest that these methods were valuable for detecting liver diseases in patients.

What percussive sounds "mean"

Percussion as a means of defining the position, and to some extent the status, of organs has a long history, with major variations in its use in Western and Oriental traditions of medicine. A wide range of sounds may be heard when percussion is employed and their interpretation has been described in numerous medical texts, but in few more thoroughly than in that of Sir Robert Hutchinson (1897), published over a century ago and still in print.

He described in detail the ways in which percussion examination can determine organ boundaries, as well as the normal and abnormal variations in resonance of individual organs. For example, in discussing thoracic percussion he describes both quantitative (ranging from hyperresonance to absolute dullness) and qualitative sound differences (various tympanic pitches, skodaic, boxy, cracked-pot, bell-sound/coin percussion, amphoric, etc.). Each of the qualitative variations is of potential diagnostic and prognostic value as it is interpreted in relation to other information available to the examiner.

Variations in sound will depend upon the relative solidity or hollowness, as well as the shape of the palpated organ, the nature and degree of intervening tissues, whether these are of bone, muscle, fat or other soft tissues, and the amount of air in the tissues being evaluated, as well as the manner in which percussion is applied (Special topic Figs 8.1 and 8.2).

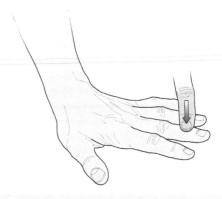

Figure ST 8.1
Distal phalanx position held horizontal against surface being evaluated.

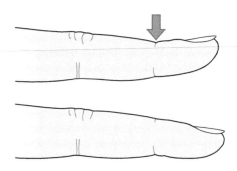

Figure ST 8.2
The arrow represents the ideal point to be struck for optimal *therapeutic* percussion efficiency, in this case using the pisiform area of the hand instead of another finger (Abrams 1910).

Method

- Hutchinson suggests that the middle finger of the left hand be used as a pleximeter.

- This is laid firmly on the tissues to be percussed, so that no air intervenes between finger and skin.

- The middle finger of the right hand then strikes this.

- The pleximeter finger can also be useful as a source of information regarding tissue resistance during percussion.

The back of the middle phalanx (of the left middle finger) is struck with the tip of the middle finger of the right hand. The stroke should be delivered from the wrist and finger-joints and not the elbow, and the percussing finger should be so bent that when the blow is delivered its terminal phalanx is at right angles to the metacarpal bones, and strikes the pleximeter perpendicularly. As soon as the blow has been given, the striking finger must be raised, lest it should impair the vibrations it has excited, just as the hammers of a piano fall back from the wires as soon as these have been struck. In cases where percussion requires to be firmer, several fingers may be used; but it is better, whenever possible to employ only one percussing finger … It is seldom necessary to deliver more than two or three strokes at any one situation. The points to be noted on percussion are the volume and pitch of the resonance elicited, and the sense of resistance experienced by the finger.

There are three cardinal percussion rules, states Hutchinson:

1. *The first is that in defining the boundaries between contiguous organs the percussion should invariably be performed from the resonant [more hollow] towards the less resonant [more solid].*

2. *The second is that the longer axis of the pleximeter [finger] should be parallel to the edge of the organ whose delimitation is being attempted, and the line of percussion should be at right angles to that edge.*

3. *The third is that the pleximeter finger must be kept in firm contact with the tissues [being evaluated].*

In abdominal percussion, Hutchinson tells us that the pitch we hear depends upon the depth of the air space, and the tension of the containing wall, of the organ, and that these two important elements vary greatly in the same viscus at different times.

For example, the presence of free gas in the peritoneal cavity causes the normal dullness elicited in liver or spleen percussion to disappear. If abnormal dullness is detected we need to find out whether this is constant in all positions or whether it shifts when the position of the patient is altered, something of particular importance if an unnatural degree of fluid presence is suspected, as in ascites. He gives the example of an unusual distension of the abdomen which could result from gas, ascites or a new growth. Both a tumor and fluid would produce a dull percussion sound, but the fluid would move (and the sound would therefore change) if the patient's position were altered, while the tumor would not.

*Special topic Exercise 8.1 **Practicing Percussion to Define the Upper and Lower Borders of the Liver***

Time suggested: 10–12 minutes

To perceive liver dullness, it is suggested that the person being palpated/percussed should be supine for anterior percussion, and seated or standing for posterior percussion.

- Percuss from the second rib downwards, to get a good lung note.

- Percuss down from rib to rib till a duller sound is detected – then repeat the process, going from space to space instead of from rib to rib.

- Percuss in this way down the mammary, midaxillary, and scapular lines.

- The upper limit of liver dullness, in the middle line, cannot be distinguished from heart dullness.

- To map it out, draw a straight line from the apex beat, to the angle where the right edge of the heart and the deep liver dullness meet.

- The upper limit of liver dullness forms an almost horizontal line around the chest.

- In defining the lower border of the liver, use very light percussion and pass upwards.

- The exact position of the lower edge of the liver is extremely variable. Usually it coincides with the costal margin in the mammary line, but may be considerably above or below this without there being any pathological change in the organ.

- In percussing the surface of the liver, where it is not covered by the lung, note that the organ has a certain degree of resistance or resilience. The normal amount of this can only be learned by practice.

- If the organ is enlarged or congested, its resistance to percussion is increased, owing to its being more firmly pressed against the chest wall.

- Percuss the liver as suggested – can you define its borders?

Therapeutic percussion

Percussion is a form of palpation that deserves to be more widely used, and the use of percussion therapeutically is a natural extension of the acquisition of this skill – aspects of which are described below.

Orthopedic/neurological percussion

In orthopedic diagnosis certain neurological problems rely for initial assessment on percussion methods. For example Tinel's sign can be elicited over any nerve root, trunk, or cord of the brachial plexus, or peripheral nerve, where they can be palpated.

In cases of carpal tunnel syndrome Tinel's test is performed by tapping the median nerve along its course in the wrist. A positive test is noted when this causes worsening of the tingling in the fingers when the nerve is tapped.

Spondylotherapy

Percussion has been used as a means of manual treatment and diagnosis for many years. The first major definitive study of the therapeutic use was that of Albert Abrams (of "Black Box" fame) whose vast text *Spondylotherapy* was first published in 1910 (Abrams 1910). The preface to that book tells us that:

In spondylotherapy the employment of mechanical vibration fills one of the most useful roles in therapeutics. It is easily controlled and is practical and effective of application in the hands of those familiar with the methods for employing spinal percussion.

Abrams described how he applied the percussive force:

For simple concussion employ a piece of soft rubber or linoleum about 6 inches [15 cm] long, 1.5 inches [4 cm] wide and about a quarter of an inch [0.5 cm] in thickness, as a pleximeter for receiving the stroke, and a plexor with a large rubber head for delivering the blow … One may also strike the spinous process with the knuckles, or better still the fingers may be used as a pleximeter and the clenched fist as a plexor … [Ideally] the strip of linoleum is applied to the spinous process or processes to be concussed, and with hammer a series of sharp and vigorous blows are allowed to fall on the pleximeter. Naturally the blows jar the patient somewhat, but beyond this no inconvenience is suffered.

CAUTION: Neither the degree of effort nor the instruments suggested by Abrams are recommended – they are reported purely out of historical interest.

Some years later, Johnson (1939) described the use of the hand or a mechanical instrument to apply percussive vibrations, "which are only effective when applied with sufficient rapidity."

Spondylotherapy (spinal percussion)

Contraindications:

- osteoporosis
- malignancy
- inflammation in the area to be treated
- recent trauma in the area to be treated
- pain during application of percussive treatment.

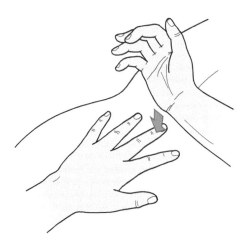

Figure ST 8.3
Percussion for reflexive effects –
spondylotherapy.

In order to stimulate organs via the spinal pathways, direct percussion techniques have long been employed by osteopathic and chiropractic practitioners. Over the past century in the USA a number of mechanical methods of percussion have evolved (Abrams 1910), as have effective manual systems in which the middle finger is placed on the appropriate spinous process(es), whilst the other hand concusses the finger with a series of rapidly rebounding blows.

This approach is known as spondylotherapy (Johnson 1939) (Special topic Fig. 8.3).

One or two percussive repetitions are applied per second. Spondylotherapy percussion is usually applied to a series of three or four (or more) adjacent vertebrae. An example of this is the treatment, as described above, of the fifth thoracic spinous process, proceeding downwards to the ninth, in the case of liver dysfunction. Treatment would only be applied if the area was painful to palpating pressure. Similarly, concussion over the 10th, 11th and 12th thoracic spinous processes would stimulate kidney function.

In order to stimulate the organ or tissues using the spinal reflexes, percussion would involve only a short amount of time: 15–30 second applications, repeated three or four times, over approximately 4–5 minutes. A mild *"flare-up"* of symptoms, and increased sensitivity in the area treated, would normally indicate that the desired degree of stimulation had been achieved.

In order to *inhibit* function, or to produce dilation of local blood vessels, Johnson (1939) suggests that percussive repetitions would be repeated for prolonged periods, in order to fatigue the reflex.

Trigger point percussion technique

Trigger points can effectively be treated using a series of percussive strokes, according to Travell and Simons (1992). They state:

1. The muscle should be lengthened to the point of onset of passive resistance.

2. The clinician or patient uses a hard rubber mallet, or reflex hammer, to hit the trigger point at precisely the same place approximately 10 times.

3. This should be done at a slow rate of no more than one impact per second, but at least one impact every 5 seconds; the slower rates are likely to be more effective.

Travell and Simons suggest that this enhances, or substitutes for, intermittent cold with stretch ("spray and stretch") methods.

The muscles that they list as benefiting most from percussion techniques include quadratus, brachioradialis, long finger extensors, and peroneus longus and brevis.

CAUTION: It is specifically suggested that the anterior and posterior compartment of the leg muscle should not be treated by percussion, due to the risk of compartment syndrome, should bleeding occur in the muscle.

TCM percussion

Contraindications:

- acute disease
- severe heart disease
- tuberculosis
- malignant tumors
- hemorrhagic disease
- skin disease in area to be treated
- poor constitutional states such as malnutrition or asthenia.

Chinese research involving percussion has dramatically added to our knowledge of the potential of these methods (Zhao-Pu 1991). In Traditional Chinese Medicine (TCM), percussion methods are incorporated into a broad heading of "acupressure."

Zhao-Pu states: "Acupressure is based on the same theory as acupuncture and uses the same points and meridians. The therapeutic effect of acupressure technique lies in the way in which it regulates and normalizes blocked functions." Included in these functions (as well as hypothesized energy transmission) are: "stimulating circulation of blood … and improving conductivity of nerves."

In TCM, percussion techniques involve one of three variations.

1. one-finger percussion using the middle finger braced by the thumb and index finger
2. three-finger percussion using the thumb, index, and middle fingers
3. five-finger percussion using the thumb and all fingers.

The degree of force applied during TCM percussion is also divided into three.

1. light, which involves a movement of the hand from the wrist joint
2. medium, which involves a movement from the elbow joint with wrist fairly rigid
3. strong, which involves a movement of the upper arm, from the shoulder, with a rigid wrist.

Treatment is offered daily, on alternate days, or once in 3 days, and a course would involve 20 sessions. Patients often receive three courses or more.

Zhao-Pu describes remarkable clinical results in patients with paralysis and cerebral birth injuries. He states:

> Research was carried out on the cerebral haemodynamics of patients with cerebral birth injury before and after acupressure (percussion and pressure techniques) therapy. Scanning techniques were used in monitoring the short half-life radioactive materials through the cerebral circulation; in almost one-third of the patients the regional cerebral blood flow was increased after acupressure therapy ranging from 28 to 60 sessions.

This approach does not produce instant results but attempts to influence, and gradually harness, the potential for recovery and improvement latent in the tissues of the patient. For more information on Oriental bodywork approaches, a complete manual of Chinese therapeutic massage (with many aspects which echo NMT methodology) edited by Sun Chengnan is highly recommended (Chengnan 1990).

References

Abrams A (1910) Spondylotherapy. San Francisco, CA: Philopolis Press.

Chengnan S (1990) Chinese bodywork. Berkeley, CA: Pacific View Press.

Gilbert VE (1996) Detection of the liver below the costal margin: Comparative value of palpation, light percussion, and auscultatory percussion. Southern Medical Journal 87 (2): 182–186.

Hutchinson R (1897) Clinical methods. London: Cassel and Company.

Johnson A (1939) Principles and practice of drugless therapeutics. Los Angeles, CA: Chiropractic Educational Extension Bureau.

Miller-Keane and O'Toole MT (2006) Miller-Keane Encyclopedia and dictionary of medicine, nursing and allied health, revised reprint, 7th edn. Philadelphia, PA: Saunders Philadelphia.

Skrainka B, Stahlhut J, Fulbeck CL, Knight F, Holmes RA and Butt JH (1986) Measuring liver span. Bedside examination versus ultrasound and scintiscan. Journal of Clinical Gastroenterology 8 (3/1): 267–270.

Travell J, Simons D (1992) Myofascial pain and dysfunction, vol 2. Baltimore: Williams and Wilkins.

Zhao-Pu W (1991) Acupressure therapy. Edinburgh: Churchill Livingstone.

Special topic 9

Joint play/"end-feel"/ range of motion: what are they?

Leon Chaitow

Joint play refers to the particular movements between bones associated with either separation of the surfaces (as in traction) or parallel movement of joint surfaces (also known as translation or translatoric gliding). Some degree of such movement is possible between most joints, restricted only by the degree of soft tissue elasticity. Any change in length of such soft tissues, therefore, automatically alters the range of joint mobility – also known as the degree of "slack" – that is available.

Joint separation or "degrees of traction"

Grades can be ascribed to the range of separation possible between joint surfaces:

- When traction is applied to a joint (at right angles to the joint surface) a slight separation, merely removing the intrinsic compressive force of surrounding tissues, is known as a Grade I degree of traction.

- When the "slack" is removed by further separation, tightening the surrounding tissues, this is a Grade II degree of traction.

- This increases to a Grade III when actual stretch of the tissues is introduced or attempted.

Glide or translation

When a gliding translation between joint surfaces occurs, this takes place with the surfaces parallel to each other (also called "rollgliding") (Special topic Fig. 9.1).

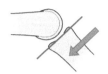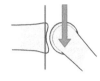

Figure ST 9.1
Parallel displacement of a bone involving translatoric gliding (after Kaltenborn). One bone is moved parallel to the treatment plane until the tissues surrounding the joint are tightened (Grade II) or the tissues crossing the joint are stretched (Grade III).

Only a portion of the joint will be able to move parallel with its opposing surface in this way, at any given time. Since the surfaces of joints are never completely flat, only one part is parallel with the other at any moment (technically this is described as due to the surfaces being incongruent).

Once again grading is possible:

- A Grade I glide involves slack being taken up and a degree of tightening of the soft tissues as barriers engage during translation.

- Grade II involves actual stretching (or attempted stretching) of these soft tissues, as translation continues.

Convex and concave rule

An important rule, relating to whether the joint surface is concave or convex, was described by Kaltenborn (1985). This states:

- If a *concave surface* moves in relation to another surface, then the direction of gliding and the direction of the movement of the bone are the same. This means that the moving bone and the concave surface of the joint are on the same side as the axis of motion (Special topic Fig. 9.2).

However:

• When a *convex joint surface* is in a gliding motion, the bone movement will be in the opposite direction to the glide. This means that the mov-

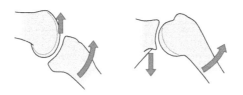

Figure ST 9.2
The direction of gliding in a joint depends upon whether the surface on which movement is occurring is concave or convex. If concave gliding occurs it is in the same direction as the bone movement (left) while convex gliding occurs in the opposite direction to the movement of the bone (right) (after Kaltenborn).

ing surface and the bone lie on opposite sides of the axis of rotation.

Therefore, when there is a joint restriction, ascertained by careful assessment of joint play (i.e., an attempt at gliding), it is essential to know the relative shape of the articulation.

• In the case of a *convex joint surface* (e.g., the *head of the humerus*) the bone will need to be moved by the therapist in a direction opposite to the direction of restricted bone motion, in order to increase or improve the range of motion in the joint.

• In the case of a *concave joint surface* (e.g., the *proximal head of the ulna*) the bone will need to be moved in the same direction as the direction of restriction of bone movement, in order to improve the range of motion in the joint (Special topic Fig. 9.3).

Importance of joint play

Just how vital joint play is to the body is made clear in the example given by Kuchera and Kuchera (1994), discussing the subtalar joint. This is a "shock-absorber," a

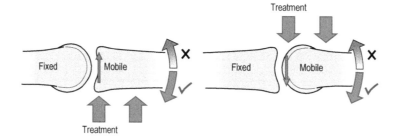

Figure ST 9.3
This figure illustrates the "convex–concave rule" in which a mobile bone moves on a fixed structure. *Left*: The joint surface is concave (as would be the case in the tibia, ulna, or a phalangeal joint). If the mobile bone was restricted in an upward direction (gray arrow), a gliding mobilization made during treatment would also be in an upward direction (as indicated by the two large arrows). *Right*: There is a mobile bone associated with a convex surface (as in the head of the humerus, the femur or talus). If this was restricted in an upward direction (gray arrow), a gliding mobilization made in treatment would be in a downward direction (large arrows) (after Kaltenborn).

designation earned, they say, because "in coordination with the intertarsal joints, it determines the distribution of forces upon the skeleton and soft tissues of the foot."

Mennell (1964) graphically describes this shock-absorbing potential:

Its most important movement is a rocking movement of the talus upon the calcaneus, which is entirely independent of voluntary muscle action. It is this movement which takes up all the stresses and strains of stubbing the toes, and that spares the ankle from gross trauma, both on toe-off and at heel-strike, in the normal function of walking, and when abnormal stresses … are inflicted on the ankle joint. If it were not for the involuntary rocking motion at the subtalar joint, fracture dislocations would be more commonplace.

Similar shock-absorbing potential exists at the sacroiliac joint (SI) which, when this is lost, as in cases where the joint has fused, can result in fractures of the sacrum (Greenman 1996).

Suggestions:

1. See discussion of "form and force" closure of the SI joint in Chapter 8.

2. See Smith's views on what he terms "foundational joints" which cannot be moved voluntarily – in Chapter 14.

Barriers

All joints have "normal" ranges of motion and palpation assessment should involve a screening of these for abnormal restriction or for hypermobility. The end of a joint's range of motion may be described as having a certain feel, and this is called "end-feel" (Special topic Fig. 9.4).

- When a joint is taken actively or passively to its end of range of normal motion, a point at which resistance is noted, it will have reached its *physiological* barrier. This has a firm but not harsh end-feel.

- Before it reaches that barrier it should be possible to recognize the very beginning of the end

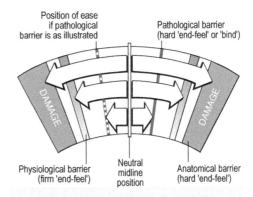

Figure ST 9.4
Schematic representation of a range of motion indicating normal restriction barriers (anatomical and physiological) as well as a pathological barrier and a position of maximal ease. The quality of the "end-feel" of each of these will vary markedly.

of range of free movement. In osteopathy this is called the "feather-edge of the barrier," where easy motion ceases and some effort is required to move the joint further (see mention of this in Chapter 5, Exercise 5.15).

- In essence once a first barrier to free movement is perceived during assessment/palpation, the barrier has been passed, and tissues will already be being loaded.

- If movement progresses past the "easy" *physiological* barrier, to its absolute limit, the anatomical barrier will have been engaged. This has a hard end-feel, beyond which any movement is likely to cause damage or irritation.

- If there is, for any reason, a restriction in the range of motion, then a *pathological* barrier would be apparent on active or passive movement in that direction.

If the reasons for the restriction involved interosseous changes (e.g., arthritis) the end-feel would be sudden or harsh. However, if – as is more usually the case – the restriction involves soft tissue dysfunction the end-feel would have a softer nature. See the views of Kappler and Jones (2003) in Special topic 6.

Kaltenborn summarizes *normal end-feel* variations thus:

- Normal soft end-feel is due to soft tissue approximation (such as in knee flexion) or soft tissue stretching (as in ankle dorsiflexion).

- Normal firm end-feel results from capsular or ligamentous stretching (internal rotation of the femur, for example).

- Normal hard end-feel occurs when bone meets bone, as in elbow extension.

However, *pathological end-feel* can involve a number of variations such as:

- a firmer, less elastic feel when scar tissue restricts movement or when shortened (dense or fibrosed) connective tissue exists

- an elastic, less soft end-feel when increased muscle tonus restricts movement

- an empty end-feel in which the patient stops the movement (or asks for it to be stopped) before a true end-feel is reached, as a result of extreme pain (fracture or active inflammation) or psychogenic factors.

Hypermobile joints

Ligaments and muscles that are hypermobile do not adequately protect joints, and therefore fail to prevent excessive ranges of motion from being achieved. Without this stability, overuse and injury stresses evolve, and muscular overuse is inevitable. Janda (1984) observes that in his experience: "In races in which hypermobility is common there is a prevalence of muscular and tendon pain, whereas typical back pain or sciatica are rare."

Logically, the excessive work rate of muscles that are adopting the role of "pseudoligaments" leads to tendon stress and muscle dysfunction, increasing tone in the antagonists of whatever is already weakened,

so complicating an already complex set of imbalances, including altered patterns of movement (Beighton et al. 1983).

What to do with abnormal barriers when you find them

One objective of palpation of restrictions is to define the degree of limitation by establishing the range of motion in various directions. Another is assessment of the nature of those restrictions through, among other factors, determination of the softness or hardness of the end-feel.

Some manipulative techniques involve engaging the pathological barrier before any of a variety of methods are employed to increase the range of motion – pushing the barrier back, so to speak. This might involve the use of isometric contractions of the agonist (shortened muscle or group of muscles) or of their antagonists, as in muscle energy technique (MET), or it might involve active high-velocity thrust (HVT) adjustment/manipulation, as in chiropractic and some osteopathic treatment. Or it might involve mobilization, using long leverage or use of joint play techniques.

A different approach would be to move towards the direction, opposite the direction of restriction, easing away from the barrier(s) of restriction, as in functional osteopathic techniques such as Strain/Counterstrain (see Chapter 5).

Whichever approach is used, there remains the importance of knowing how to "feel" the end of range of motion in any direction, without provoking sensitive tissues further. Practicing on normal tissues and joints makes recognition of restricted ones simpler. Kaltenborn states: "The ability to see and feel the quality of movement is of special significance in manual therapy, as slight alterations from the normal may often be the only clue to a correct diagnosis."

Active and passive movements

If pain occurs anywhere in a range of movement (active or passive) which is both preceded and followed by pain-free motion, the range in which the pain is noted is called a *painful arc*. Deviations of normal pathways during such a painful arc indicate avoidance strategies, and are important diagnostically.

As a rule, active movements test all anatomical structures as well as the psychological willingness of the patient to move the area. Passive movements test only non-contractile tissues, with such movements being compared with accepted norms as well as the corresponding opposite joint. End-feel, painful arcs, shortened muscles, restricted or exaggerated joint function are all assessed in this way. As a general rule, a greater degree of motion is achieved passively rather than actively.

Many of the exercises in Chapter 8 will provide the opportunity for you to refine your skills in "reading" end-feel.

Special topic Exercise 9.1 *Assessing Joint Play at the Proximal Tibiofibular Joint*

Time suggested: 3–4 minutes

- Your palpation partner should be supine with hip and knee flexed, so that the sole of the foot is flat on the table.

- You sit so that your buttock rests on the patient's toes, stabilizing the foot to the table.

- The head of the fibula is grasped between thumb and index finger of one hand, as the other hand holds the tibia firmly, inferior to the patella.

- Care should be taken to avoid excessive pressure on the posterior aspect of the fibula head, as the peroneal nerve lies close by (Kuchera & Goodridge 1997).

- The thumb, resting on the anterior surface of the fibula, should be reinforced by placing the thumb of the other hand over it.

- A movement that takes the fibular head firmly posteriorly and anteriorly, in a slightly curved

manner (i.e., not quite a straight backward and forward movement, but more back and slightly curving inferiorly, followed by forward and slightly curving superiorly, at an angle of approximately 30°), determines whether there is freedom of joint glide in each direction.

If restriction is noted in either direction, repetitive rhythmical – but gentle – springing of the fibula, at the end of its range, should restore normal joint play.

It is worth noting that when the fibular head glides anteriorly there is automatic reciprocal movement posteriorly at the distal fibula (lateral malleolus), while posterior glide of the fibula head results in anterior movement of the distal fibula. Restrictions at the distal fibula are, therefore, likely to influence behavior proximally and vice versa.

- Are you able to feel the glide?

References

Beighton P, Grahame R and Bird H (1983) Hypermobility of joints. Berlin: Springer Verlag.

Greenman P (1996) Principles of manual medicine, 2nd edn. Baltimore: Williams and Wilkins.

Janda V (1984) Low back pain – trends, controversies. Presentation, Turku, Finland, 3–4 September.

Kaltenborn F (1985) Mobilization of the extremity joints. Oslo: Olaf Norlis Bokhandel.

Kappler RE and Jones JM (2003) Thrust (high-velocity/low-amplitude) techniques, in Ward RC (ed) Foundations for osteopathic medicine, 2nd edn. Philadelphia, PA: Lippincott, Williams and Wilkins, pp 852–880.

Kuchera M and Goodridge J (1997) Lower extremity, in Ward R (ed) Foundations for osteopathic medicine. Baltimore, MD: Williams and Wilkins.

Kuchera W and Kuchera M (1994) Osteopathic principles in practice. Columbus, OH: Greyden Press.

Mennell J (1964) Joint pain. Boston, MA: T and A Churchill.

Before starting on the exploration of joint palpation and assessment, it is worth reflecting on the advice of several osteopathic authorities. Their words are designed to make us think outside of the obvious ... although once reflected on, and accepted, the advice should hopefully become obvious!

Kappler and Jones (2003) have attempted to define the nature of what it is that we are feeling, when a restriction barrier is noted during assessment of a joint:

As the barrier is engaged, increasing amounts of force are necessary and the distance decreases. The term barrier may be misleading if it is interpreted as a wall or rigid obstacle to be overcome with a push. As the joint reaches the barrier, restraints in the form of tight muscles and fascia, serve to inhibit further motion. We are pulling against restraints rather than pushing against some anatomic structure.

Mitchell (1998) makes a similarly thought-provoking observation:

Treating a joint motion restriction as if the cause were tight muscle(s) helps to restore normal joint motion.

Regardless of the cause of restriction ... treatment, based on a "short muscle" paradigm, is usually completely effective in eliminating blockage, and restoring normal range of motion, even when the blockage is due to non-muscular factors.

The assessment of the functional integrity, or otherwise, of joints has been exhaustively covered in many osteopathic, orthopedic, and chiropractic textbooks over the past century or more. The intent in this chapter is not to duplicate such information, but rather to summarize some important elements of joint palpation, together with the provision of guides as to what some "normal" ranges of motion might be expected to be, and how to assess these.

In addition, some novel, sequential assessment approaches will be covered, as will an approach, developed in the context of osteopathic medicine, that claims to evaluate the *current degree* of structural adaptive potential of the individual (Zink & Lawson 1979).

Serious students of joint palpation should seek elsewhere for more comprehensive descriptions of clinical joint assessments, as well as studying Whitney Lowe's orthopedic assessment discussions, in Chapter 9.

Observe, palpate, actively and passively test

Dysfunction of joints can be demonstrated in three different ways, all of which form part of a comprehensive assessment of the musculoskeletal system:

1. observation

2. palpation

3. testing of function (which is itself separated into active and passive movements).

We have already seen in earlier chapters that there exist useful sequential screening approaches for uncovering evidence of shortened muscles (e.g., see Chapter 5 for postural muscle screening), or changes within those muscles (such as NMT assessment, Nimmo's method, etc.).

Mitchell et al. (1979) provide further useful guidance on succinct methods for eliciting information as to where to focus attention or where more detailed examination is required. Such an approach is necessary, since it is patently impossible during any normal consultation examination to cover each and every muscle, joint and test. As Mitchell puts it: "The purpose ... is to identify a body region, or body regions, which deserve(s) more detailed evaluation."

Notes

Each of the segments and numbered exercises below can be seen as individual opportunities for developing and practicing palpation and observational skills. Note that not all joints, or their functions, are covered, since this book is not meant to provide detailed instruction in structural and functional analysis, but rather to *enhance the skills* needed to do so.

Symptoms

When palpating and assessing dysfunction it is important to identify what eases symptoms, as well as what aggravates them, as this may reveal patterns that "load" and "unload" the biomechanical and neurophysiological features, out of which so many symptoms emerge.

The patient's own viewpoint as to what helps and what worsens symptoms, as well as the practitioner's evaluation as to where restrictions and abnormal tissue states may exist, and how dysfunction manifests during standard testing and palpation, should, together with the history, form the basis for arriving at a provisional judgment as to the nature of the dysfunction being assessed. Such a judgment does not necessarily mean that a diagnosis has been made, only that a working hypothesis has been formulated, based on a mix of objective and subjective evidence.

Repetitions are important

In performing assessments (testing a shoulder for internal rotation, for example), if a particular action produces no symptom, it may be useful to have the movement performed a number of times. As Jacob and McKenzie (1996) explain: "Standard range of motion examinations and orthopedic tests do not adequately explore how the particular patient's spinal [or other area of the body] mechanics and symptoms are affected by specific movements and/or positioning."

Perhaps the greatest limitation of many examinations and tests is the supposition that each test movement needs to be performed only once in order to fathom how the patient's complaint responds. The effects of repetitive movements, or positions maintained for varying periods of time, may best approximate what occurs in the "real world".

Assessments should evaluate symptoms in relation to posture and position, as well as to function or movement. Function needs to be evaluated in relation to quality, as well as symmetry, and the ranges (and quality) of movement involved (see Chapters 9 and 10).

Any assessment needs to take account of the gender, age, body type, and health status of the person being assessed, as all these factors can influence a comparison with the "norm." Attention should also be paid to the effect of movement on symptoms (does it hurt more or less when a particular movement is performed?), as well as to the degree of functional normality revealed by the movement.

Exercise 8.1 *Observation of the Patient*

Time suggested 10–12 minutes (reducing to 3–5 minutes with practice)

Observe your palpation partner walking, both slowly and briskly. Look for:

1. normal and equal length of stride

2. good weight transfer from heel to lateral foot, to metatarsal joints, with a push-off from the big toe

3. evidence of external or internal rotation of the legs

4. normal flexion and extension of hips, knees and ankles.

Pay particular attention to the presence, or otherwise, of a well-developed arch during mid-stride on the weight-bearing foot.

Normal gait should involve the following.

- Weight placed evenly on each foot.

- Pelvis virtually horizontal, with a slight sway being normal (more so in women).

- The spinal column curves, when observed from behind, should move from side to side, in a wave-like manner, with the greatest range in the mid-lumbar area.

- The thoracolumbar junction should remain above the sacrum at all times (see notes on long leg/short leg later in this chapter).

- A swing of the arms should come from the shoulder with little head motion.

- Asymmetry of arm position.

- The upper shoulder fixators should appear relaxed.

Overall you should look for:

1. asymmetrical patterns, stiffness, and any tendency to rock or limp

2. symmetrical levels of knees and malleoli

3. morphological asymmetries – scars, bruises, etc.

Exercise 8.1 *Continued*

Lewit (1992) suggests listening to the sounds made as the patient walks. He also points out that "certain faults become more marked if the patient closes her eyes, walks on tiptoe or on the heels, and these should be examined as required."

Always ask patients to adopt their typical work posture as part of the evaluation.

Try to read any body language that hints at unresolved or somatized emotional issues – inhibited/withdrawn, extrovert, "military," depressed, or other stereotypical postures.

Record all findings.

Exercise 8.2 *Postural Observation – Posterior and Lateral Aspects*

Time suggested   **10–12 minutes (reducing to 3–5 with practice)**

Posture should then be viewed from behind, attention being given to:

- head balance (are ear lobes at the same height?)
- neck and shoulder symmetry
- levels of scapulae
- any lateral spine curves
- the distance the arms hang from the side of the body
- the levels of the folds at waist level (are they symmetrical?)
- gluteal folds (are they the same height from the floor?)
- morphological changes.

The side view is then examined for:

- normality of anteroposterior spinal curves
- head position relative to the body
- abdominal ptosis
- winging of the scapulae
- the angle of the feet
- morphological changes.

Record and chart all findings.

Exercise 8.3 *Postural Observations and Range of Spinal motion*

Time suggested   **10–12 minutes (reducing to 3–5 with practice)**

Posture and symmetry are then observed from the front and the following are observed and recorded, evaluating symmetry or otherwise of:

- stance (foot placement)
- patella height
- intercostal angle
- clavicles.

The side view is then evaluated again.

- Is the head/center of gravity over the body or forward or backwards of it?

The person is asked to bend backwards – range should be around 35°, with a sharp bend at the lumbosacral junction or at the thoracolumbar junction (in cases of increased mobility).

Anteflexion has a normal range of around 60° when the knees are extended.

Hamstring shortness affects this test so seated anteflexion is a more accurate assessment of lumbar flexibility.

Side bending, with strict care that no ante- or retroflexion accompanies this, should achieve a range of 20° to each side.

Note that hypermobility of the lumbar spine is, according to Lewit (1992), indicated most strongly by hyperlordosis when standing relaxed, together with exaggerated lumbar kyphosis when sitting relaxed.

Record all findings.

Exercise 8.4 *Crest Height Palpation*

Time suggested   **2–4 minutes**

The barefoot person stands erect, with back to you (your eyes at the level of the iliac crests).

Feet should be a little apart, ankles directly below the hip sockets (heels 10–15 cm (4–6 inches) apart), toes pointing straight ahead.

Exercise 8.4 *Continued*

Place the radial border of your index finger (hands palm down) just inferior to the iliac crests and push firmly in a superomedial direction, until the index fingers rest on the pelvic crest.

If your hands are level, there is no anatomical leg length difference.

If there is a difference (and there is no iliac rotation or spinal scoliosis), then an anatomical leg length difference is possible (see later in this chapter for discussion of leg length discrepancy).

A slim book should be placed under the heel of the short side, to equalize leg length, until symmetry of pelvic crest heights is achieved, so that the following tests (below) can be performed.

- Could there be an anatomical leg length difference?
- Can you balance the iliac crest heights by "building up" the short leg?

Exercise 8.5 *Palpation of PSIS Position*

Time suggested 2–3 minutes

Assessment of the posterior superior iliac spine (PSIS) position is achieved by palpating just below the sacral dimples, for osseous prominences. These are palpated for symmetry.

Is one anterior or posterior, in relation to the other?

If one PSIS is anterior to the other, then there is shortness of either

- the ipsilateral external rotators, possibly including iliopsoas, quadratus femoris, gemellus (superior and/or inferior) and obturator (internal and/or external) if the hip is not flexed, and piriformis, if the hip is flexed, or
- the contralateral internal rotators, possibly including gluteus medius and minimus and hamstrings (if the hip is not flexed) or adductor magnus and hamstrings (if the hip is flexed).

Posterior displacement indicates the possibility of precisely the opposite pattern of shortening.

- Is one PSIS superior or inferior to the other, as you palpate?

Inferior displacement may involve short hamstrings, iliac or pubic dysfunction.

Record whether one PSIS is anterior or posterior in relation to the other and whether either PSIS appears superior or inferior when compared with the other.

Thoughts on sacroiliac palpation assessment

In practice, apparently retricted SI joints may – or may not – be reported as painful (Freburger & Riddle 2001). Therefore, tests for motion dysfunction/restriction (see below) cannot be assumed to identify sources of pain, and similarly pain provocation tests (some such tests are described in Chapter 9, but not for the SI joint) cannot be assumed to correlate with identified motion dysfunction (Laslett 2008).

Current evidence suggests that a single test cannot be sufficient for diagnosing SIJ dysfunction, so that a cluster of tests should be applied (as in Exercises 8.6, 8.8, 8.10A and B) – with more than one being positive in order to suggest the presence of restriction/dysfunction (Robinson et al. 2007).

Exercise 8.6 *Standing Flexion Test*

Time suggested 3 minutes

Your palpation partner should be standing as in Exercise 8.4 above (i.e., iliac crests having been leveled by placing a slim book under the short leg if asymmetry was discovered). Your thumbs should be placed firmly on the inferior slopes of the PSIS. Your partner keeps his knees extended as he bends forwards towards the toes, while your contact thumbs retain their positions on the same tissues overlying the PSIS (Fig. 8.1).

Is there movement of your thumbs?

You should observe, especially near the end of the excursion of the bend, whether one or other PSIS "travels" more anterosuperiorly than the other.

If one thumb moves a greater distance anterosuperiorly during flexion, it indicates that the ilium is "fixed" to the sacrum, on that side (or that the contralateral hamstrings are short, or that the ipsilateral quadratus lumborum is short: therefore, *all these muscles should have been assessed prior to the standing flexion test*, as shown in Chapter 5).

Exercise 8.6 *Continued*

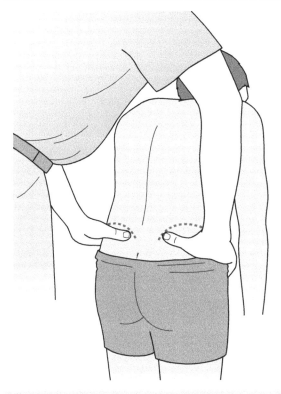

Figure 8.1
Standing flexion test for iliosacral dysfunction. The restricted side is the one on which the thumb moves during flexion.

Notes

If both hamstrings are excessively short this may produce a false negative standing flexion test result, with the flexion potential limited by the muscular shortness, preventing an accurate assessment of iliac movement.

At the end of the flexion excursion, Lee (1999) asks the patient to come back to upright and bend backward, in order to extend the lumbar spine. "If normal, the PSISs should move equally in an inferior [caudad] direction."

The standing flexion test indicates *iliosacral dysfunction,* because the muscular influences from the lower extremity determine iliac relationships with the sacrum, when standing.

That influence disappears when the patient is seated (see Exercise 8.8 below), at which time a positive test would indicate *sacroiliac dysfunction* (i.e., if asymmetry of PSIS movement occurs during seated flexion, as evidenced by thumb movement).

- Did your thumbs move symmetrically during standing flexion or not at all?

- Which iliosacral joint, if any, is dysfunctional?

Notes

Both the standing flexion test (above) and the "stork" test (see Exercise 8.10 below) are only capable of demonstrating *which side* of the pelvis is most dysfunctional, restricted, or hypomobile. They do not offer evidence as to what *type* of dysfunction has occurred (i.e., whether it is an anterior or posterior innominate rotation, internal or external innominate flare dysfunction, or something else).

The nature of the dysfunction needs to be evaluated by other means, some of which are described below.

Exercise 8.7 *Observation of Rotoscoliosis During Standing Flexion*

Time suggested 2–3 minutes

With the person standing fully flexed, you should move to a position so that the spine may be viewed from directly in front (looking down the spine), for paravertebral (erector spinae) symmetry.

Record what is found, for comparison with subsequent evidence noted when the patient is seated (Exercise 8.9).

Mitchell (1998) suggests that:

- If there is greater paravertebral fullness on one side of the spine, this is probably evidence of a degree of rotoscoliosis, caused by the transverse processes being more posterior on the side of greater fullness.

- If this is more evident in standing flexion than in seated flexion, muscular tightness/shortness (postural muscles of the leg/pelvis, for example) is probably a primary factor, with the rotoscoliosis a compensatory feature.

Chapter 8

Exercise 8.7 *Continued*

- If, however, greater paraspinal fullness is displayed during seated flexion, then rotoscoliosis is probably primary, with pelvic imbalance and postural muscle shortness being compensatory.

- If the evidence of fullness on one side during flexion is the same when both seated and standing, then rotoscoliosis is primary (as in scoliosis), with no leg muscle compensation.

- Is there increased "fullness" in the paraspinal muscles during flexion?

- If so, what does it relate to, according to Mitchell's guidelines described above?

Exercise 8.8 *Seated Flexion Test*

Time suggested   2–3 minutes

The seated flexion test evaluates sacroiliac dysfunction and adds to evidence relating to erector spinae tightness.

Your palpation partner should be seated on a low, firm surface, legs apart, hands behind neck. You should be behind, eyes at the level of the PSISs, while your thumbs palpate the inferior aspect of each PSIS (Fig. 8.2). The person goes into a slow forward bend, as far as possible, as you observe the behavior of your thumbs.

You should observe, especially near the end of the excursion of the bend, whether one or other PSIS "travels" more anterosuperiorly than the other.

If one thumb moves a greater distance anterosuperiorly during flexion, it indicates that the sacrum is "fixed" to the ilium, on that side. It is therefore a sacroiliac restriction.

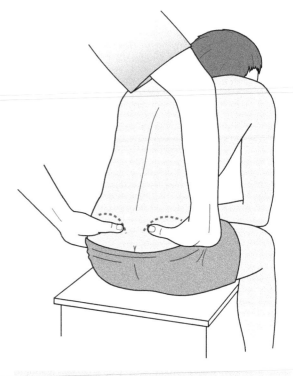

Figure 8.2
Seated flexion test for sacroiliac dysfunction. The restricted side is the one on which the thumb moves during flexion.

Box 8.1 Difference between iliosacral, and sacroiliac restrictions

If you conceive the ilia as a frame, and the sacrum as a wedge surrounded by that frame on two sides, it is easy to understand how what appears to be one part of a joint surface "stuck" to another part of that joint surface , may have quite different causes.

Take for example a door and a doorframe. If a door moves with difficulty when opened, the problem may relate to distortion of the frame, or warping of the door, or both.

Exercise 8.9 *Observation of Rotoscoliosis During Seated Flexion*

Time suggested 2–3 minutes

In this same position (seated flexion) the fullness of the paravertebral muscles is again observed as you move to the front of the patient, with findings being interpreted as described in Exercise 8.7, above.

If paraspinal fullness is more apparent on one side, during seated flexion, and there is no appreciable degree of rotoscoliosis, suspect quadratus lumborum shortening on that side.

This can produce a pelvic tilt, as well as interfering with respiration (through its influence on both the 12th rib to which it is attached, or the diaphragm with which its fascia merges).

The side-lying hip abduction test described in Chapter 5, and/or direct palpation of the lateral border of quadratus, can give evidence of overactivity and therefore shortness of QL, as well as possible spasm or trigger point activity above the iliac crest (see Exercise 5.13, Figs 5.18 and 5.19).

- Is there asymmetry in the paraspinal muscles during this test?
- If so, how do you interpret it?

Confirmation of standing flexion test findings

It is seldom wise to rely on a single test result as evidence of dysfunction (see Chapter 2 for discussion of this). Therefore, if there is an indication of iliosacral or sacroiliac dysfunction, based, for example, on the standing or seated flexion tests, it is wise to also confirm dysfunction using other methods.

The tests described in Exercises 8.10A and B, as well as 8.11A and B, offer opportunities to support – or challenge – the accuracy of previously gathered information.

Lee (2002) has noted that while individually, in isolation, some tests may fail evaluation as to their reliability and validity, *when such tests are combined into a sequence, involving a number of evaluation strategies, and especially when "a clinical reasoning process is applied to their findings", they offer a logical biomechanical diagnosis and, "without apology, they continue to be defended."*

As you perform the exercises in this (and other) chapters, you are urged to re-read Chapter 2 with its in-depth discussion of the value and validity of palpation tests, and the importance of ensuring that more than one piece of evidence is used, when deciding on the significance of tests.

Clinical reasoning should be used as you weigh the relative importance of test and assessment results, in relation to each other, in relation to symptoms, and in relation to the person's personal and medical history.

Exercise 8.10A *Standing Iliosacral "Stork" or Gillet Test (Fig. 8.3)*

Time suggested 3–4 minutes

You are behind your standing partner. Place one thumb on the PSIS and the other thumb on the ipsilateral sacral crest, at the same level.

Your partner flexes the knee and hip and lifts the tested side knee, so that he is standing only on the contralateral leg.

The normal response would be for the ilium on the tested side to rotate posteriorly as the sacrum rotates toward the side of movement. This would bring the thumb on the PSIS caudad and medial. Lee (1999) states that this test (if performed on the right), "examines the ability of the right innominate to posteriorly rotate, the sacrum to right rotate, and the L5 vertebrae to right rotate/sideflex."

If, however, upon flexion of the knee and hip, the ipsilateral PSIS moves cephalad in relation to the sacrum, this is an indication of ipsilateral pubic symphysis and iliosacral dysfunction.

This finding can be used to confirm the findings of the standing flexion test (above).

Petty and Moore (1998) also suggest that a positive Gillet test indicates ipsilateral sacroiliac dysfunction.

Lee (1999) reminds us that this test also allows assessment of "the patient's ability to transfer weight through the contralateral limb and to maintain balance."

The innominate should rotate anteriorly and the thumb on the PSIS should displace superolaterally, relative to the sacrum.

Failure to do so suggests a restriction of the innominate's ability to rotate anteriorly and to glide inferoposteriorly on the sacrum.

- Did your thumb on the PSIS move appropriately, superolaterally?

- If not, what does it mean?

Notes on form and force closure of the SI joint

Two mechanisms lock the SI joint physiologically, known as "form closure" and "force closure" mechanisms (Vleeming et al. 2007):

- *Form closure* represents stability that occurs when the close-fitting joint surfaces of the SI joint approximate, in order to reduce movement opportunities.

    The efficiency and degree of form closure varies with the particular characteristics of the joint (size, shape, age) as well as the level of loading involved. Lee (1999) explains:

    In the skeletally mature, S1, S2 and S3 contribute to the formation of the sacral surface [of the SI joint] and each part can be oriented in a different vertical plane. In addition the sacrum is wedged anteroposteriorly. These factors provide resistance to both vertical and horizontal translation. In the young, the wedging is incomplete, such that the SI joint is planar at all three levels and is vulnerable to shear forces until ossification is complete (third decade).

- *Force closure* relates to the support offered to the SI joint by the ligaments of the area, directly, as well as the various muscular and ligamentous sling systems (see discussions in this chapter and also Fig. 8.4) (Vleeming et al. 1997).

    Examples of force closure are:

- during anterior rotation of the innominate, or during sacral counternutation, the SI joint is stabilized by a tightening of the long dorsal sacroiliac ligament (LDSIL) (Fig. 8.5).

- during sacral nutation, or posterior rotation of the innominate, the SI joint is stabilized by the sacrotuberous and interosseous ligaments.

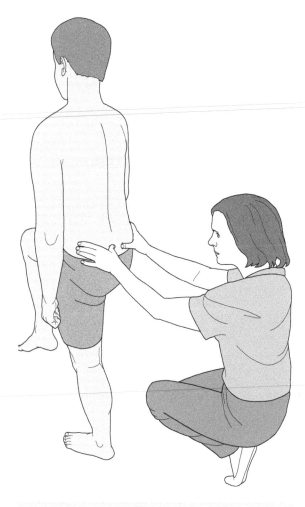

Figure 8.3
Standing iliosacral "stork" or Gillet test.

Exercise 8.10B *Standing Hip Extension Test*

Time suggested   3–4 minutes

The person stands with weight on both feet equally.

You palpate the PSIS and sacral base, as in the stork/Gillet test (Exercise 8.10A) above.

The person extends the leg at the hip, on the side to be tested.

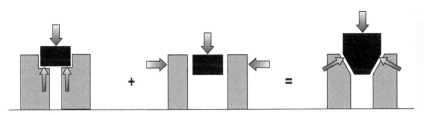

Figure 8.4
Schematic illustration of force and form closure of the sacroiliac joint.

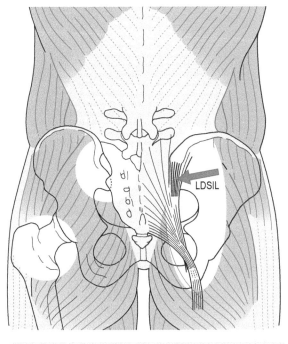

Figure 8.5
The long dorsal sacroiliac ligament (LDSIL).

Exercise 8.11 *Form and Force Tests*

Time suggested **3 minutes**

8.11A: Prone active straight leg raising test

This functional assessment enhances information deriving from the seated flexion test (Exercise 8.8).

- The prone person is asked to extend the leg at the hip by approximately 10°.

- Hinging should occur at the hip joint and the pelvis should remain in contact with the table throughout.

- Excessive degrees of pelvic rotation in the transverse plane (i.e., anterior pelvic rotation) indicate possible dysfunction.

- *Force* closure may be enhanced during the exercise if latissimus dorsi can be recruited to increase tension on the thoracolumbar fascia. Lee (1999) states: "This is done by [the practitioner] resisting extension of the medially rotated [contralateral] arm prior to lifting the leg."

Interpretation

If *force closure* enhances more normal SI joint function, the prognosis for improvement is good, to be achieved by means of exercise and reformed use patterns (Fig. 8.6A).

If *form closure* (i.e., structural components) of the SI joint are at fault, the prone straight leg raise will be more normal when medial compression of the joint is applied on the innominates, during the procedure (Fig. 8.6B).

8.11B: Supine leg raising test for pelvic stability

This functional assessment enhances information deriving from the seated flexion test (Exercise 8.8).

- The person is supine and is asked to raise one leg.

If there is evidence of compensating rotation of the pelvis toward the side of the raised leg during performance of the leg raising, dysfunction is confirmed.

The same leg should then be raised as you impart compressive force, directed medially across the pelvis, with a hand on the lateral aspect of each innominate, at the level of the ASIS (this augments form closure of the SI joint).

To enhance *force* closure, the same leg is raised with the person slightly flexing and rotating the trunk toward the side being tested, against your resistance, which is applied to the contralateral shoulder. This activates oblique muscular forces and force-closes the ipsilateral SI joint (which is being assessed) (Fig. 8.7A).

Exercise 8.11 *Continued*

If this *form* closure enhances the person's ability to easily raise the leg, this suggests that structural factors within the joint (form) may require externally enhanced support, such as a supporting belt (Fig. 8.7B).

Interpretation

If the initial leg raising effort suggests SI dysfunction and this is reduced by means of force closure, the prognosis is good, if the patient engages in appropriate rehabilitation exercise.

- Did either the prone or supine leg raising test suggest sacroiliac dysfunction?

- Were any such indications reduced when form closure was applied by you?

- Were any such indications reduced when force closure was created by resisted muscular efforts, as described?

- Do any of these findings support suggested SI joint dysfunction findings, based on the seated flexion test, the stork or standing hip extension tests?

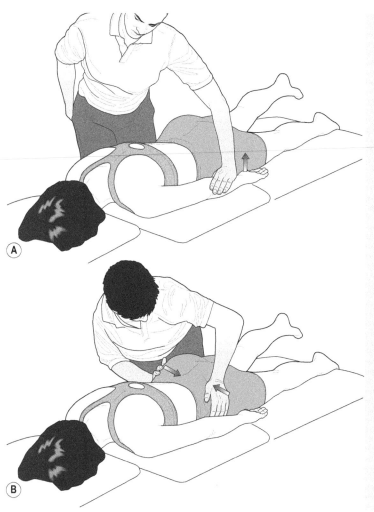

Figure 8.6
(A, B) Force and form test in prone.

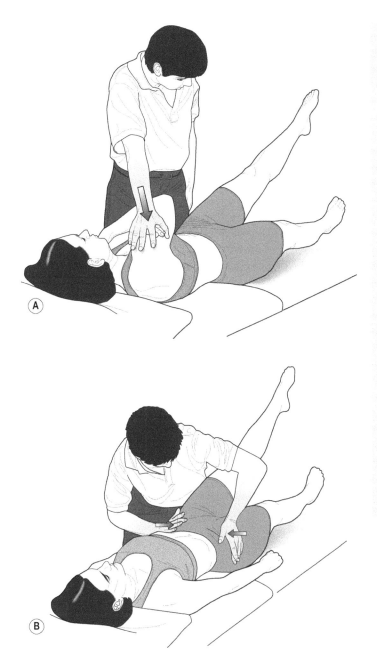

Figure 8.7
(A, B) Form and force test in supine.

Exercise 8.12 *The F-Ab-ER-E Test*

Time suggested   **3–4 minutes**

You should now perform the F-Ab-ER-E test, so called because it simultaneously assesses flexion–abduction–

external rotation–extension of the hip, in that sequence. This test pinpoints hip pathology.

Your palpation partner lies supine, and you stand on the side of the table closest to the leg being tested. The person flexes the hip, allowing external rotation, so that the foot of that leg rests just above the opposite knee.

Chapter 8

Exercise 8.12 *Continued*

The knee on the tested leg is allowed to drop towards the table. It should reach a position where the lower leg is horizontal with the table. If this is not possible, carefully try to take it to that position by depressing the knee towards the floor (Fig. 8.8).

Compare the range with the other side.

- If there is pain in the hip as the knee drops (or is taken) towards the floor, there is probably hip pathology.
- Is there any hip dysfunction evidenced by this test in your patient (model)?

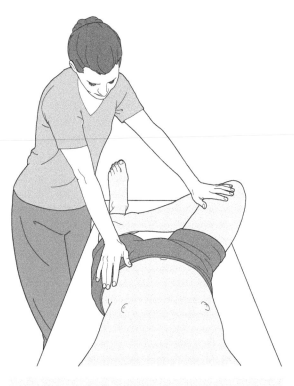

Figure 8.8
The F-Ab-ER-E test.

Exercise 8.13 *Pubic Tubercle Palpation*

Time suggested   3–4 minutes

Mitchell and his colleagues (1979) also suggest other assessments be made of this region, specifically for pubic tubercle height.

Ask the supine person to find the pubic crest on himself, and to maintain a finger-pad contact on the superior surface of the bone, close to the symphysis.

You should stand to one side, at upper thigh level, facing cephalad.

Once the superior surface of the pubic bone has been located, the palm of your table-side hand should be placed on the lower abdomen, finger tips close to the umbilicus. The heel of your hand is slid caudally, until it comes into contact with the superior aspect of the pubic bone.

Having located this landmark, you place both index fingers on the anterior aspect of the symphysis pubis and slide each of these laterally (to opposite sides) approximately 1–2 finger-tip widths, in order to evaluate the positions of the pubic tubercles.

- Is one tubercle more cephalad or caudad than the other?
- Is there evidence of increased tension one side or the other at the attachment of the inguinal ligament?
- Is one side more tender than the other?
- If one side is more cephalad it is only possible to discover which side is dysfunctional (i.e., is one side too cephalad or is the other too caudad?) by referring to the standing flexion test (Exercise 8.6 above).
- The side of dysfunction is shown by relative motion of the palpating PSIS (thumb) in that test.
- Does one side of the pubis palpate as being nearer the head than the other?
- If so, is that side superior or is the other side inferior?

Exercise 8.14 *Palpation of Ischial Tuberosity Height*

Time suggested 3–4 minutes

Place the heels of your hands over the ischial tuberosities, fingers directed towards the head of your prone palpation partner.

The most inferior aspect of the tuberosities is located with your thumbs and the relative height is assessed with your eyes directly above them. (See notes in Special topic 3, on use of the dominant eye.)

If the tuberosities are level there is no dysfunction. If one side is more cephalad than the other, it is presumed to involve a superior dysfunction on that side.

This can be confirmed by assessment of the status of the sacrotuberous ligaments. To test these, the thumbs now slide in a medial and superior direction (towards the coccyx) bilaterally, until they meet the resistance of the sacrotuberous ligament.

If there is a superior ischial subluxation/dysfunction, the ligament on that side will palpate as being slack compared with its pair.

- Are the ischial tuberosities level?
- If not, which is superior?

Exercise 8.15 *Palpation of Internal Malleoli*

Time suggested 3–4 minutes

Apparent ("functional") short leg assessment is based initially on assessment of the levels of the internal malleoli.

Stand at the foot of the table and compare the levels of the internal malleoli, with your palpation partner supine. If there is a discrepancy in the levels of the malleoli this may signify a short leg due to iliosacral and pubic dysfunction.

Ask the person to lie prone and re-examine the internal malleoli. If there is a discrepancy when prone, the short leg is likely to be due to sacroiliac or lumbar dysfunction.

Notes

These concepts and others will be expanded on later in this chapter when the short leg/long leg question will be examined in more detail.

- Is there an apparent short leg? If so, is this due to iliosacral or sacroiliac problems?
- Do these findings tally with the standing/seated flexion tests? Or the stork/standing leg extension tests? Or the form/force closure tests?

Exercise 8.16 *ASIS Palpation*

Time suggested 5 minutes each

Tests of ASIS positions indicate iliac rotation dysfunction and iliac flare patterns. The side of dysfunction, when comparing the levels of the ASISs, relates to the side on which the thumb moved cephalad during the standing flexion test.

8.16A

Your palpation partner lies supine and straight. You should locate and palpate the inferior slopes of the ASISs with your thumbs and view from directly above the pelvis with your dominant eye (see Special topic 3 on eye dominance) in order to compare the levels for superior/inferior symmetry/asymmetry (Fig. 8.9A). If the ASISs are level, there is no imbalance.

Conversely, if there was a right-side dysfunction indicated by the standing flexion test and the left-side ASIS is inferior in this assessment, it indicates a right-sided posteriorly rotated ilium.

Spend a little time (draw a sketch or examine the patient) working out why this is so, if it appears confusing.

If one ASIS is more superior than the other it could indicate a posterior iliac restriction on that side or an anterior iliac restriction on the other side. This is differentiated by comparison with the results of the standing flexion test (Exercise 8.6 above; Fig. 8.9B&C).

- Is one ASIS more superior than the other?
- If so, does it relate to a posterior iliac lesion on that side or to an anterior iliac lesion on the other side ?

Chapter 8

Exercise 8.16 *Continued*

8.16B

Now compare the distances from the umbilicus (if scars make this unreliable use the xiphoid as a landmark instead) to ASIS contacts on both sides.

If the distances are equal there is no imbalance (Fig. 8.10A).

If there is a difference it could mean that on the greater side (longer distance from umbilicus to ASIS) an *outflare of the ilium* has occurred or that an *inflare* has occurred on the shorter distance side.

Once again, reference to the standing flexion test (8.6) gives the answer.

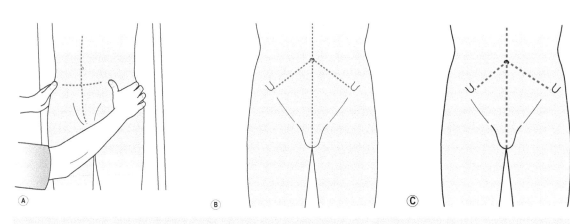

Figure 8.9
(A) Practitioner adopts a position offering a bird's-eye view of ASIS prominences on which to rest the thumbs. (B) The ASISs are level and there is no iliosacral rotational dysfunction. (C) The right ASIS is higher (more cephalad) than the left (more caudad). If a thumb "traveled" on the right side during the standing flexion test this would represent a posterior right iliosacral rotation dysfunction. If a thumb "traveled" on the left side during the test this would represent an anterior left iliosacral rotation dysfunction.

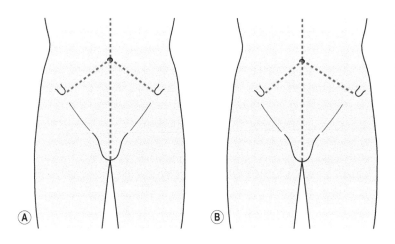

Figure 8.10
(A) The ASISs are equidistant from the umbilicus and the midline, and there is no iliosacral flare dysfunction. (B) The ASIS on the right is closer to the umbilicus/midline which indicates that either there is a right side iliosacral inflare (if the right thumb moved during the standing flexion test) or there is a left side iliosacral outflare (if the left thumb moved during the standing flexion test).

Exercise 8.16 *Continued*

If the flexion test showed an iliosacral restriction on the right and the ASIS umbilicus distance is less on the right, there is indeed an iliac inflare on that side (Fig. 8.10B).

- What would it indicate if the flexion test (Exercise 8.6) had shown an iliosacral restriction on the right and the ASIS–umbilicus distance was greater on the left side?

- What difference, if any, is there in the distances from ASIS to umbilicus (or other landmark) as you view them?

- What does this indicate in relation to your palpation partner, if there was an indication of a iliac dysfunction when you performed Exercise 8.6?

Discussion regarding Exercises 8.1–8.16

If you have comfortably and competently completed the exercises in this chapter up to this point, then you should be able to observe your patient for signs of asymmetry and functional imbalance and decide whether or not an iliosacral or sacroiliac restriction exists – and what type it is.

Your confidence in the assessment results will be amplified by various tests confirming each other. If there are contradictions between the various test results, the possibility exists that either the tests are not being carried out well, or that any dysfunctional pattern that is present does not relate to anything these tests might reveal.

The variations in the presence or otherwise of increased paraspinal muscle fullness in seated and standing flexion tests may have alerted you to the presence of rotoscoliosis, and the possible influence of postural muscle shortness on whatever patterns you have observed or palpated.

Spinal dysfunction

The next few test exercises focus on identification of spinal dysfunction.

Individual spinal segments may be assessed for a variety of restrictions and motions: flexion, extension, side bending (left and right), rotation (left and right) as well as such translatory movements as separation (traction), compression and lateral and anteroposterior translations.

General observation assessment is made by viewing the patient standing upright, standing flexed, seated and seated flexed, as well as in such other positions (extension for example) as you may think useful.

The following exercises, *which are not meant to provide a completely comprehensive spinal assessment, but are designed to improve both general and specific palpation skills*, include methods derived from a number of texts, including: Sutton (1977), Lewit (1992) and Grieve (1984). Also much consulted in the devising of these exercises were the words of William Walton (1971).

Exercise 8.17 *Spinal Palpation Assessment Sequence*

Time suggested **7–12 minutes for each method**

8.17A: Upper thoracic spine, seated assessment

Your palpation partner should be seated.

You place both thumbs on the transverse processes of T1 to T3 successively, as the person first flexes, returns to neutral, and then extends the head/neck repetitively, slowly, until evaluation is complete.

- Was there any asymmetry or one-sided or bilateral sense of excessive bind during any of the movements?

8.17B: Mid-thoracic spine, prone assessment

Your palpation partner should be prone, with his chin resting on the table, head in the midline.

Your thumbs should be placed sequentially on the transverse processes of T4 to T9. Firm ventral pressure is exerted, after soft tissue slack has been removed, in order to evaluate resistance of each segment to hyperextension.

- Any sense of unilateral or bilateral resistance or bind should be noted.

- A rotation restriction, towards the side of maximum resistance, may be suspected.

8.17C: Sphinx position, mid-thoracic palpation

The prone person arches his back by supporting the upper body on the elbows, chin resting on the heels of hands.

Exercise 8.17 *Continued*

You are at the head of the table, palpating the tips of the transverse processes from T7 to L5 with your thumbs, noting any increased posteriority, which may indicate rotation towards that side of the involved segment.

Note also any sense of tissue tension/bind.

8.17D: Seated thoracic assessment/palpation

- An alternative or additional evaluation might involve having the seated person straddling the table for stability or on a high, fixed stool. The patient then places the hands behind the neck, elbows together in front of the face. Both elbows are grasped in one of your hands, from above. The elbows are then held from above and sequential flexion is introduced as the tension of the end of the range of movement of each segment is palpated with your other hand. The person is taken from neutral into anteflexion (forward bending) and back to neutral. This allows you to evaluate the quality of flexion movement between the thoracic segments as you move down the spine. At the same time tissue texture may be noted, and questions asked regarding tenderness. Periosteal pain points on the spinous processes (see Chapter 5) indicate chronically increased tonus in the attaching muscles (Fig. 8.11A).

- The patient then places the hands behind the neck, elbows together in front of the face. Both elbows are grasped in one of your hands, from below, allowing spinal extension to be easily introduced, as a finger of the other hand palpates between the spinous processes for the degree of movement and the quality of the end of the range of motion, at each segment sequentially. The person is taken from neutral into retroflexion (backwards bending) and back to neutral, repetitively, slowly, until evaluation is complete. If the spinous processes fail to "close," then a flexion restriction is probable (i.e., it cannot extend) (Fig. 8.11B).

- For side bending assessment you stand behind, palpating the segment to be tested – on either a spinous process or transverse processes, while the other hand introduces caudad pressure through the contralateral shoulder, to produce side bending. This palpating hand therefore acts as a fulcrum. The end range of motion of each segment is assessed in the thoracic spine. Any sense of increased bind or altered quality of "end-feel" may indicate an inability to side bend and therefore a restricted segment (Fig. 8.11C).

- Rotation is examined with the person seated astride the table, hands behind the neck. You stand to one side and pass a hand across the chest to grasp the opposite shoulder, forearm lying across the chest. Flexion is introduced and the trunk is sequentially rotated, as the individual segments are palpated. (Note that rotation must be around the body's axis, so that the palpating fingers – one each side of the spine – can palpate accurately the degree of rotation available in each direction.) Any sense of bind or altered end-feel might indicate a rotation restriction in the segment being evaluated.

- What restrictions in normal motion or altered quality of end-feel did you find in this region using these methods?

Record your findings.

8.17E: Denslow's thoracic palpation

Denslow (1960) suggests the following thoracic palpation exercise.

The patient is sitting. Palpate the spinous processes of T1, T6 and T12 and note whether or not bony prominences appear to be hard and clean cut (as would be felt if a similarly shaped piece of metal with rounded edges were palpated through a velvet cloth) or if the tissues over, and investing the spinous processes appear to be thickened ... Examination for motion under voluntary control is achieved by placing the tip of the middle finger of one hand between the spinous processes at the cervicothoracic area. With the other hand flex and extend the patient's neck. Move the finger from interspace to interspace until the spines of C7 and T1 are identified. Check for the ease and range of motion ... Examination for motion not under voluntary control is achieved by repeating the procedure described above, and at the end of the range of motion, which is under voluntary control, spring the joint to produce further flexion or extension and check for "give" in the restraining tissues.

This last element, the springing of the joint, allows you to evaluate the quality of the end of the range of motion. Is it elastic, hard, spongy, firm but not excessively so ... or what?

- Which of the diagnostic methods gave you the best results?

- Which of the positions allowed you the most sensitive assessment contacts?

Record your findings.

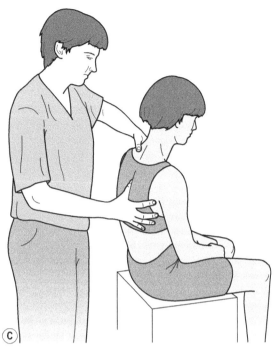

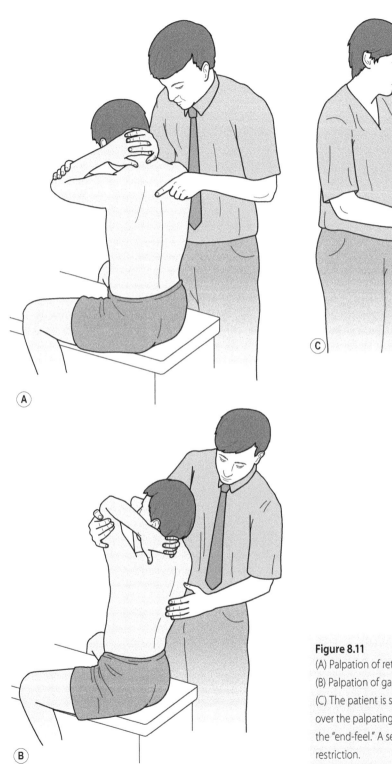

Figure 8.11
(A) Palpation of retroflexion (extension) of the thoracic spine.
(B) Palpation of gapping of spinous processes during flexion.
(C) The patient is side bent (towards the right in this instance)
over the palpating thumb which assesses the nature of
the "end-feel." A sense of unusual "bind" might indicate a
restriction.

Exercise 8.18 *Lumbar Palpation*

Time suggested   7–10 minutes

Your palpation partner should lie prone.

This palpation exercise involves sequential "springing" of individual segments and is performed with two fingers of one hand resting on the transverse processes of a segment, while the hypothenar eminence of the other (extended) arm rests over them.

Slack is taken out and a springing movement to the floor is made as the intrinsic resistance of the segment is assessed. A yielding springiness should be felt.

If, however, resistance is sensed and if there is pain, a restriction exists. If only pain is felt, a disc lesion is possible.

With the person side-lying these segments are again palpated by gentle springing of each lumbar segment, first with the patient anteflexed and then retroflexed.

This palpation method tells you whether a segment is not moving freely, i.e., that it is "blocked," but does not tell you what form that restriction takes (locked in flexion, rotation, etc.).

● What restrictions in normal motion did you find in this region so far?

Discussion regarding Exercises 8.17–8.18

These exercises provide palpation possibilities for evaluating whether localized segmental dysfunction is present, as well as ways of identifying what the nature of such dysfunction is.

This text does not comprehensively describe all methods for such evaluation. It does, however, provide the tools that can enhance the skills necessary for using these, or other, methods of evaluation, in spinal assessment.

Semantics

In spinal palpation and evaluation, you should aim to be able to assess and describe the characteristics of a restricted spinal segment in a manner that other healthcare professionals can understand.

The terminology used to describe a restricted spinal joint may include the words "blocked," "stuck," "dysfunctional," "lesioned," or "subluxated", depending upon whether the description emerges from physical medicine, osteopathy or chiropractic.

The use of language extends to specifics as well. For example, when a flexion restriction exists in the thoracic spine (i.e., the segment is unable to extend fully or is "locked in flexion"), you should be able to determine and to describe:

● the degree to which the spinous process of the vertebra in question is able to approximate to and/or to separate from the vertebrae above and below it

● whether there is a greater degree of protuberance of the spinous process of the vertebra in question, compared with those above and below it

● whether there is an overall increase in the degree of flexion in the area being evaluated

● whether there is an overall decrease in the degree of extension in the area in question

● whether there are any associated motion restrictions evident (side bending, rotation, etc.)

● whether there is any muscular hypertonicity, or spasm, or other palpable tissue changes (e.g., fibrotic, edema, inflammation) in the area

● whether there is tenderness on palpation

● whether there is pain without palpation in the area

● the effect of the restriction, if any, on the associated ribs.

It should be possible to answer these questions during the sequence of assessment described above in all the joints of the spine, almost without thought, once your palpation skills are sufficiently sensitive.

Refer back to the previous chapter and those methods that focus on more "functional" approaches and that ask the palpating hand to recognize both normal and abnormal responses in the region being assessed, when a normal function is being performed – whether this involves a movement or a function such as breathing.

Breathing

(See Chapter 12 for more on this topic.)

Our attention now turns toward evaluation of one aspect of breathing function, and of rib restrictions.

Exercise 8.19 *Breathing Wave Assessment*

Time suggested   2–3 minutes

Your palpation partner should first sit on a firm surface, feet on the floor, and adopt a fully slumped position:

- If the spine is flexible the profile of the spine should appear as a "C" shaped curve (see Fig. 5.25A).

- If areas of the thoracic spine are relatively inflexible a profile such as seen in Fig. 5.25D will be observed.

- The "flat" areas in such a spine will be associated with degrees of rib restriction, and when lying prone on a firm surface (with a suitable pillow beneath the abdomen to prevent undue lumbar extension), on inhalation, a breathing "wave" should be observed (Fig. 8.12). When the spine

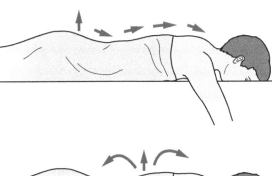

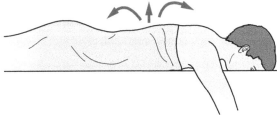

Figure 8.12
Functional (top) and dysfunctional breathing wave patterns as the spine responds to inhalation.

is flexible, that wave-like motion starts in the lumbar region, and spreads in a wave up to the upper thoracic spine.

- However, if there is restriction, either intrinsically or by virtue of the paraspinal musculature in any of the spinal segments, as shown in the previous thoracic spine assessment exercises, or in the slump position, the wave movement will be different (see Fig. 8.12) and those restricted segments are likely to rise as a "block" on inhalation, and will possibly be the part of the spine that moves first on inhalation.

- Observe the wave and if areas move in a block-like manner, palpate these to assess their tone and tissue status (fibrotic, etc.). Compare what you palpate with tissues in more functional areas, where the wave moves sequentially rather than as a block.

- Does the wave start at the sacrum?

- Does it start elsewhere?

- Do some parts of the spine move as a block?

Chart this, as well as the directions in which the wave moves, after its commencement (cephalad, caudad, both directions?). Where does the wave cease – mid-thoracic area, base of neck?

Compare what is observed with findings of restriction during palpation, as in the previous spinal assessment exercises or the observed paraspinal "fullness" in earlier assessments or particularly in relation to areas of flatness as observed in Chapter 5, Exercise 5.18A and B, and Fig. 5.25D.

The breathing wave is not diagnostic but provides a "snapshot" of the current response of the spine to inhalation and exhalation. It can be used to evaluate progress as restricted areas are treated, and the wave alters to a more normal pattern over time.

Exercise 8.20 *Palpation for Depressed Ribs*

Time suggested   5–7 minutes

Ribs restricted in exhalation are depressed (they cannot freely move into the inhalation phase).

Depressed ribs are identified by palpation, which should be performed from the side of the table that brings the dominant eye over the center line (see Special topic 3 on the dominant eye). The eyes should be focused between the palpating digits, so that peripheral vision picks up any variation in the movement of the ribs (Fig. 8.13).

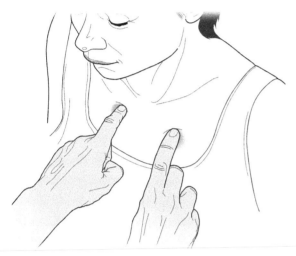

(A)

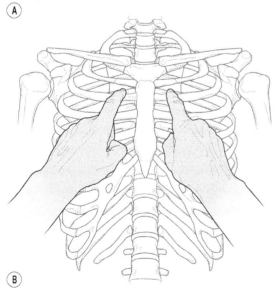

(B)

Figure 8.13
(A, B) Placement of fingers during rib palpation.

Motion of both bucket (up and down motion of upper ribs) and pump-handle (lateral and medial movement of lower ribs) movements should be assessed.

Examination is performed while the supine (knees flexed) patient breathes deeply and steadily. The rib positions (right and left, same level) at full inhalation and exhalation are compared for relative rise and fall (upper ribs), as well as lateral excursion (lower ribs).

Place your index fingers on the superior surface of a pair of ribs. If one of the pair fails to rise as far as the other (or to move laterally, if below the fifth rib), it is depressed.

There will usually be a series of such ribs forming a compensating group, rather than a single rib, unless it has been traumatically jarred. It is necessary to identify the most cephalad of a group of ribs that fails to rise normally on exhalation. This is regarded as the key rib, which is locked in its exhalation position (i.e., it is depressed).

Just as such a rib can affect those below it, so can one locked in inhalation (i.e., an elevated rib, see below) affect those above it, making the most caudad of a group of elevated ribs the key one.

First and second ribs are often depressed and may be associated with pain and numbness in the shoulder, suggesting thoracic outlet syndrome or scalene anticus syndrome (anterior and medial scalene insert into the first rib and posterior scalene inserts into the second rib).

Such depressed ribs are often found in patients with asthma or obstructive pulmonary problems or where there is a tendency to hyperventilation.

In Jones's SCS methodology (see Chapter 5), tender points for depressed ribs lie on the mid-axillary line, in the intercostal spaces above and/or below the rib in question.

- What restrictions in normal rib motion did you find in this region?

- Are there any depressed ribs?

- Did you find a group of these and if so, did you identify the most cephalad of that group?

- Do these findings correlate with tender points on the mid-axillary line at the same level?

- Can you identify associated scalene and/or pectoral shortness relating to any depressed rib dysfunction, if you palpate these muscles?

Exercise 8.21 *Palpation for Elevated Ribs*

Time suggested **5–7 minutes**

Ribs restricted in inhalation are described as "elevated." These are identified by palpation using one fingertip placed on the superior surface of the pair of ribs being assessed (as in the previous exercise). Slightly exaggerated breathing effort is called for, in both inhalation and exhalation, during testing.

Motion of both bucket (up and down motion of upper ribs) and pump-handle (lateral and medial movement of lower ribs) movements should be assessed. Your eyes should be focused between the palpating digits, so that peripheral vision picks up any variation in the movement of the ribs (see Fig. 8.13).

If a rib on one side fails to return to neutral to the same degree as its pair, it is an elevated rib, locked in an inhalation position.

When an elevated rib is identified, all pairs of ribs below should be checked until a normal pair are identified (i.e., both rise and fall equally). The abnormal rib cephalad to the normal pair is the key rib (this being the most caudad of the elevated group).

The intercostal muscles superior to an elevated rib will usually be sensitive and will palpate as tense.

The fifth rib is commonly noted to be locked in elevation. There may be an associated deep radiating chest pain on deep breathing and tightness in the pectoralis minor. Cardiac or pulmonary disease may need to be excluded. There may be swelling indicating costal chondritis.

Tender points for elevated ribs lie at the angles of the ribs posteriorly.

- What restrictions in normal motion did you find in the ribs palpated?

- Did you identify an elevated rib? If so, did you identify a group of these and, most importantly, the most caudad of this group?

- Did these findings correlate with tender points in the intercostal spaces around the angles of the ribs, posteriorly?

- Did you palpate any interspace sensitivity, especially in the space above an elevated rib and close to the sternum?

Exercise 8.22 *Greenman's Rib Palpation Method*

Time suggested **3–5 minutes**

Philip Greenman (1989) suggests additional palpation processes for assessment of rib dysfunction.

Sitting behind the seated or standing person, palpate the most posterior aspects of the ribcage, from above downwards, feeling for a "smooth" convexity that gets wider from above downwards.

What is being felt for is any rib angle that seems to be more or less posterior than others. At the same time, any increase in tone in the muscles overlying or between the ribs (as well as pain) is sought.

The muscles that attach to the angles of the ribs are the iliocostalis group and they become hypertonic when rib dysfunction occurs.

- Can you identify any rib dysfunction using this form of palpation?

Exercise 8.23 *Rib Palpation Seated*

Time suggested **5–7 minutes**

Your palpation partner is seated or prone and you sit behind or stand to one side.

With fingertips, palpate along the shafts of the ribs, feeling for differences one from the other. The inferior margins of ribs are more easily palpated than the superior ones.

Assess the intercostal width (space between the ribs), evaluate differences in symmetry and feel for changes in tone in the intercostal muscles. Trigger points and fibrous changes may be found.

Move towards the spine and locate the articulation between the ribs and the transverse processes. Palpate these, as the patient deeply inhales and exhales.

Assess intercostal motion as well as rib mobility in relation to its spinal articulation.

- Could you palpate all the elements described in this assessment?

● Compare your findings with those established in your previous rib function assessments as outlined above.

Notes on acromioclavicular and sternoclavicular dysfunction

Whereas spinal/neck and most other joints are moved by (and under the postural influence of) muscles, and therefore to an extent are capable of having their function modified by muscular influences, articulations such as those of the sternoclavicular, acromioclavicular, and iliosacral joints are far less amenable to such influences. Nevertheless, muscle energy techniques are widely used in the osteopathic profession to help restore the functional integrity of these joints. Review the ideas of Fritz Smith in Chapter 14, regarding *foundational joints*, and also Special topic 9, on joint play.

Exercise 8.24 *Assessment of Acromioclavicular Dysfunction*

Time suggested 3–5 minutes

Begin evaluation of acromioclavicular (AC) dysfunction at the scapula, the mechanics of which closely relate to AC function.

Your palpation partner sits erect and the spines of both scapulae are palpated by you, standing behind.

Make finger contact with the medial borders of the scapulae and then identify the inferior angle. Using your palpating fingers on these landmarks, check the levels to see whether they are the same. Asymmetry suggests AC dysfunction, although the side of dysfunction remains to be determined.

To test the right-side AC joint, you stand behind the person, with your left hand palpating over the joint. Your right hand holds the patient's right elbow.

The arm should be lifted in a direction 45° from the sagittal and frontal planes and as the arm approaches 90° elevation,

the AC joint should be carefully palpated for hinge movement between the acromion and the clavicle. When there is no restriction, the palpating hand/finger should move slightly caudad as the arm is abducted beyond 90°.

If the AC joint is restricted the palpating digit will move cephalad as the arm goes beyond 90° elevation.

The relative positions of the scapulae become important once dysfunction at the AC joint has been identified, as this determines the position the arm is held in when soft tissue manipulation is used – in either internal or external rotation of the shoulder (Chaitow 2001).

● Were the scapulae symmetrically positioned or was one more cephalad than the other?

● Do both your partner's AC joints respond normally to abduction of the arm, as described?

● If not, is the scapula on the dysfunctional side superior or inferior to the normal side?

Exercise 8.25 *Assessment of Restricted Abduction of the Sternoclaviclar Joint ("Shrug Test") (Figure 8.14A)*

Time suggested 3–5 minutes

As the clavicle abducts, it rotates posteriorly.

To test for this motion the person lies supine or is seated, with arms at the side.

You place your index fingers on the superior surface of the medial end of the clavicle and ask the person to shrug the shoulders as you palpate for the expected caudal movement of the medial clavicle.

If either clavicle fails to fall caudad there is a restriction preventing normal.

Do your patient's sternoclavicular joints respond normally to a shrug or does the joint remain static or even rise rather than fall as this action occurs?

Exercise 8.26 *Assessment of Restricted Horizontal Flexion of the Upper Arm (Sternoclaviclar Restriction – "Prayer Test") (Figure 8.14B)*

Time suggested 1–2 minutes

Your palpation partner should lie supine and you stand to one side with your index fingers resting on the anteromedial aspect of each clavicle.

The person is asked to extend the arms forwards, palms together, pointing to the ceiling in a "prayer" position.

On pushing the hands forwards towards the ceiling, the clavicular heads should drop towards the floor and not rise up to follow the hands

If one or both fail to drop, there is a restriction (Fig. 8.14B).

● Do your patient's sternoclavicular joints respond normally to the prayer test?

Discussion regarding Exercises 8.19–8.26

This series of exercises started with breathing taking center stage, first with an appreciation of the breathing wave, as

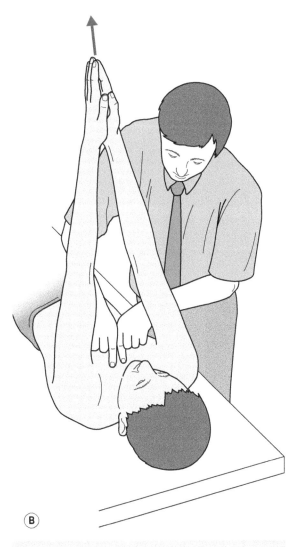

(B)

Figure 8.14B
Assessment ("prayer test") for restricted horizontal flexion of the sternoclavicular joint.

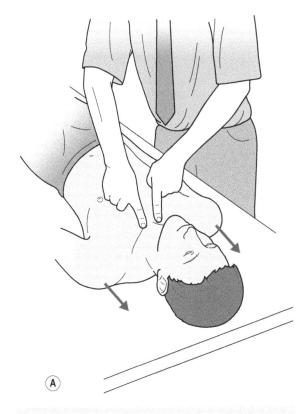

(A)

Figure 8.14A
Assessment ("shrug test") for restriction in clavicular mobility.

a means of seeing how muscular and spinal restrictions might impinge on a normal function pattern, and then by introducing specific rib restriction characteristics, which can be both palpated and observed. The possibility of the presence of clavicular restrictions can be elicited by observation or palpation or both.

In this chapter, overall, it should have become clear that observation and palpation go together intimately and that general evaluation needs to provide a background to specific local restrictions and dysfunctions. You can also see that functional (such as the breathing wave observation) and structural (such as rib restriction) evaluations are inseparable.

Palpation of the skull

The next palpation exercise is a structural one, pure and simple, and focuses on the anatomy and landmarks of the skull.

In earlier chapters some of the exercises assessed elements of cranial and sacral rhythm function. The next palpation exercise is aimed specifically at learning more about cranial sutures and articulations. Whether or not you intend to use cranial osteopathic (or craniosacral or sacro-occipital/SOT) methods, the exercise provides a useful way to enhance your palpatory skills and familiarize yourself with the amazing landscape of the skull.

This exercise should be performed on a living person, but in order to derive maximum benefit it is suggested that a good reference manual and a disarticulated skull (human or plastic), be kept handy for reference and comparison of anatomical landmarks, suture patterns, and general familiarization with individual articulations.

Extensive osteopathic research has shown that the sutures of the skull permit a minute degree of plasticity, or motion, and that the sutures themselves, in life, contain connective tissue fibers, arranged in specific patterns related to the functional motions of the area. There are also blood vessels and small neural structures (including free nerve endings and unmyelinated fibers) in the sutures.

The following palpation is not comprehensive, as it leaves out most of the face and orbital structures. *It is meant as a palpation exercise, not as a lesson in cranial work* (Chaitow 1999).

Exercise 8.27 *Palpation of the Cranial Sutures and Landmarks (Figure 8.15)*

Time suggested **15–20 minutes**

Start by having your palpation partner lie supine, without a pillow. You are seated at the head of the table, forearms supported on the table, as you palpate, with pads of fingers, the vertex of the skull just over halfway posteriorly for the sagittal suture.

Before commencing the palpation, observe the symmetry of the head and face from the perspective you now have.

- Does the nose seem centrally directed or does it slant one way or the other?
- Are the ears symmetrical?
- Are the eyebrows symmetrical?
- Is the slope of the forehead acute or fairly flat?
- Is the center of the jaw in the midline or angled?
- Is the head as a whole symmetrical or distorted in any observable way?

Now begin to trace the path of the sagittal suture and note its pattern of serration, which is wider posteriorly and narrows anteriorly.

A suture may be palpated by very lightly running the pad of a single digit from side to side, so as to sense the path of the meandering joint.

As you move from side to side along this suture, anteriorly, you will come to a depression or hollow, known as the bregma, where the coronal suture meets the sagittal suture.

- Was one side of the suture more prominent than the other?
- Were there any areas of unexpected rigidity?

Now, using one hand on each side (using the finger pads), palpate laterally from the bregma along the coronal suture (asking the same questions as to symmetry and rigidity or any unusual tissue changes) until you reach the articulation between the frontal and parietal bones.

- Ask yourself also whether or not the sutures are symmetrical.

Exercise 8.27 *continued*

As your finger pads reach the end of the coronal sutures, they will palpate a slight prominence, after which the pterion is reached. This is the meeting point of the temporal, sphenoid, parietal, and frontal bones.

Review these landmarks, sutures, and bones on an atlas or model of the skull. Are the depressions and prominences symmetrical, on each side of the skull?

Moving slightly more inferiorly you will palpate, at the temple, the tip of the greater wing of the sphenoid, a most important contact in cranial work.

● Is one great wing (temple) more prominent than the other?

● Is one side higher or lower than the other?

● Are there any areas of unusual rigidity?

Return to the pterion in order to follow the articulation between the parietal bone and the temporal squama

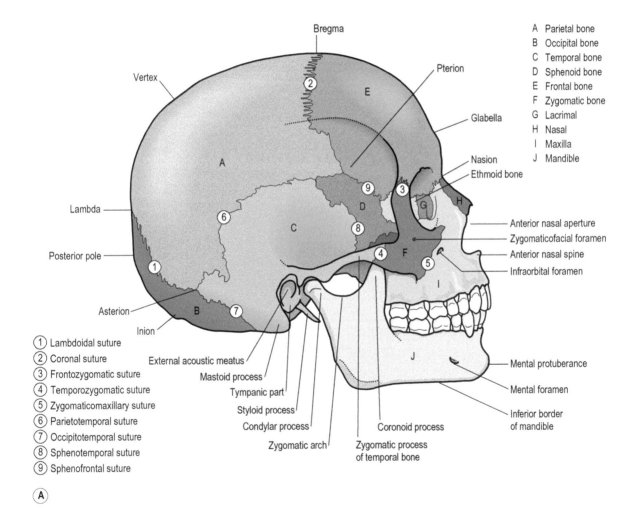

A Parietal bone
B Occipital bone
C Temporal bone
D Sphenoid bone
E Frontal bone
F Zygomatic bone
G Lacrimal
H Nasal
I Maxilla
J Mandible

① Lambdoidal suture
② Coronal suture
③ Frontozygomatic suture
④ Temporozygomatic suture
⑤ Zygomaticomaxillary suture
⑥ Parietotemporal suture
⑦ Occipitotemporal suture
⑧ Sphenotemporal suture
⑨ Sphenofrontal suture

Figure 8.15
(A) Cranial sutures and landmarks.

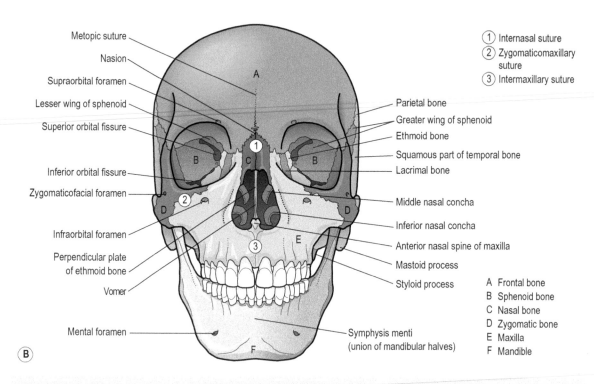

Metopic suture
Nasion
Supraorbital foramen
Lesser wing of sphenoid
Superior orbital fissure
Inferior orbital fissure
Zygomaticofacial foramen
Infraorbital foramen
Perpendicular plate of ethmoid bone
Vomer
Mental foramen

A

① Internasal suture
② Zygomaticomaxillary suture
③ Intermaxillary suture

Parietal bone
Greater wing of sphenoid
Ethmoid bone
Squamous part of temporal bone
Lacrimal bone
Middle nasal concha
Inferior nasal concha
Anterior nasal spine of maxilla
Mastoid process
Styloid process

A Frontal bone
B Sphenoid bone
C Nasal bone
D Zygomatic bone
E Maxilla
F Mandible

Symphysis menti
(union of mandibular halves)

Figure 8.15 *Continued*
(B) Cranial sutures and landmarks.

Exercise 8.27 *continued*

(review your textbook or disarticulated model). This curves backwards over the ear (the temporal squama is beveled on its interior surface to glide slightly over this articulation).

Follow this very subtle articulation on each side; these are best palpated by repetitively running a finger pad (very) lightly from the parietal bone down towards the ear (and so onto the temporal bone) and back again, noting the slight bump as you pass over the articulation.

As your finger pads progress posteriorly along the temporo-parietal articulations, they eventually reach the asterion on each side. The asterion is a star-shaped (hence its name) junction where the occipital, temporal, and parietal bones meet.

● Ask yourself constantly the same questions regarding symmetry, prominences, depressions, rigidity. Make sure you identify each of the named landmarks and sutures.

Pass from the asterions superiorly (and medially) along the lambdoidal sutures, until you once again reach the midline. As you palpate the individual sutures, you should constantly compare side with side.

The lambdoidal sutures meet the sagittal suture at the L-shaped lambda. Now move each finger pad back again to the asterion and palpate your way towards the mastoid processes, along the occipitomastoid sutures, which will vanish below soft tissues as you approach the neck.

Palpate this and become aware of the powerful muscular attachments inserting into the cranium from below (including upper trapezius and sternocleidomastoid) as well as the huge and powerful muscles that attach only to the cranium, such as temporalis. Have your partner activate some of these muscles as you palpate the sutures, in order to evaluate the slight movements they produce.

Now return up the lambdoidal sutures to the lambda, from where this palpation journey began, for it is from here that the sagittal suture runs anteriorly toward the bregma.

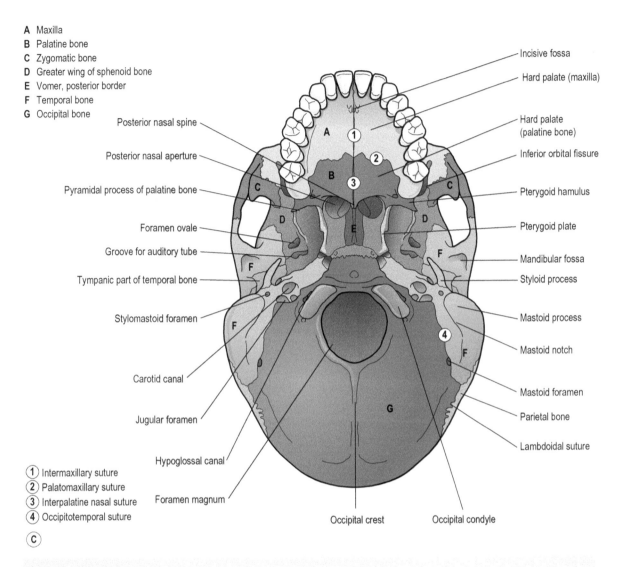

A Maxilla
B Palatine bone
C Zygomatic bone
D Greater wing of sphenoid bone
E Vomer, posterior border
F Temporal bone
G Occipital bone

Posterior nasal spine
Posterior nasal aperture
Pyramidal process of palatine bone
Foramen ovale
Groove for auditory tube
Tympanic part of temporal bone
Stylomastoid foramen
Carotid canal
Jugular foramen
Hypoglossal canal
Foramen magnum

Incisive fossa
Hard palate (maxilla)
Hard palate (palatine bone)
Inferior orbital fissure
Pterygoid hamulus
Pterygoid plate
Mandibular fossa
Styloid process
Mastoid process
Mastoid notch
Mastoid foramen
Parietal bone
Lambdoidal suture

Occipital crest   Occipital condyle

① Intermaxillary suture
② Palatomaxillary suture
③ Interpalatine nasal suture
④ Occipitotemporal suture
Ⓒ

Figure 8.15 *Continued*
(C) Cranial sutures and landmarks.

Exercise 8.27 *continued*

CAUTION Never use more than a few grams of pressure on any sutures when palpating.

The time needed to perform this palpation exercise well is at least 15 minutes. Repeat the exercise many times, until these landmarks are familiar to you and you are instantly aware of the answers to the questions raised.

Assessing the body's compensation potential : Zink and Lawson's method

In some of the tests associated with leg length imbalance, Lewit included evaluation of the manner in which the spine responds to the challenge of a short leg. In a very real way this provides a picture of the current degree of compensation potential of the spinal and pelvic structures, when faced with adaptive demands.

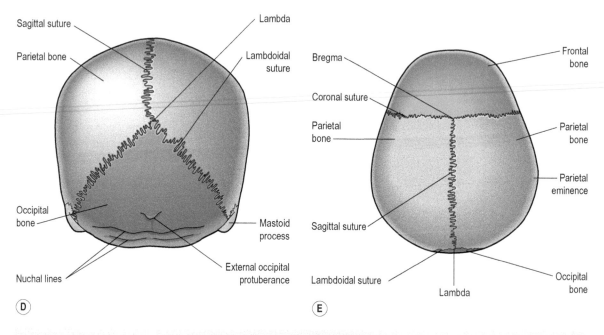

Figure 8.15 *Continued*
(D,E) Cranial sutures and landmarks.

How well can the spine cope with being shoved off balance in this way?

If it cannot cope very well (by virtue of not meeting Lewit's criteria), how well or badly might you expect it to cope with other demands, such as therapeutically designed modifications involving lengthening, strengthening, mobilization, manipulation, etc.?

Zink and Lawson (1979) described methods for testing tissues' rotational preference at four crossover sites where fascial tensions can most usefully be noted:

- occipitoatlantal (OA) (see Fig. 8.17)

- cervicothoracic (CT) (see Figs 8.18 and 8.19)

- thoracolumbar (TL) (see Fig. 8.20)

- lumbosacral (LS) (see Fig. 8.21).

They report that most people display alternating patterns of rotatory preference, with about 80% having a common pattern of L-R-L-R, which they termed the "common compensatory pattern" (CCP), reading from the OA region downwards.

Zink and Lawson observed that the 20% of people whose CCP did not alternate had poor general health histories. Treatment of either CCP or uncompensated fascial patterns has the objective of trying, as far as is possible, to create a symmetrical degree of rotatory motion at these key crossover sites.

Fascial compensation is seen as a useful, beneficial, and above all functional response (i.e., no obvious symptoms result) on the part of the musculoskeletal system, for example as a result of anomalies such as a short leg or overuse. Decompensation describes the same phenomenon, where adaptive changes are seen to be dysfunctional, producing symptoms, evidencing a failure of homeostatic mechanisms (i.e., adaptation and self-repair).

Zink and Lawson (1979) have therefore described a model of postural patterning, resulting from the progression towards fascial decompensation. By testing the tissue "preferences" (loose/tight) in these different transitional areas, Zink and Lawson maintain that it is possible to classify patterns in clinically useful ways:

Well compensated ✓ **Poorly compensated** ✗

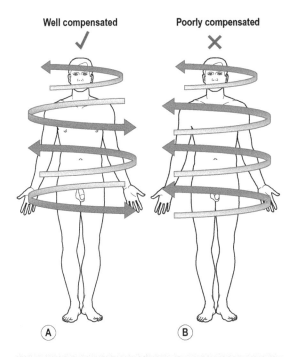

(A) (B)

Figure 8.16

(A, B) Zink's common compensatory postural (fascial) patterns. Tissue "preferences" in different areas identify adaptation patterns in clinically useful ways: ideal = minimal adaptive load transferred to other regions; compensated (A) = patterns alternate in direction from area to area; atlanto-occipital, cervicothoracic, thoracolumbar, lumbosacral; uncompensated (B) = patterns that do not alternate. Therapeutic objectives that encourage better compensation are optimal. (Adapted from Zink & Lawson 1979.)

- ideal patterns, which are characterized by minimal adaptive load being transferred to other regions, as evidenced by more or less symmetrical degrees of rotation potential

- compensated patterns, which alternate in direction from area to area (e.g., atlanto-occipital–cervicothoracic–thoracolumbar–lumbosacral) and which are commonly adaptive in nature (Fig. 8.16A)

- uncompensated patterns, which do not alternate and are commonly the result of trauma (Fig. 8.16B).

Exercise 8.28 *Assessment of Common Compensatory Patterns*

Time suggested **3–5 minutes**

Occipitoatlantal area (Fig. 8.17)

Your palpation partner is supine and you stand at the head. Cradle the head as the neck is fully (but painlessly) flexed, so that any rotatory motion will be focused into the upper cervical area only.

Carefully introduce rotation left and right of the occipito-atlantal structures.

Is there a preference to turn easily to the left or the right or is rotation symmetrically free?

Cervicothoracic area (Fig. 8.18)

The person is supine and relaxed. You sit or kneel at the head of the table and slide your hands under the patient's scapulae. Each hand independently assesses the area being palpated for its "tightness/looseness" preferences, by easing first one and then the other scapula area towards the ceiling.

Is there preference for the upper thoracic area to turn right or left?

OR:

- Place your index and middle finger under the transverse processes of the first thoracic vertebra (Fig. 8.19).

- Gently test the amount of "give" when you use one finger and then the other to lift that side anteriorly – effectively rotating the segment to the other side.

- To which side does the segment move most easily?

- Does this finding agree with the method described above, in which your hands were under the scapulae?

Thoracolumbar area (Fig. 8.20)

The person is supine and you stand at their waist level facing cephalad. Place your hands over the lower thoracic structures, fingers lying along the lower rib shafts, directed laterally.

Treating the structure being palpated as a cylinder, your hands test the preference of the cylinder to rotate around its central axis, one way and then the other.

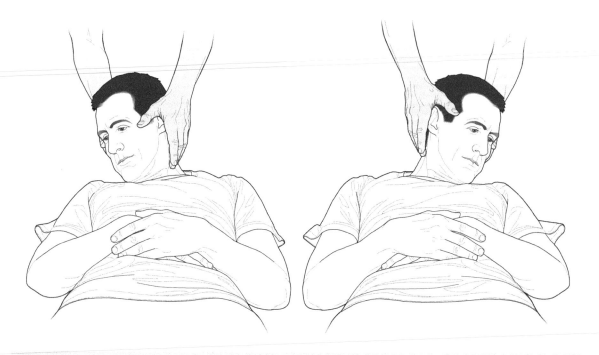

Figure 8.17
Assessment of tissue rotation preference in occipitoatlantal transitional area.

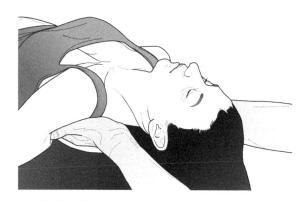

Figure 8.18
Assessment of tissue rotation preference in cervicothoracic transitional area.

● In which direction does the thoracic "cylinder" prefer to rotate?

Lumbosacral area (Fig. 8.21)

Time suggested **3–5 minutes**

The person is supine and you stand below their waist level, facing cephalad, and place your hands on the anterior pelvic structures. This contact is used as a "steering wheel" to evaluate tissue preference, as the pelvis is rotated around its central axis, seeking information as to its "tight/loose" preferences.

In which direction does the pelvis prefer to rotate?

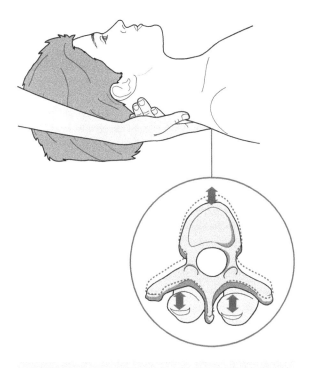

Figure 8.19
Index and middle fingers independently test rotational preference of first thoracic segment.

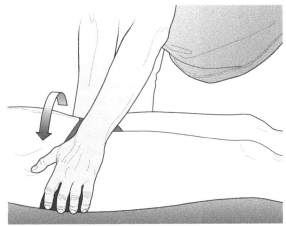

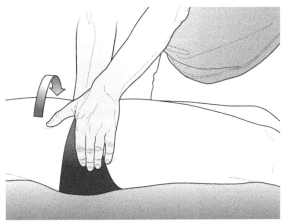

Figure 8.21
Assessment of tissue rotation preference in lumbosacral (pelvic diaphragm) transitional area.

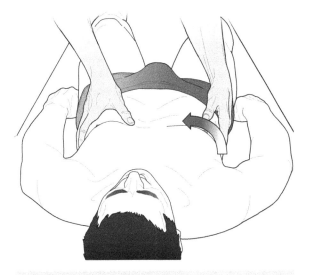

Figure 8.20
Assessment of tissue rotation preference in thoracolumbar (respiratory diaphragm) transition area.

Reflections on possible learning outcomes from Exercise 8.28

- Was there *asymmetry* in terms of the rotational preference of tissues, in any of the four tested regions? If so, record these.

- Based on Zink and Lawson's hypothesis, what are the implications of your findings regarding the rotational preferences of these four regions, in terms of the individual's adaptive capacity and overall health status?

● Did you ensure that you were using the *least possible effort* to induce smooth and comfortable rotational movements?

Conclusion

This chapter has attempted to involve you in discovering ways of extracting information by means of palpation assessment. If you have worked through the exercises you should now be able to see the need for both "gross" and detailed observation, palpation, and assessment of structure and function, in order to feel more confident in your decision making, as to treatment choices.

The next chapter, by Whitney Lowe, offers ways of "Accurately identifying musculoskeletal dysfunction".

References

Chaitow L (1999) Cranial manipulation: Theory and practice. Edinburgh: Churchill Livingstone.

Chaitow L (2001) Muscle energy techniques, 2nd edn. Edinburgh: Churchill Livingstone.

Denslow J (1960) Palpation of the musculoskeletal system. Journal of the American Osteopathic Association 60: 1107–1115.

Freburger J and Riddle D (2001) Using published evidence to guide the examination of the sacroiliac joint region. Physical Therapy 81 (5): 1135.

Greenman P (1989) Principles of manual medicine. Baltimore: Williams and Wilkins.

Grieve G (1984) Mobilisation of the spine. London: Churchill Livingstone.

Jacob A and McKenzie R (1996) Spinal therapeutics based on responses to loading, in Liebenson C (ed) Rehabilitation of the Spine. Baltimore: Williams and Wilkins.

Kappler RE and Jones JM (2003) Thrust (high-velocity/low-amplitude) techniques, in Ward RC (ed) Foundations for Osteopathic Medicine, 2nd edn. Philadelphia: Lippincott, Williams and Wilkins, pp 852–880.

Laslett M (2008) Evidence-based diagnosis and treatment of the painful sacroiliac joint. Journal of Manual and Manipulative Therapy 16 (3): 142–152.

Lee D (1999) The pelvic girdle. Edinburgh: Churchill Livingstone.

Lee D (2002) The palpation reliability debate. Journal of Bodywork and Movement Therapies 6 (1): 18–37.

Lewit K (1992) Manipulation in rehabilitation of the locomotor system, 2nd edn. London: Butterworths.

Mitchell F, Moran P and Pruzzo N (1979) An evaluation of osteopathic muscle energy procedures. Valley Park, MO: Mitchell, Moran, and Pruzzo Associates.

Mitchell F Jr (1998) Muscle energy manual, vol 2. East Lansing, MI: MET Press, p 1.

Petty N and Moore A (1998) Neuromusculoskeletal examination and assessment. Edinburgh: Churchill Livingstone.

Robinson H, Brox JI, Robinson R, Bjelland E, Solem S and Telje T (2007) The reliability of selected motion and pain provocation tests for the sacroiliac joint. Manual Therapy 12 (1): 72–79.

Sutton S (1977) An osteopathic method of history taking and physical examination. Colorado Springs: Yearbook of the Academy of Applied Osteopathy.

Vleeming A, Snijders C, Stoeckart R and Mens J (1997) The role of the sacroiliac joints in coupling between spine, pelvis, legs and arms, in Vleeming A, Mooney V, Dorman T, Snijders C and Stoeckart R (eds) Movement, Stability and Low Back Pain. Edinburgh: Churchill Livingstone.

Vleeming A, Mooney V and Stoekart R (eds) 2007 Movement, Stability and Lumbopelvic Pain, 2nd edn. Edinburgh: Churchill Livingstone/Elsevier.

Walton W (1971) Palpatory diagnosis of the osteopathic lesion. Journal of the American Osteopathic Association 70 (12): 1295–1305.

Zink G and Lawson W (1979) Osteopathic structural examination and functional interpretation of the soma. Osteopathic Annals 7 (12): 433–440.

Accurately identifying musculoskeletal dysfunction

Whitney Lowe

Musculoskeletal disorders (MSDs) are exceptionally prevalent and are the second most common reason for a person to seek medical care (Craton & Matheson 1993). The importance of developing effective evaluation skills for MSDs is highlighted by the fact that people are seeking the care of soft-tissue manual therapists in ever-increasing numbers (Sherman et al. 2005). The lack of focus on MSDs in traditional as well as complementary and alternative medicine (CAM) programs highlights the need for practitioners to take a self-directed approach in enhancing their own physical examination skills (DiCaprio et al. 2003; Matzkin et al. 2005; Stockard & Allen 2006). Exercises and concepts presented in this text are designed to address this training deficiency so practitioners are more prepared to treat the plethora of soft-tissue pain and injury conditions presented to them.

The locomotor soft tissues of the body make up the largest portion of the body's mass. Due to their rich innervation, they are also responsible for a surprisingly large amount of neurological input to the central nervous system. Schleip (2003), in his paper on fascial plasticity, states:

It commonly comes as a big surprise to many people to learn that our richest and largest sensory organ is not the eyes, ears, skin, or vestibular system but is in fact our muscles with their related fascia. Our central nervous system receives its greatest amount of sensory nerves from our myofascial tissues.

The tremendous amount of sensory input from locomotor soft tissues, combined with their responsibility for governing all aspects of movement, makes them crucial structures for detailed examination in any condition of soft-tissue pain or dysfunction. And yet, despite advances in diagnostic capabilities through advanced technology, the ability to identify soft-tissue disorders accurately is still limited. The majority of high-tech diagnostic tests are effective at evaluating abnormalities in tissue *structure*, but are not similarly effective in identifying aberrations in tissue *function*.

There are instances, such as intervertebral disc herniations, where there is an alteration of tissue structure, but no guarantee that the alteration is the source of pain for the patient (Boden et al. 1990; Borenstein et al. 2001). The absence of any gold standard in high-tech diagnostic studies for MSDs emphasizes the importance of the physical examination, which focuses greater attention on locomotor tissue function.

There is no substitute for a thoroughly performed physical examination when evaluating function of the locomotor soft tissues. Palpation and assessment skills, such as those described in this text, provide valuable information about soft-tissue function that gives the practitioner guidance on how to proceed with appropriate treatment or referral.

It is easy to see the importance of physical examination skills for identifying the nature of soft-tissue pathology when first evaluating a patient. However, their importance extends well beyond the initial evaluation. The evaluation of soft-tissue dysfunction continues throughout the duration of treatment to adjust treatment approaches and measure the success of treatment against desired outcomes. Especially in manual therapies that involve direct soft-tissue manipulation, the practitioner's hands use highly refined palpation skills to assess tissue quality at the same time. The ability to simultaneously evaluate qualities of soft tissue while directing and/or changing treatment approaches and immediately adjusting to the tissue's response is a remarkable advantage for the manual therapist.

Clinical reasoning and the evaluation process

Assessment of MSDs is both an art and a science. There are no easy testing procedures that when used alone can identify most of these pathologies. Instead, a combination of basic anatomical knowledge, clinical skill, experience, and sound reasoning is crucial for the practitioner. These qualities build on each other, and there is continual interplay between them during the evaluation process.

An ability to recognize and discern various states of health or pathology in soft tissues is grounded in a fundamental understanding of how those tissues work under normal circumstances. A practitioner should also understand the most common types of pathology that occur to each of the major soft tissues. Assessment of soft-tissue pathology relies on comparing the current state of the dysfunctional tissue to how it should be operating under normal circumstances.

The primary function of the locomotor soft tissues is to create and limit movement in the body. During movement all tissues of the body are subjected to specific mechanical forces. Locomotor soft tissues are primarily subjected to forces of compression and tension. Consequently, biomechanical analysis plays a fundamental role in the evaluation of MSDs. The practitioner must be able to recognize, understand, and apply concepts of kinesiology and biomechanics to each unique clinical presentation because identifying forces to which the tissue is subjected is fundamental to the orthopedic evaluation process.

Due to the unique nature of the human anatomical structure, MSDs are common. These pathologies include disorders such as carpal tunnel syndrome, rotator cuff tears, or lateral ankle sprains. The practitioner who is familiar with some of the more common disorders affecting the musculoskeletal system has a distinct advantage in identifying any existing tissue pathology. Recognizing signs and symptoms that are characteristic of these common clinical problems helps the practitioner organize the large amount of information derived from the physical evaluation process.

As with many clinical decisions for the healthcare professional, definitive conclusions about a patient's condition can be elusive. A good starting point is the accumulation of specific knowledge about soft-tissue pathologies. But accumulation of knowledge alone is not enough. Physical examination procedures that shed more light on the current pathology are used along with knowledge of anatomy, physiology, kinesiology, and pathology. The glue that holds these processes together is *clinical reasoning*. Clinical reasoning is used to guide an interpretation of the results from the examination process.

Clinical reasoning allows us to examine signs and symptoms and evaluate their relationship to the patient's complaint. For example, a patient that reports shoulder pain would be questioned about the onset of the pain. Through questioning in the initial intake, it is established that there is a history of repetitive overhead motion with the upper extremity on the involved side. There is reproduction of pain during certain active, passive, and resistive movements of the shoulder in the physical examination. It is the practitioner's use of clinical reasoning that helps interpret the findings from the history and physical examination. Throughout the evaluation process the practitioner considers anatomical structures in the region, biomechanical factors during various shoulder motions, and awareness of several common soft-tissue disorders. The analytical process of digesting all this information to derive an accurate conception of the soft-tissue pathology is what clinical reasoning, orthopedic assessment, and evaluation of MSDs is all about.

Orthopedic assessment skills
What is orthopedic assessment?

Orthopedic assessment is a systematic process of gathering information in order to make informed decisions about treatment (Lowe 2006). Information is gathered in numerous ways. Some of it comes through the oral history or comments that the patient offers. However, a great deal of this information comes from the various aspects of the physical examination itself. It is the job of the clinician to effectively sift through and interpret the gathered information. Some pieces of clinical information derived during the assessment are more important than others. As the practitioner's assessment skills develop, their ability to prioritize information from the evaluation improves.

The most effective way to manage the great amount of information derived from a detailed assessment is to have a structured system for gathering and deciphering the results of the examination. There are numerous assessment systems or strategies. This chapter focuses on one of those systems, the HOPRS protocol, which is highly effective for manual therapy practitioners (Lowe 2006). The HOPRS assessment protocol is a slight modification of the HOPS assessment model, which is routinely used in orthopedic and sports medicine environments.

This model has five component parts: history, observation, palpation, range of motion and resistance testing, and special orthopedic tests. In this chapter, the components of this assessment protocol are explored along with exercises that help refine the practitioner's assessment skills.

History

Taking a comprehensive case history from the patient is one of the most important aspects of effective assessment. Hearing the patient's description of their pain or injury complaint in their own words can yield valuable clues about the nature of the soft-tissue disorder. Foundational knowledge of anatomy, kinesiology, pathology, and various pain or injury conditions helps guide questions during the history. There is no substitute for a well-taken history and it provides some of the most valuable information in the assessment process (Woolf 2003).

Observation

Relevant causes of soft-tissue injury are sometimes evident with visible alterations in body structure. Postural distortion is a good example. An exaggerated anterior pelvic tilt or forward head posture are indicative of altered biomechanical balance and may be the cause of soft-tissue distress. Atrophy, swelling, bruising, discoloration, or alterations in relative position of adjacent body regions indicate the likelihood of soft-tissue dysfunction. Any characteristics evident during observation are evaluated in conjunction with information from other portions of the assessment process.

Palpation

Palpatory skills are of primary importance in the assessment process. Any of the exercises in this text used to enhance palpatory literacy are a great advantage in the soft-tissue examination process. Because manual therapists spend more time palpating soft tissue than any other healthcare professional, they have a distinct advantage when it comes to the use of the hands for examination purposes. Presence of swelling, tissue texture abnormalities, muscle tightness, myofascial trigger points, muscle strains, ligament sprains, and numerous other disorders are more easily pinpointed with highly refined palpation skills.

Palpation is used for both assessment and treatment simultaneously. During treatment, the practitioner receives immediate feedback through touch about tissue texture, consistency, a muscle's response to treatment, etc. Soft-tissue treatment can be immediately adjusted based on the way the tissue is responding to the treatment. This immediate assessment–treatment feedback loop is a primary reason for the effectiveness of so many different treatment approaches in manual therapy.

Range of motion and resistance testing

This section of the assessment process is comprised of active range of motion (AROM), passive range of motion (PROM), and manual resistive tests (MRT). As described elsewhere in this text, active movements are those initiated by the patient without any help from the practitioner. Passive movements are those in which the practitioner moves some region of the patient's body with no assistance from the patient. In an MRT, the patient engages a muscle contraction against resistance offered by the practitioner, but no motion occurs at the joint. The cross-referenced results from these three tests can produce information helpful in identifying the existing soft-tissue dysfunction.

Palpation during AROM, PROM and MRT evaluations

One of the very important factors being examined during these three procedures is how the patient's tissues respond to active and passive movement and resisted motions. Palpation is used to evaluate the quality of movement during these tests. This form of palpation differs slightly from that used in most palpatory activities.

Generally, the practitioner does not perform any palpation during active movement tests. Active movement uses the least palpatory activity because the patient is performing the entire movement without assistance from the practitioner. However, sometimes additional information can be elicited if a joint, limb, or body region is palpated during active motion. In many cases, light palpation is more valuable than heavier pressure as it allows the practitioner to feel subtle tissue qualities during movement. An example is crepitus or grinding sensations felt under the patella when the surface of the patella is palpated during flexion and extension of the knee (Fig. 9.1).

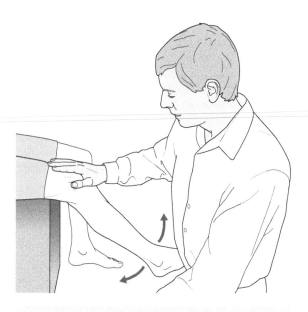

Figure 9.1
Palpating the patella during active motion.

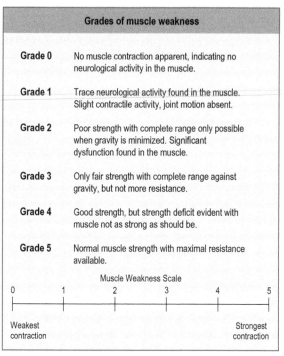

Figure 9.2
Manual resistive tests grading scale.

In PROM evaluations, the practitioner is in contact with the patient throughout the test. While the practitioner's hands are holding and moving a body segment, they are also sensitive evaluation instruments that can pick up cues to pathology including resistance to movement, crepitus, muscular compensations, or apparent obstructions such as loose bodies in a joint cavity. In addition to feeling the quality of motion during passive evaluation, an important characteristic called the *end-feel* is identified during passive motion. The end-feel is the descriptive quality of how motion ends during a particular passive movement. It is a valuable means of identifying specific types of joint pathology. See Special topic 9 for more information on types of end-feel.

In an MRT, the practitioner is resisting the patient's effort to perform a specific joint motion. Because the practitioner is resisting the movement, an isometric muscle contraction is used. The practitioner attempts to identify if the resisted movement causes pain or weakness. Pain is usually indicative of some dysfunction within the muscle–tendon unit and it may be accompanied by weakness of the resisted motion due to reflex muscular inhibition.

The practitioner is looking for muscle weakness through palpatory sensitivity and comparison to the unaffected side. Weakness could be the result of neurological dysfunction. In either case, it is the practitioner's sensitivity to the amount of muscle contraction used when compared to the unaffected side or to another established norm that indicates muscular dysfunction. A helpful guide for measuring the degree of muscular strength is given in Figure 9.2.

Exercise 9.1 *Recognizing Muscle Resistance in MRTs*

Time suggested 5–7 minutes

An MRT evaluation is performed to identify pain or weakness in the tissues that produce a contractile force. Identifying whether or not muscle weakness exists requires that the

Exercise 9.1 *Continued*

patient's muscle contraction be measured against a norm or standard. When a unilateral dysfunction is being examined, the degree of muscle contraction can be measured against the unaffected side. The unaffected side represents the normal contractile capability, which the dysfunctional side is then measured against. Sometimes muscle contractions cannot be measured against a healthy norm in the same individual because both sides are affected or central trunk muscles are being examined and there is no way to test one side against the other effectively. In these situations, having a guideline such as the one presented in Figure 9.2 to measure a muscle's strength by itself is particularly helpful.

Select three resisted actions that will be tested on each side of the body (e.g., lateral rotation of the shoulder, extension of the knee, and dorsiflexion of the ankle). Perform a manual resistive test for all the motions on the right side of the body first. Assign each action a grade based on the scale in Figure 9.2. Then perform the same resisted actions on the left side of the body and grade them as well. Go back to examine the grades given to each of the muscle actions and see if there is any difference in grade between the same actions on the left and right sides of the body. If there is a difference, go back and test those actions again but this time test one side and then immediately test the other side using the same resisted action. Does measuring the strength difference by grades give the same result as when measuring one side to the other? Is the strength difference between each side evident when you perform these tests right after each other?

Interpreting results from AROM, PROM, and MRT evaluations

What makes AROM, PROM, and MRT examination procedures so valuable is the amount of information about soft-tissue dysfunction that can be gleaned from them. In his seminal text on orthopedic evaluation, Cyriax (1982) introduced the concept of categorizing soft tissues as *contractile* or *inert*. Contractile tissues are those that are actively involved in the delivery of tensile force to the bones in order to produce movement. Muscles and tendons are the two tissues initially categorized as contractile. While tendons do not contract, they are still involved in the delivery of the muscle contraction force.

Recent physiological studies have confirmed that fascial tissue has contractile properties (Schleip et al. 2006). Fascia is also responsible for aiding in the transmission of high tensile loads during movement (Gracovetsky 2007; Yahia et al. 1993). In view of these recent findings it seems appropriate to modify Cyriax's original classification of contractile tissues to include fascia as well.

Inert tissues make up the remaining locomotor soft tissues that are not involved in transmitting tensile loads to the bones in order to produce movement. While they do not produce mechanical forces to create movement, inert tissues are stretched or compressed in the midst of various movements. The locomotor inert tissues include cartilage, nerve, dura, joint capsule, ligament, and bursa.

Cyriax developed a comprehensive evaluation process to discriminate which of these various contractile or inert tissues might be responsible for a specific pain complaint. His idea was to selectively apply stress to the different tissues to see if a patient's primary pain could be reproduced, thereby indicating which tissue was the source of pain. He referred to this system as the *selective tissue tension* paradigm (Cyriax 1982). Effective use of the selective tissue tension paradigm requires the practitioner understand the potential effects each of the three different types of evaluation procedures (AROM, PROM, and MRT) has on the contractile or inert tissues.

Contractile tissues are used to generate the force of any movement. Therefore, during AROM evaluations, contractile tissues that produce the desired movement when engaged are under selective tension. For example, during active shoulder abduction from a standing position the shoulder abductors (supraspinatus and deltoid) are actively engaged to produce the motion. Inert tissues near the shoulder are either compressed or stretched during active movement. Because both contractile and inert tissues are engaged during active motion, pain produced in active movement could be originating from either of these two categories of tissues. Clearly, taken alone, AROM evaluations do not provide significant assistance in discriminating the tissues at fault. It is only when the results from this procedure are combined with the PROM and MRT tests that the valuable clinical benefits are evident.

To perform a passive movement the practitioner moves the patient's limb or body without assistance from the patient. Because the patient is not contributing muscular effort to produce the passive movement, contractile tissues are not engaged in a PROM evaluation. Yet, the inert tissues are still under some degree of compression or tension as the joint is moved through its full range of motion. If pain is produced during a PROM procedure and the same pain is also present during AROM, it is likely an inert tissue is responsible for the pain because only the inert tissues are involved in both these evaluation procedures.

In order to further clarify and validate the locomotor soft tissue responsible for the patient's pain, a third evaluation procedure is used to cross-reference the previous two. Inert tissues are stretched or compressed during movement in both AROM and PROM. An MRT uses muscle contraction so there is engagement of the contractile tissues, but there is no motion occurring at the joint. With no motion at the joint, the inert tissues are no longer being compressed or stretched by movements through the joint's range. Consequently, if there is pain with AROM and with a resisted movement in the same direction, a contractile tissue is the likely source of the pain. If a contractile tissue is the source of the pain, it is also likely that there would be no pain during the passive movement in the same direction because the muscle is not engaged.

Performing AROM, PROM, or MRT evaluations by themselves can provide some helpful information, but the real advantage of Cyriax's selective tissue tension paradigm is using all three testing procedures and comparing the results from each. A helpful way to visualize the interpretation of results from these three testing procedures is shown in Figure 9.3.

Exceptions with test results

Most guidelines have exceptions – situations under which the general guideline does not apply. There are two important exceptions to the interpretation of AROM, PROM, and MRT results. It was stated previously that during a PROM evaluation the contractile tissues are not engaged. However, contractile tissues that perform the action opposite the action being evaluated will be stretched at the end of a PROM test. For example, when performing a passive elbow flexion, the elbow flexor muscles are not used. However,

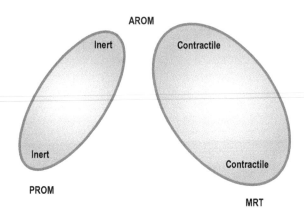

Figure 9.3
Triangle of active range of motion (AROM), passive range of motion (PROM), and manual resistive tests (MRT). If pain is present with AROM and PROM, but not with MRT, an inert tissue is the most likely cause for the problem. If pain is present with AROM and MRT, but not with PROM, a contractile tissue is most likely the cause.

near the end range of passive elbow flexion the antagonist contractile tissues begin to be stretched, in this case the triceps (elbow extensors). Stretching the antagonist triceps could therefore produce pain in contractile tissue in a PROM evaluation if there was an injury to that muscle group. If the triceps are involved and pain occurs at the end of elbow flexion, pain is likely to be felt on the posterior side of the arm. Clearly, it would not be the elbow flexors producing pain at the end of elbow flexion.

Another possible exception with contractile tissues can occur during AROM and MRT evaluations. In some cases, there will be no pain with AROM in a specific direction. However, pain might occur when that same motion is attempted with resisted action. The reason there may be no pain with AROM and pain with MRT is that fewer fibers are recruited during AROM than in the resisted action.

For example, there may be no pain with active motion in wrist flexion but pain with resisted wrist flexion. In this case, the contractile tissues appear to be at fault because of the pain with resisted wrist flexion. At the same time, lack of pain with active wrist flexion suggests the contractile tissues are not involved. Knowledge of the structure and function of the hand, in this case, should instruct the practitioner to put greater emphasis on the resisted wrist flexion test. When performing wrist flexion, only the weight of the hand is being lifted. Therefore, not many muscle fibers are required to perform the action. With so few fibers recruited to perform the action, there is not sufficient tensile load generated to reproduce the primary pain complaint. When the MRT is performed, however, there is a much greater load on the muscle, fascia, and tendon fibers and consequently pain is felt during that test procedure.

Exercise 9.2 *AROM, PROM, and MRT Evaluations*

Time suggested **5–7 minutes**

Pick a particular extremity joint for the evaluation process. Determine the normal single-plane motions that occur at that joint. For example, if the ankle is selected the motions used in the evaluation process include dorsiflexion, plantarflexion, inversion, and eversion. Perform an AROM, PROM, and MRT evaluation for each of the motions that occur at the joint selected. Make note of any differences in the subject's response between active and passive movements for the same motion. If there are differences, what might that mean? Compare the findings in active and passive motion with the MRTs performed. What has the information gathered suggested about the nature of any soft-tissue dysfunction?

Special tests

A special orthopedic test is a particular testing maneuver (frequently named after the originator) that is designed to produce a particular sign or symptom when the maneuver is performed. Common examples of special orthopedic tests are Phalen's test for carpal tunnel syndrome, Lachman's test for anterior cruciate ligament injury, or the Neer impingement test for shoulder impingement syndrome.

While special orthopedic tests are designed to improve accuracy in identifying various pathological disorders, the tests are not equally reliable. Recognizing which tests are more accurate is crucial because there is a bewildering array of special tests that can be used (Coady et al. 2004).

The accuracy of any special orthopedic test is based on two primary factors: its *sensitivity* and its *specificity*. The sensitivity of a testing procedure is how accurate it is at producing a positive result in each person that has the condition for which the test is designed. Specificity is how accurate the test is at ruling out all those that do not have the particular dysfunction for which it is being used. The most accurate special tests have a high degree of sensitivity and a high degree of specificity.

Special tests are designed to put selective stress on an anatomical structure or exaggerate the features of a particular pathological disorder. A greater understanding of anatomy, kinesiology, biomechanics, and common pathological conditions gives the practitioner the option of altering some of these special tests to glean more information from them or better understand their application. Traditional orthopedic tests are sometimes modified or enhanced, in cases creating completely new testing procedures, which may then become a more commonly used standard. An example of modifying a traditional orthopedic test to increase its sensitivity is the addition of neural tension to the upper extremity while performing a standard nerve compression evaluation procedure, such as Phalen's test (Lowe 2008).

Special orthopedic tests are designed to produce a variety of results. Some elicit or exaggerate a patient's pain complaint while others may be designed to evaluate limitations in range of motion or other symptomatic factors. Most special tests can fit into one of four general categories of testing:

- pain provocation

- positional or postural

- hypermobility

- neurodynamic.

Each of these categories is explored in greater detail below. Under each category is a description of the general principles for tests that fall into that category followed by two special test examples and illustrations that describe the particular test. Important considerations that could modify or affect the results from tests in each category are also included.

Pain provocation tests

When a patient seeks the help of a practitioner for addressing a pain or injury condition, the first step in the process is to identify the cause of the pain. In many cases, finding what movements or positions exactly reproduce the pain is the most effective way to identify which tissue(s) are the source. A special test that is designed to reproduce or exaggerate the patient's initial pain complaint is called a *pain provocation test*.

With a pain provocation test it is important to clarify if the pain felt during the test procedure is the *same* pain or discomfort that comprised the initial complaint. Some special test maneuvers can cause stress to multiple tissues so just indicating that pain is produced during a test is not sufficient.

If it is suspected that a particular pain provocation test is going to increase the patient's pain, it is best to leave that test until the end of the evaluation process. Leaving the pain provocation test until the end of the evaluation process decreases the likelihood that those sensations will influence or interfere with other tests.

Another factor to consider with pain provocation tests is that in many cases the testing process will exaggerate the patient's pain to a degree higher than before the test. It is important to perform these tests with a degree of both confidence and compassion. Performing a pain provocation test with a strong sense of compassion can help decrease the degree of lingering discomfort for the patient.

Exercise 9.3 *Empty Can Test*

Time suggested **1–2 minutes**

The empty can test is usually performed bilaterally, even when one shoulder is symptomatic. The non-affected side is used for comparison. If pain is reproduced at any point during the test, continuing the test is unnecessary. The patient faces the practitioner. From this position the patient brings both arms into 45° of horizontal adduction. The patient is asked about pain or discomfort as the position is held. With the arms in partial horizontal adduction, the patient is instructed to medially rotate the arms, as if emptying cans held in the hands (Fig. 9.4). At the end of this motion, the practitioner asks about pain or discomfort. The patient holds the arms

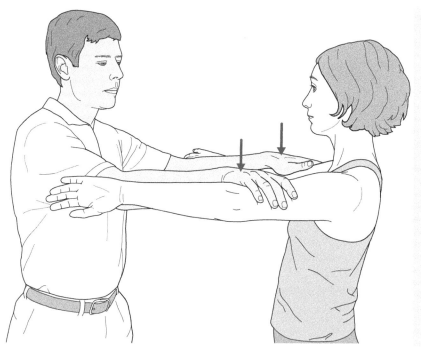

Figure 9.4
Empty can test.

Exercise 9.3 *Continued*

in the final position while the practitioner attempts to push both arms down with moderate effort. Pain that reproduces the primary complaint is a positive result (Lowe 2006).

This test is designed to elicit increased pain if the patient has impingement of soft tissues in the subacromial space. There are a number of tissues that could be compressed in this test, thereby reproducing pain when the test is performed. Possible involved tissues include the subacromial bursa, supraspinatus tendon, biceps tendon long head, and the upper portions of the joint capsule. What this test does not tell the practitioner is which of those different tissues is responsible for the pain increase. Additional evaluation procedures are required to clarify further which tissue is the primary one at fault. However, if when performing this test, pain is not exaggerated until the very last step when pressure is applied to the abducted arms, there would be a strong indication that the supraspinatus muscle–tendon unit was involved because the only factor that changed in the final step was additional load on that contractile tissue (the supraspinatus).

Exercise 9.4 *Tennis Elbow Test*

Time suggested **1–2 minutes**

The patient is standing or seated. The practitioner wraps one hand around the patient's elbow so the thumb is pressing on the extensor tendons just distal to the lateral epicondyle of the humerus. Be careful not to press on the ulnar nerve on the posterior side of the elbow while holding the elbow. The practitioner's other hand grasps the patient's hand and uses it to resist the patient's wrist extension (Fig. 9.5). Only offer resistance to wrist extension and do not push the patient's arm toward the floor, as this recruits other muscles that may confuse the test. This test is simply a manual resistive test for wrist extension with pressure being placed simultaneously on the affected tendons (Lowe 2006).

This test is designed to reproduce and increase symptoms resulting from tendinosis in the proximal wrist extensor tendons. It is simply a manual resistive test with additional compression of the affected tendons. Palpating the tendons during the initial evaluation is likely to reveal exaggerated tenderness. When there is additional tensile load on the tendons from a muscle contraction the palpation more

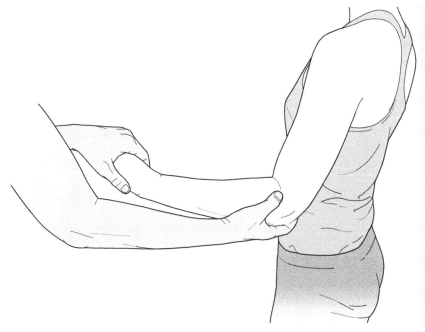

Figure 9.5
Tennis elbow test.

Exercise 9.4 *Continued*

easily reproduces the patient's discomfort. It is common for asymptomatic individuals to have some discomfort with this test. Consequently, the practitioner is looking for pain that is greater than the unaffected side or out of proportion to the amount of pressure being applied. It is also important to determine if the pain is the same as that in the initial complaint.

Positional or postural tests

Pain provocation tests are the most common type of special test but some tests employ other indicators such as alterations in position, movement, or range of motion. When using a positional special test the practitioner is not attempting to reproduce the patient's specific symptoms. Positional special tests examine the patient's posture or position and attempt to determine its relationship to the current complaint. These tests are somewhat indirect, but their value should not be ignored.

Exercise 9.5 *Modified Thomas Test*

Time suggested 1–2 minutes

The patient leans on the edge of the treatment table without fully sitting on the table. The patient brings the knee that is not being tested to the chest. Once the knee is drawn to the chest, the practitioner assists the patient in rolling back onto the treatment table. The thigh being held to the chest should be at about a 45° angle to the table. The practitioner observes the patient's extended thigh from a lateral view (Fig. 9.6). If the thigh is at horizontal or above, hypertonicity in the iliopsoas is indicated. If the thigh drops below horizontal, the iliopsoas is considered within normal parameters for flexibility. If the rectus femoris is at normal length, the lower leg should drop toward the floor at a vertical angle. If the lower leg is not vertical some hypertonicity in the rectus femoris is evident (Lowe 2006).

This test is for a hypertonic iliopsoas. Tightness in the iliopsoas can contribute to low back pain, postural distortions, sacroiliac joint dysfunction, and a number of other conditions. It is unlikely that a tight iliopsoas muscle would be the exclusive cause of any of these disorders. Consequently, this test is not designed to indicate a specific pathology. Yet, it is highly valuable when examining the relative contribution of the iliop-

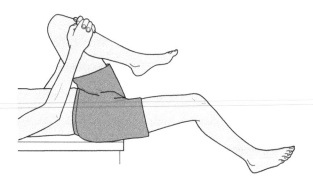

Figure 9.6
Modified Thomas test.

soas to various other conditions. The depth of the iliopsoas in the abdomen and its proximity to sensitive vascular structures makes direct palpation of the muscle challenging. When direct palpation is not an easy option, a muscle length test such as this one is a helpful evaluation method.

Exercise 9.6 *Apley Scratch Test*

Time suggested 1–2 minutes

The patient is standing and brings one arm as far as possible into abduction and lateral rotation as if scratching the upper back between the scapulae. The other arm is brought into adduction and medial rotation as if scratching the upper to mid-back (Fig. 9.7). Position of the hands is observed and compared bilaterally. Each shoulder is tested in the upper position (abduction and lateral rotation) and the lower position (adduction and medial rotation). Problems with the abduction and lateral rotation are usually greater than adduction and medial rotation (Lowe 2006).

This procedure is used to evaluate range of motion limitations in the glenohumeral joint. Glenohumeral capsular restrictions are especially likely to cause limited motion in the combined motions of abduction and lateral rotation. As with the modified Thomas test described above, this test does not necessarily produce pain, but it is valuable to identify any particular movement restrictions. Combined with other evaluation procedures it can help the practitioner understand altered glenohumeral biomechanics and their contribution to pain or injury in the patient.

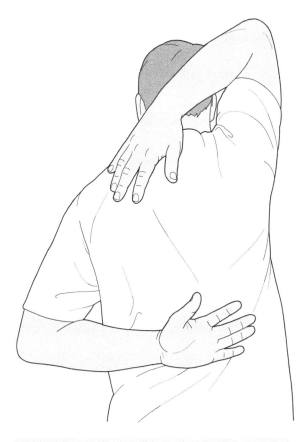

Figure 9.7
Apley scratch test.

Hypermobility tests

Joint mobility is primarily controlled by ligaments that span the joint. Damage to those ligaments can produce pain as well as excessive joint motion. When there is excess joint motion, altered joint mechanics result and gradual joint degeneration may produce an early onset of arthritis, bone spurs, or other pathologies.

Ligamentous laxity is the primary cause of joint hypermobility. Laxity in the ligaments can result from genetics or from injury where the ligament was stretched or torn. In some conditions a ligament injury is painful at the time of injury but not painful later, although significant joint hypermobility has resulted from the injury. An example of

this situation is a third degree sprain where a ligament has completely ruptured. It may be very painful at the time of injury, but no pain occurs later because the two ends of the ligament are completely torn away from each other. However, there will be excessive mobility in the joint. Damage in the joint is likely to result from the sprain and the resultant hypermobility. Tests for joint hypermobility are primarily looking for excess joint motion, but could also elicit pain depending on the nature of the existing pathology.

Exercise 9.7 *Valgus Stress Test*

Time suggested **1–2 minutes**

The patient is supine on the table. The practitioner stabilizes the distal medial tibia with one hand, while applying valgus force to the lateral knee with the other hand (Fig. 9.8). The amount of valgus force to apply will vary but is best described as moderate. Make sure the middle of the hand applying the valgus force is placed directly over the joint line and not superior or inferior. If the hands are not in the right position, the practitioner cannot adequately feel movement in the joint. Pain or a mushy end-feel indicates

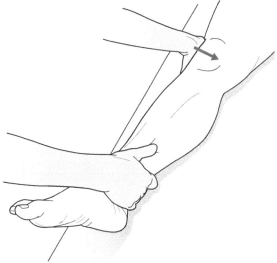

Figure 9.8
Valgus stress test.

Exercise 9.7 *Continued*

damage to the medial collateral ligament (MCL). A small amount of gapping over the medial joint line may be visible as the valgus force is applied (Lowe 2006).

The MCL is designed to resist valgus forces to the knee. A valgus force at the knee is one that is applied from the lateral side of the knee and aimed in a medial direction. Ligament sprains resulting in hypermobility often occur from a valgus force or from excessive rotary stress to the knee. In this test an additional valgus force is applied to the knee. A healthy knee should feel firm and resistant when the valgus force is applied. The soft or mushy end-feel compared to the non-injured side indicates excess joint mobility. Depending on severity of the injury there may be pain associated with the end-feel as well.

Exercise 9.8 *Ankle Drawer Test*

Time suggested 1–2 minutes

The practitioner stabilizes the anterior distal tibia with one hand while pulling the posterior calcaneus in an anterior direction with the other hand (Fig. 9.9). Forward shifting or a soft, mushy end-feel suggests ligamentous laxity. The procedure may cause pain with a first or second degree sprain. In a third degree sprain there is significant movement, but limited pain due to complete rupture of the affected ligament. Do not mistake the slight amount of dorsiflexion that occurs during the test for forward translation of the foot (Lowe 2006).

Damage to the anterior talofibular ligament is the most common lower extremity soft-tissue injury (Garrick & Requa 1988). With the entire body weight resting on the foot with each foot strike, hypermobility in the ankle joint can lead to significant degenerative changes. With an injury such as the ankle sprain being so common, many people may have some degree of excess mobility when tested with this procedure. The important clinical question is whether or not excess mobility is contributing to existing joint or soft tissue distress.

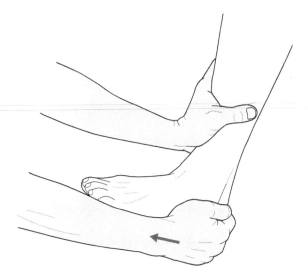

Figure 9.9
Ankle drawer test.

Neurodynamic tests

Compression of peripheral nerves by soft tissue, between soft tissue and bone, or between adjacent bones is a frequent cause of pain. While nerve compression syndromes such as carpal tunnel syndrome and piriformis syndrome are well documented, they are not the only type of mechanical stress on nerve structures, especially in the extremities. Recent attention has focused on the necessity of mobility in the nervous system and the role that lack of proper neural mobility can play in soft-tissue dysfunction (Butler 2000; Shacklock 2005).

Neurodynamic tests are designed to stress nerve tissues to see if the patient's symptoms are reproduced. Pain is a common symptom of neural dysfunction so many of these procedures could also be considered pain provocation tests. However, neural dysfunction can also produce symptoms such as numbness, paresthesia, or motor weakness, which are not pain sensations, so these tests are not always pain provoking. Continuing to hold a nerve in a position that irritates it can significantly aggravate symptoms. In neurodynamic tests, once a positive sign is indicated by symptom increase the compression or tension should be relieved from the nerve by releasing the test position.

Exercise 9.9 *Straight Leg Raise*

There are several steps in this test. The patient is asked about changes in sensation or increases in symptoms after each step is performed (the position is usually held for about 30–60 seconds). Increases in neurological symptoms indicate the likelihood of nerve root compression in the lumbar region. The patient is supine on the treatment table. The practitioner raises the leg of the affected side (the side where symptoms are felt) as if attempting to stretch the hamstring muscles. The practitioner continues to raise the leg on this side until the patient reports a reproduction of symptoms (Fig. 9.10). The sciatic nerve is fully stretched at about 70° of hip flexion, so symptoms are usually present by this point. The leg is slightly lowered to determine if symptoms decrease. This slight movement helps differentiate the symptoms from hamstring tightness when the next step is performed. At this position, the patient dorsiflexes the foot and the head and neck are then flexed (Lowe 2006). If symptoms in the distribution of the sciatic nerve are increased at any of these steps the test is considered positive.

This test is used to examine for obstructions in the lower lumbar region that could be pressing on nerve roots. Neurological symptoms are usually felt down the lower extremity in the distribution of the sciatic nerve. The nature of many nerve pathologies is such that it can be difficult to identify accurately where along the length of a nerve the actual compression or mobility restriction is located. Nerve root pathology can produce symptoms anywhere within its associated dermatome. A peripheral neuropathy generally produces symptoms distal to the site of compression, but it still makes accurate identification of the nerve pathology's location challenging.

Exercise 9.10 *Elbow Flexion Test*

The patient is standing or seated and brings both elbows into full flexion with the forearms supinated and the wrists hyperextended (Fig. 9.11). The patient should adopt the position on both sides at the same time so a comparison with the unaffected side can be made. If symptoms are reproduced within about 60 seconds, compression of the ulnar nerve in the cubital tunnel is likely (Lowe 2006).

In this test, the ulnar nerve is compressed within the cubital tunnel because the elbow is held in flexion. Elbow flexion also stretches the nerve at the same time it is being compressed. Numerous neurodynamic tests have elements of both compression and tension in them. The symptoms of neural compression and tension are the same so there is no way to distinguish the two simply by symptom pattern. Because of the difficulty in pinpointing the exact location of neural pathology in many cases, treatment approaches encourage a reduction in compression and tension along the whole length of the nerve. Soft-tissue manual therapies are an excellent treatment approach to accomplish that goal.

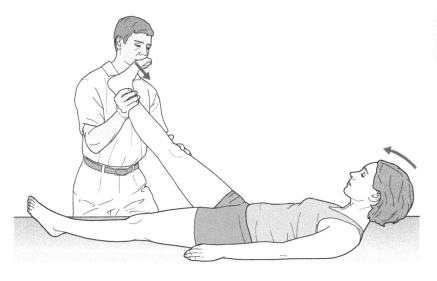

Figure 9.10
Straight leg raise (SLR).

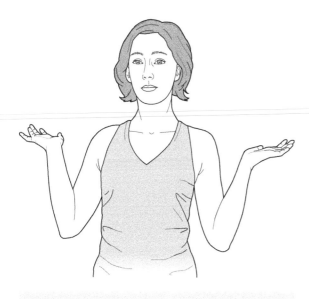

Figure 9.11
Elbow flexion test.

There are numerous textbooks on orthopedic assessment and each is filled with a plethora of special tests such as the ones described above. It is a common error made when first learning about orthopedic assessment to put too much emphasis on memorizing and applying a large number of these named orthopedic tests. Running through a laundry list of testing procedures will not allow the practitioner to land on an accurate evaluation of the patient's condition. Coady et al. (2003) state that medical students report being confused by the different tests and attempting to memorize large numbers of them was overwhelming. Focusing too much attention on memorizing all the conceivable tests misses the entire point of integrating the whole physical examination process presented through the HOPRS protocol and developing effective clinical reasoning.

Clinical reasoning in action

In some cases, the practitioner is faced with situations where multiple tissues could be the source of pain or discomfort. These are situations where the clinical reasoning skills described above are of crucial importance. The practitioner must effectively apply knowledge of anatomy and kinesiology to discern the cause of the disorder. A good example of the importance of clinical reasoning and analysis is illustrated in the following example.

A patient reports pain in the gluteal region that extends into the lower extremity. The pain is described as sharp, with periodic sensations of paresthesia. Performance of the straight leg raise causes a slight reproduction of symptoms in the lower extremity. However, it would be premature to assume that the cause of discomfort is primarily neurological, even though symptoms were reproduced with the straight leg raise test (a neurodynamic test). While the straight leg raise does increase tension on the sciatic nerve and increases symptoms for neural pathologies in this region, those are not the only effects of this test.

In the straight leg raise, the hamstring muscles are also being stretched. The hamstrings attach to the ischial tuberosity and are contiguous with the sacrotuberous ligament and lumbodorsal fascia (Vleeming et al. 1999). Tension generated in the hamstrings during the straight leg raise is transmitted through the sacrotuberous ligament and can pull on the sacrum's position. Sacroiliac joint dysfunction can produce sciatic-like lumbopelvic and lower extremity symptoms. Tension on the sacrotuberous ligament can pull the sacrum enough to irritate a sacroiliac joint pathology. Consequently, additional evaluation is necessary to discriminate between these different potential causes of the patient's complaint.

The physical examination components of orthopedic assessment are similar to other palpation skills; they only improve through continual applied practice. Yet, effective orthopedic assessment must also include clinical reasoning, and knowledge of soft tissue structure and function, common pathologies, applied anatomy, and kinesiology. The greater the practitioner's skill in integrating these various elements, the faster and more accurately is that practitioner able to evaluate the nature of soft-tissue dysfunction. Accurate identification of tissue dysfunction is the ground from which any effective soft-tissue treatment approach is built.

References

Boden SD, McCowin PR, Davis DO, Dina TS, Mark AS and Wiesel S (1990) Abnormal magnetic-resonance scans of the cervical spine in asymptomatic subjects. A prospective investigation. Journal of Bone and Joint Surgery American volume 72 (8): 1178–1184.

Borenstein DG, O'Mara JW Jr, Boden SD et al. (2001) The value of magnetic resonance imaging of the lumbar spine to predict low-back pain in asymptomatic subjects: A seven-year follow-up study. Journal of Bone and Joint Surgery American volume 83-A (9): 1306–1311.

Butler D (2000) The sensitive nervous system. Adelaide, Australia: Noigroup Publications.

Coady D, Kay L and Walker D (2003) Regional musculoskeletal examination: What the students say. Journal of Clinical Rheumatology 9 (2): 67–71.

Coady D, Walker D and Kay L (2004) Regional Examination of the Musculoskeletal System (REMS): a core set of clinical skills for medical students. Rheumatology (Oxford) 43 (5): 633–639.

Craton N and Matheson GO (1993) Training and clinical competency in musculoskeletal medicine. Identifying the problem. Sports Medicine 15 (5): 328–337.

Cyriax J (1982) Textbook of orthopaedic medicine, vol 1: Diagnosis of soft tissue lesions, 8th edn. London: Baillière Tindall.

DiCaprio MR, Covey A and Bernstein J (2003) Curricular requirements for musculoskeletal medicine in American medical schools. Journal of Bone and Joint Surgery American volume 85-A (3): 565–567.

Garrick JG and Requa RK (1988) The epidemiology of foot and ankle injuries in sports. Clinics in Sports Medicine 7 (1): 29–36.

Gracovetsky S (2007) Is the lumbodorsal fascia necessary. Paper presented at the Fascia Research Congress, Harvard Medical School, Boston, MA.

Lowe W (2006) Orthopedic assessment in massage therapy. Sisters, OR: Daviau-Scott.

Lowe W (2008) Suggested variations on standard carpal tunnel syndrome assessment tests. Journal of Bodywork and Movement Therapies 12 (2): 151–157.

Matzkin E, Smith EL, Freccero D and Richardson AB (2005). Adequacy of education in musculoskeletal medicine. Journal of Bone and Joint Surgery American volume 87-A (2): 310–314.

Schleip R (2003) Fascial plasticity – a new neurobiological explanation. Journal of Bodywork and Movement Therapies 7 (1): 11–19.

Schleip R, Naylor IL, Ursu D et al. (2006) Passive muscle stiffness may be influenced by active contractility of intramuscular connective tissue. Medical Hypotheses 66 (1): 66–71.

Shacklock M (2005) Clinical neurodynamics. Edinburgh: Elsevier.

Sherman KJ, Cherkin DC, Kahn J et al. (2005) A survey of training and practice patterns of massage therapists in two US states. BMC Complementary and Alternative Medicine 5: 13.

Stockard AR and Allen TW (2006) Competence levels in musculoskeletal medicine: Comparison of osteopathic and allopathic medical graduates. Journal of the American Osteopathic Association 106 (6): 350–355.

Vleeming A, Mooney V, Dorman T, Snijders C and Stoeckart R (1999) Movement, stability, and low back pain. New York: Churchill Livingstone.

Woolf AD (2003) How to assess musculoskeletal conditions. History and physical examination. Best Practice and Research. Clinical Rheumatology 17 (3): 381–402.

Yahia LH, Pigeon P and DesRosiers EA (1993) Viscoelastic properties of the human lumbodorsal fascia. Journal of Biomedical Engineering 15 (5): 425–429.

Movement health

"Transforming society by optimizing movement to improve the human experience."

This simple and clear sentence was adopted in 2013 by the American Physical Therapy Association (APTA) as their vision statement (Websource 1). It puts "movement" as a single tenet at the foundation of physical therapies. To attain "movement health" is therefore a key goal of therapists for their patients (McNeill & Blandford 2015; Sahrmann 2014). APTA's broad view of movement in their guiding principles to their vision statement, points out that the ramifications of "movement" reaches beyond health and "is key to optimal living and quality of life" as it allows people "to participate in and contribute to society."

Movement health has been defined as "a desired state that is not only injury free and absent of the presence of uncontrolled movement but also a state that allows the exerciser to choose how to move" (Blandford 2014a; McNeill & Blandford 2015).

Movement health includes high quality "functional movement," which is itself made up of smaller component parts of the movement of joints, limbs, girdles and spine, throughout the kinetic chain.

Assessing for *movement health* may involve looking at the whole patterns that create functional movements, but a movement fault may occur at only one joint within this movement, and in only one direction. Finer assessment may also be interested in the *threshold* at which that fault occurs (Comerford & Mottram 2012).

To remain in, or re-attain, movement health Blandford (2014b) suggests an individual needs:

1. *awareness* of the body, movement, and movement quality

2. *control* of the software (central nervous system (CNS)) and hardware (musculature and structure) of the neuromusculoskeletal system

3. varied *intensity*: a postural task needs to be achieved at a low intensity of physical work and a strength-based

task needs to be met with an appropriate high intensity of muscular effort

4. *variability*: a wide choice of movement strategies should be available for use for a single movement task.

A therapist can approach a movement-related problem by influencing individual or combined elements of these four points.

- Somatic therapies aim to improve movement health by increasing body *awareness*: put simply, improving movement output by influencing input.

- Sporting drills or repeated functional exercises within neuromusculoskeletal rehabilitation can be thought of as attempts to improve *control*.

- Principles around the use of repetitive maximums in weight training, using an appropriate number of repetitions in a physical challenge so that the *intensity* of an exercise matches the desired goal (along with cardiovascular training), form the foundation of the fitness industry.

- Perhaps the least understood element is *variability*, but this factor is what is practiced in dance, gymnastics, and Pilates training, amongst other disciplines, when the same or very similar movements are repeated over and over, perhaps in a different plane or a reversed sequence but giving the movement control center of the brain the chance to develop many engramic choices for similar movements, thereby improving the robustness of the movement system both neurologically and structurally.

Movement "*dis-ease*" can be viewed through the lens of Sahrmann's (2014) focus on the order of the syllables in the words pathokinesiologic and kineseopathologic. The former word indicates that pathology and pain can alter movement patterns and the latter describes that faulty movement patterns can create pathology.

Hodges and Tucker (2011) suggest theories to deepen the pathokinesiologic explanations of why people move differently in pain but indicate that that they do is self-evident.

Research published in 2015 by Dingenen et al. compares the gold standard and research laboratory three-dimensional multijoint assessment with more clinic friendly two-dimensional sagittal plane vertical jump landing strategies (video analysis). They identify that a more erect landing strategy associated with a smaller degree of knee and hip flexion places greater forces through the quadriceps and knee joint. Other landing strategies can be knee flexion dominant (with reduced hip flexion) or the most knee protective strategy involving a greater degree of trunk, hip, and knee flexion. They found that looking for a decreased degree of hip flexion in the two-dimensional test correlated with the three-dimensional findings.

Dingenen et al. suggest that this possibly adopted decreased hip flexion movement strategy may be *predictive* of risk of knee injury, and therefore be kinesiopathologic.

This test is described later in the text as a practical example (see Exercise 10.3).

People in pain show changes in motor control due to reorganization of the motor cortex. If – as an example – the infraspinatus muscle's motor representation in the brain is assessed bilaterally, using transcranial magnetic stimulation (fMRI) (Ngomo et al. 2015), a single-sided rotator cuff tendinopathy shows an asymmetrical decrease in the corticospinal excitability on the affected side. This, the researchers suggest, is related to the *chronicity* of pain but not its *intensity*. They state: "while cortical reorganisation correlates with magnitude of pain in neuropathic pain syndromes, it could be more related to chronicity in the case of musculoskeletal disorders."

This link between chronicity and motor cortex changes observed using fMRI has been confirmed in numerous studies, including studies of:

- osteoarthritis of the knee (Shanahan et al. 2015).
- lateral epicondylalgia (Shanahan et al. 2015).
- non-specific chronic low back pain (Schabrun et al. 2015).

People in pain also show changes in muscle function through changes in motor recruitment.

- Worsley et al. (2013) showed that prior to a motor control exercise intervention, in young adults with pain and signs of shoulder impingement, the subjects presented with a recruitment impairment of serratus anterior and lower trapezius. The change in the motor recruitment in this study was reversed by a 10-week motor control exercise regime concentrating on scapular orientation by retraining motor recruitment about the shoulder. Not only was scapular orientation improved but there was significantly increased function and reduced pain.

- In non-specific chronic low back pain (NSCLBP) research authors Van Damme et al. (2014) reference O'Sullivan (2000, 2005): "Motor Control Impairment (MCI) is estimated to appear in 30% of patients with low back pain (2005) and flexion-related MCIs are the most common disorders observed in clinical practice (2000)." Van Damme et al. found they could differentiate a lumbar flexion movement control impairment (MCI) subject from a healthy subject using surface electromyography.

The changes in motor recruitment that occur in those in pain indicate that there is a loss of variability, a loss of choice in motor planning for that individual.

Moseley and Hodges suggested in (2006) that a normal postural strategy does not return after an individual's low back pain resolves. A robust motor system allows for an exploratory variation in motor tasks and when this is lost due to pain, adaptation is prevented, increasing the risk of chronicity.

Movement evaluation

It is therefore becoming increasingly evident that movement faults, whether causative of pain and injury, or as the result of pain or injury, need to be assessed. Precise assessment and the findings can suggest precise rehabilitative interventions aimed at optimizing the control of movement, thereby maximizing a patient's recovery rate and reduction of risk of first episode injuries or re-injury.

Control of movement can be evaluated with tests that challenge the cognitive ability of an individual to control movement (Comerford & Mottram 2012; McNeill 2014b; Mischiati et al. 2015). For movement evaluation to be successful tests need to be reliable, valid and easily reproducible.

Visual rating has been shown to be both a valid and reliable tool for identifying young athletes with poor frontal plane dynamic pelvis and knee alignment (Whatman et al. 2013). Mischiati et al. (2015) have also found this to be so in the "battery of tests" approach taught in The Performance Matrix. If a therapist is experienced this appears to further improve reliability (Gribble et al. 2013; Luomajoki et al. 2007).

Pre-season screening in sport is now routine and often looks at measuring joint mobility, muscle extensibility, endurance and strength, as well as fitness tests and physiological testing (Butler et al. 2010). Such tests have a role in providing benchmarks for re-screening reference during the season and post injury, and provide some indication of limitations that need addressing – but many do not predict injury (Butler et al. 2010).

- Modern thought on movement evaluation has its basis in the early work on muscle function by Kendall et al. (2005). Kendall and colleagues' focus was on "the graded testing of muscle strength and analysing the interrelationship of strength and function" (Comerford & Mottram 2012).

- Janda too was initially interested in individual muscle testing; his first book, published in Czech in 1949 when he was 21, was on this subject. But he became interested in movement patterns, muscle imbalance and patterns of dysfunction with his classically reported finding that subjects who do not use gluteus maximus in hip extension, instead use increased anterior pelvic tilt to help create the movement.

- So Janda focused his attention on testing *muscle function* not *individual muscle strength* and his treatment strategies became focused on sensorimotor training, using simple exercises and unstable surfaces, as opposed to the more usual strength-training approaches of the day (Page et al. 2010).

- Janda also focused on increasing the extensibility of the shortened musculature (Janda 1996).

- Sahrmann developed a diagnostic framework for movement impairments using the relative flexibility concept, looking for a movement direction susceptible to motion (Sahrmann 2002). Her treatment approach uses exercise to improve the stiffness of the motion segments and regions that move too much.

> **Notes**
>
> See Chapter 5 for more on Janda's work.

Quality of movement, and the control of movement is now regarded as an important element of movement efficiency (Roussel et al. 2009) and focus is now looking at assessment protocols that examine uninjured subjects, looking at non-symptomatic deficits within the kinetic chain that might predispose to injury (Mischiati et al. 2015).

Movement assessment systems all utilize movement tests, but to gain enough useful information the tests need to be grouped into a battery of tests. As yet only some individual tests are being identified as being valid and reliable. Carlsson and Rasmussen-Barr (2013) report that tests that focus on examining only one factor – such as pelvic tilt or lateral shift of the trunk – show very good agreement in inter- and intra-observer testing, but as the number of factors increase, such as deviating the spine or pelvis, or compensatory movement from limbs, it becomes harder to attain such agreement.

It appears that entire system validation may be a long way off yet, though promising results on nine selected tests from The Foundation Matrix report acceptable inter- and intra-rater reliability on selected tests (Mischiati et al. 2015).

Recent initial research has been undertaken looking at synergy and divergence between different methods of movement-based subgrouping. Some overlap was found between elements of the movement assessment systems meaning that subgroups found in one system may be able to be further subdivided using another. The authors suggest that an integrated assessment model may refine treatment targeting (Karayannis et al. 2015).

Using movement evaluation findings in treatment

Assessment of movement on its own will not effect change in the patient; it is the management suggested by the findings that give the assessment its worth, so understanding a movement evaluation's treatment strategies is extremely important.

Undertaking a movement assessment returns greater information to the therapist giving more choice in their treatment strategies. It also suggests that findings about specific movement faults can create specific exercise choices which may eventually supplant the current more general exercise guides, as provided by institutions such as the UK's National Institute for Health and Care Excellence (NICE), who suggest that exercise programs may include: aerobic activity, movement instruction, muscle strengthening, postural control, and stretching (NICE Guidelines 2009).

Notwithstanding the biopsychosocial factors associated in non-specific chronic low back pain (NSCLBP) that may alter therapeutic approach, specific exercise for specific movement faults should be taught as well, rechecked at intervals, and the patient be compliant to the regime (McNeill 2014a).

Differentiating evidence-based therapeutic exercise, individualized to a specific patient from a pathoanatomical diagnosis-based protocol (such as those designed for patellar malalignment) can mean reducing a number of potentially unnecessary exercises. These "extra" exercises are required by protocol-based exercise interventions as they need to cater for a wide range of variables that may not even be present in an individual with that condition, since most individuals vary from a textbook case. Clinical reasoning, therefore, must be used during exercise design.

Aims and goals must be considered and should shift in response to changes through the rehabilitative period. A non-linear approach should be made (Box 10.1).

Box 10.1 A therapist must ask:

- Why this exercise?

- What level of effort should be set?

- What dose of exercise – how long, how many repetitions, how often?

- When can it be progressed?

- When should it be stopped?

- How do I know if it is working?

- In what timeframe should changes be seen?

- What are the risks (Comerford & Mottram 2012)?

Therapist skills and practical examples

It is likely that all therapists in the musculoskeletal sphere use movement evaluation to some degree within their day-to-day practice. Exhaustively testing the whole kinetic chain, though desirable, can be time consuming, but the layering of recognition of common patterns of uncontrolled movement, or direction susceptible to movement, can over time inform management choice, to the point that a therapist can be primarily engaged managing their patients' movement quality.

A therapist will need to develop a sound background in the concepts of *movement health* and ideally be conversant with one system of *movement evaluation*, so that as research continues to clarify both movement assessment and management, the therapist can refine their skillset, adapting their approach to accept best practice.

Observation

Acute observation of a patient's movement patterns is fundamental (see also Special topic 3, on visual assessment).

Exercise 10.1 *Prone Knee Bend Test*

Take for example the *prone knee bend test* (Fig. 10.1).

This movement test is described by Sahrmann (2002) as an example of her "relative flexibility" concept. An understanding that the passive or active stiffness of muscle and soft tissues as they cross joints can influence at which joint that movement can be seen is important.

A muscle that is increasing in bulk due to an effect of training can become stiffer throughout its range of motion. Sahrmann uses the analogy of tighter and looser springs in series which indicate that movement is likely to be observed to occur in an area that is loosely held and less likely to occur in an area that is more tightly held.

- The subject to be tested lies prone and one knee is passively flexed to 135°.

- The knee should be able to flex to 135° without any anterior tilt of the lumbar spine or pelvis.

- If anterior tilt does occur this can be an example of compensatory relative flexibility – where the soft tissue structures controlling anterior tilt are less stiff than the rectus femoris, as it extends.

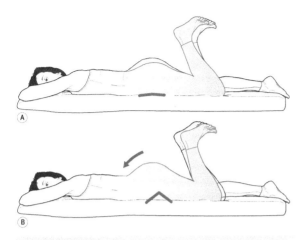

Figure 10.1
Prone knee bend. (A) Active prone knee flexion without anterior tilt of the pelvis. (B) Active prone knee flexion of a "stiff" hip flexor creating a compensatory anterior tilt of the pelvis. In this example of relative flexibility the active knee flexion gets to approximately the same range. In (A) the stiffness of the anterior tilt stabilizing muscles, the lower obliques, and gluteus maximus are in balance but in (B) the lumbopelvic region anteriorly tilts due to either an under-recruitment of the gluteal and abdominal stabilizers of the pelvis, or an excessive stiffness of the rectus femoris muscle.

● If the rectus femoris is stiff, not short, the therapist stabilizing the pelvis to prevent anterior tilt should still find the knee flexes to 135°; however, if the rectus femoris is short, the knee will stop flexing before achieving that range.

● If the test is actively applied with the subject generating the knee bend themselves, this can test the subject's ability to generate an automatic stabilization effect controlling pelvic tilt while allowing the knee to flex to the 135° benchmark.

Interpretation of the test may lead a therapist to choose to apply cognitive control to increasing the muscular stiffness of the muscles that prevent anterior tilt during the knee flexion – or to apply techniques to increase extensibility of the rectus femoris.

Observation of where movement occurs, and in what part of the range, and the ability to interpret the findings are important elements of evaluating movement.

Van Dillen et al. (2003) showed that lumbar extension with rotation, lumbar extension, and lumbar rotation in a variation of this test were able to relate direction to patient's pain, while Loumajoki et al. (2008) were able to show a difference between the response of patients and healthy controls.

● When you apply this test to different subjects can you identify the variable responses described above?

● Were you able to identify different rectus femoris states? Normal? Stiff? Short and stiff?

● What therapeutic choices might this lead you towards?

Exercise 10.2 *Standing Bow Test*

Tests of dissociation of movement are frequently applied.

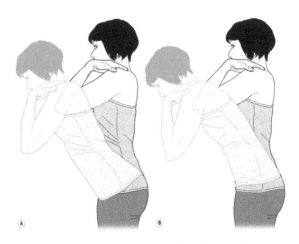

Figure 10.2
Standing bow. (A) A correct dissociation pattern showing the maintenance of a lumbar lordosis during a hip flexion movement. A therapist may help the patient be aware of how to maintain the lumbar lordosis during the hip flexion/lumbar flexion dissociation exercise through the use of physical cueing. The therapist could touch each of the patient's lower four lumbar spinous processes and the top of their sacrum with their fingertips to help enhance the patient's proprioception. (B) A lumbar (and thoracic flexion) during the standing bow "associating" the spinal flexion with the hip flexion.

A *standing bow test* (Fig. 10.2) was shown by Roussel et al. (2009) to be predictive of an increased risk of developing lower extremity or lumbar spine injuries in dancers.

- The subject stands with a neutral lumbar spine, that is, in the mid-range between anterior and posterior pelvic tilt.

- (S)he is then instructed to flex the hips to 50° without flexing or extending the lumbar spine.

- The ability to disassociate hip flexion from lumbar flexion (or extension) can be created by the stabilizing muscles of the trunk activating isometrically to keep the spine in its neutral position.

- For the test to show a failure of control, the movement should not be able to be improved by instruction and correction (Luomajoki et al. 2007).

- When you apply this test involving different subjects, what are your findings?

- Were you able to identify instances where the lumbar spine could not be kept neutral during hip flexion to 50°?

- If so, what treatment/rehabilitation strategies might you employ?

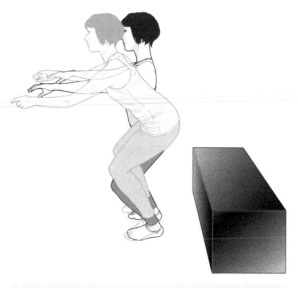

Figure 10.3
Landing a "double leg drop vertical jump." This example superimposes two landing strategies – the minimal hip and knee flexion "erect" landing posture versus the more desirable "hip and knee flexion" strategy, in which the landing force is primarily absorbed into the gluteal musculature with additional absorption into the knee extensor musculature.

Exercise 10.3 *Double-Leg Drop Vertical Jump Test*

This test uses higher loading forces, meaning that muscular strength is required to pass the test.

Due to the width of the female pelvis, female athletes are at an increased risk of knee injury during dynamic lower limb movements.

These three-dimensional movements can be pared down to an easier two-dimensional movement assessment – if viewed from the side during the *double-leg drop vertical jump test* (DVJ) (Fig. 10.3).

Dingenen et al. (2015) suggest it is the deepest part of the landing strategy that may help an assessor work out whether the complex three-dimensional lower limb movements involved in the landing are desirable to reduce risk of injury at the knee.

- The subject is asked to drop off a box 30 cm (12 inches) in height, with two legs, with their feet positioned 20 cm (8 inches) apart, immediately followed by a maximal vertical jump.

- If the test is videoed the measurement should occur at the deepest part of the landing – prior to the vertical jump.

Three typical landing strategies can be employed, including:

1. an erect landing stance with reduced hip and knee flexion

2. a deep knee flexion landing strategy with reduced hip flexion

3. a flexed landing pattern with hip and knee flexion, with ankle dorsiflexion.

It is the latter which Dingenen et al. suggest is the more protective of the knee.

The absorption of the load into the gluteal musculature is regarded as important and therefore the hip flexion is the most important element for the assessor to keep an eye on during the test.

For injury prevention programs, Dingenen et al. suggest that movement re-education should aim at increasing the amount of hip and trunk flexion during DVJ, to avoid high-risk knee movements.

A single leg version off a 10 cm (4 inch) box produced similar results and advice.

- When applying this test are you able to observe the various landing strategies?

- Using a video recording is likely to be the best way of making this judgement.

- If you do observe less desirable landing strategies, how might this inform your therapeutic choices?

Shoulder dysfunction

A therapist also needs to problem-solve and use movement solutions to help generate the basis of appropriate exercise prescription. The following shoulder girdle example helps illustrate this.

Rotator cuff-related shoulder pain (RCRSP) is a term used by Lewis (2016) to encompass a spectrum of shoulder conditions that include subacromial (impingement) pain, rotator cuff tendinopathy, and rotator cuff tears – both partial and full thickness.

Lewis's assessment of accepted theories of etiology suggest that localizing a shoulder problem to a single structure is fraught due to the basic design of the rotator cuff which fuses the tendons into one structure.

He also questions the view that acromial irritation leads to rotator cuff symptoms, or that the shape of the distal end of the acromion correlates with symptoms, or indeed that a subacromial decompression surgery is more effective than a structured and supervised exercise program (Ketola et al. 2013).

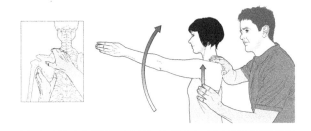

Figure 10.4
Shoulder symptom modification procedure. In this example the therapist tests if the patient's usual pain provocation movement of shoulder flexion is reduced if the scapula is elevated gently during the active shoulder flexion.

Lewis suggests that a RCRSP patient wants less pain and better function. To that end he proposed the shoulder symptom modification procedure (Lewis 2009) (Fig. 10.4) in which the patient's presenting symptomatic movement, often shoulder flexion, is repeated while the therapist adds movement, or taping, to the thoracic spine to reduce kyphosis, or alters the scapular position by adding scapular elevation, depression, protraction, retraction, posterior tilt, anterior tilt, internal rotation, or external rotation, or changes the humeral head position during the movement.

The movement that reduces the symptom becomes the basis of a specific gentle exercise regime.

The current focus on the movement system, its evaluation, and its management is a growing field that is here to stay. Hopefully these examples and tests offer insights that can be explored through additional study and/or training.

References

Blandford L (2014a) Injury prevention and movement control. Core values and posture, vol 1. London: YMCAed.

Blandford L (2014b) Injury prevention and movement control. Warm up, flexibility and resistance training, vol 2. London: YMCAed.

Butler RB, Plisky P, Southers C, Scoma C and Kiesel BK (2010) Biomechanical analysis of the different classification of the functional movement screen deep squat test. Sports Biomechanics 9 (4): 270–279.

Carlsson H and Rasmussen-Barr E (2013) Clinical screening tests for assessing movement control in non-specific low-back pain. A systematic review of intra- and inter-observer reliability studies. Manual Therapy 18: 103–110.

Comerford M and Mottram S (2012) Kinetic control: The management of uncontrolled movement. Edinburgh: Elsevier, Churchill Livingstone.

Dingenen B, Malfait B, Vanrenterghem J, Robinson MA, Verschueren SMP and Staes FF (2015) Can two-dimensional measured peak saggital plane excursions during drop vertical jumps help identify three-dimensional measured joint movements? Knee 22 (2): 73–79.

Gribble PA, Brigle J, Pietrosimone BG, Pfile KR and Webster KA (2013) Intrarater reliability of the functional movement screen. Journal of Strength and Conditioning Research 27 (4): 978–981.

Hodges PW and Tucker K (2011) Moving differently in pain: A new theory to explain adaptation to pain. Pain. 152 (3 Suppl): S90–S98.

Janda V (1996) Evaluation of muscle imbalance, in Liebenson C (ed), Rehabilitation of the Spine. Baltimore: Williams and Wilkins.

Karayannis NV, Jull GA and Hodges PW (2015) Movement-based subgrouping in low back pain: Synergy and divergence in approaches. Physiotherapy 102 (2): 159–169.

Kendall F, McCreary EK, Rovance PG, Rodgers MM and Romani WA (2005) Muscles testing and function with posture and pain, 5th edn. Baltimore: Lippincott Williams and Wilkins.

Ketola S, Lehtinen J, Rousi T, Nissinen M, Huhtala H, Konttinen YT and Arnala I (2013) No evidence of long-term benefits of arthroscopic acromioplasty in the treatment of shoulder impingement syndrome: Five-year results of a randomised controlled trial. Bone and Joint Research 2 (7): 132–139.

Lewis J (2009) Rotator cuff tendinopathy/subacromial impingement syndrome: Is it time for a new method of assessment? British Journal of Sports Medicine 43: 259–264.

Lewis J (2016) Rotator cuff related shoulder pain: Assessment, management and uncertainties. Manual Therapy 23: 57–68.

Luomajoki H, Kool J, Bruin ED and Airaksinen O (2007) Reliability of movement control tests in the lumbar spine. BMC Musculoskeletal Disorders 8: 90.

Luomajoki H, Kool J, Bruin ED and Airaksinen O (2008) Movement control tests of the low back: Evaluation of the difference between patients with low back pain and healthy controls. BMC Musculoskeletal Disorders 9: 170.

McNeill W (2014a) Pilates: Ranging beyond neutral. [Editorial]. Journal of Bodywork and Movement Therapies 18: 119–123.

McNeill W (2014b) The double knee swing test: A practical example of the performance matrix movement screen. Journal of Bodywork and Movement Therapies 18: 477–481.

McNeill W and Blandford L (2015) Movement health. Journal of Bodywork and Movement Therapies 19: 150–159.

Mischiati C, Comerford M, Gosford E et al. (2015) Intra and inter-rater reliability of screening for movement impairments: Movement control tests from The Foundation Matrix. Journal of Sports Science and Medicine 14: 427–440.

Moseley GL and Hodges PW (2006) Reduced variability of postural strategy prevents normalisation of motor changes induced by back pain: A risk factor for chronic trouble? Behavioural Neuroscience 120 (2): 474–476.

Ngomo S, Mercier C, Bouyer LJ, Savoie A and Roy J-S (2015) Alterations in central motor representation increase over time in individuals with rotator cuff tendinopathy. Clinical Neurophysiology 126: 365–371.

NICE Guidelines (CG88) (2009) Low back pain adults: Early management. Available at: www.nice.org.uk/guidance/cg88/chapter/1-guidance#physical-activity-and-exercise (accessed October 19, 2016).

O'Sullivan P (2000) Lumbar segmental instability: Clinical presentation and specific exercise management. Manual Therapy 5 (1): 2–12.

O'Sullivan P (2005) Diagnosis and classification of chronic low back pain disorders: Maladaptive movement and movement control impairments as underlying mechanism. Manual Therapy 10: 242–255.

Page P, Frank C and Lardner R (2010) Assessment and treatment of muscle imbalance. The Janda approach. Champaign, IL: Human Kinetics.

Roussel NA, Nijs J, Mottram S, Van Moorsel A, Truijen S and Stassijns G (2009) Altered lumbopelvic movement control but not generalized joint hypermobility is associated with increased injury in dancers. Manual Therapy 14 (6): 630–635.

Sahrmann S (2002) Diagnosis and treatment of movement impairment syndromes. St Louis, MO: Mosby.

Sahrmann SA (2014) The human movement system: Our professional identity. Physical Therapy 94: 1034–1042.

Schabrun S, Elgueta-Cancino EL and Hodges PW (2015) Smudging of the motor cortex is related to the severity of low back pain. Spine. Epub ahead of print. DOI: 10.1097/BRS.0000000000000938.

Shanahan C, Hodges PW, Wrigley TV, Bennell K and Farrell M (2015) Organisation of the motor cortex differs between people with and without knee osteoarthritis. Arthritis Research and Therapy 17 (1): 164.

Van Damme B, Stevens V, Perneel C et al. (2014) A surface electromyography based objective method to identify patients with nonspecific chronic low back pain, presenting a flexion related movement control impairment. Journal of Electromyography and Kinesiology 24: 954–964.

Van Dillen LR, Sahrmann SA, Norton BJ, Caldwell CA, McDonnell MK and Bloom NJ (2003) Movement system impairment-based categories for low back pain: Stage 1 validation. Journal of Orthopaedic and Sports Physical Therapy 33 (3): 126–142.

Websource 1 Available at: http://www.apta.org/Vision/ (accessed October 19, 2016).

Whatman C, Hume P and Hing W (2013) The reliability and validity of physiotherapist visual rating of dynamic pelvis and knee alignment in young athletes. Physical Therapy in Sport 14: 168–174.

Worsley P, Warner M, Mottram S et al. (2013) Motor control retraining exercises for shoulder impingement: Effects on function, muscle activation, and biomechanics in young adults. Journal of Shoulder and Elbow Surgery 22 (4): 11–19.

Special topic 10

Fibromyalgia palpation assessment
Leon Chaitow

Not everyone agrees with the current protocol of the American College of Rheumatology for assessing/ diagnosing fibromyalgia syndrome (FMS) (Dommerholt & Issa 2009). However, it is what it is, and until a consensus emerges as to a different set of criteria it is useful to know how rheumatologists, and others, come to the decision that an individual meets the current criteria for a diagnosis of what is commonly known as fibromyalgia.

NOTE: The term 'fibromyalgia' is likely to change, just as chronic fatigue syndrome has recently morphed into SEID or 'systemic exertion intolerance disease' (Clayton 2015).

In 1990, the American College of Rheumatology (ACR) developed the following criteria for FMS (Wolfe et al. 1990):

- widespread bilateral pain above and below the waist of at least 3 months' duration

- the presence of *excessive* tenderness on applying pressure to 11 of 18 muscle/tendon sites – tender points.

A positive report of pain in the area being depressed indicates a tender point. Tender points should not be confused with trigger points, such as those commonly seen in myofascial pain syndrome (although the tender points may in fact be trigger points).

Patients who have fewer tender points than the number required by the tender point criteria are still often diagnosed with fibromyalgia, as long as they have had widespread pain in all four quadrants of the body for at least 3 months – and not necessarily at the actual tender point sites themselves. However, in fibromyalgia patients, the rest of their physical examination is often normal, including muscle strength and range of motion.

Fibromyalgia tender point palpation protocol

1. Locate each of the nine bilateral points to be palpated (Special topic Fig. 10.1).

2. Also test three control points – one on the mid-forehead, another on the patient's left thumbnail, and another on the dorsum of the forearm. These are useful to gauge the individual's general pain tolerance as 4 kg applied to any of these will not normally evoke a report of pain.

3. Before applying pressure say something such as this to the patient: "Various areas of your body will be examined for pain as I apply moderate pressure to them. Please say 'yes' or 'no' if there is any pain when I press."

4. Apply pressure with the dominant thumb, perpendicular to the palpated site, for 4 seconds, with 4 kg of pressure (or preferably use an algometer or dolorimeter).

5. Manually applied 4 kg of pressure is usually sufficient to whiten the nailbed.

6. If the response on pressure is "yes", ask for a numeric pain intensity rating out of 10.

7. If 11 out of 18 points are positive an FMS diagnosis might be appropriate – if there has been widespread pain for at least 3 months affecting all quadrants of the body.

8. A number of associated conditions make the diagnosis more probable.

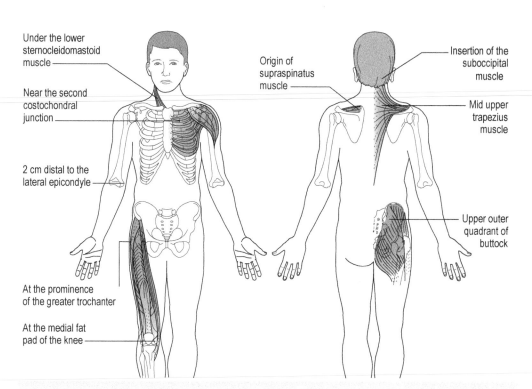

Figure ST 10.1
Recommended sites to evaluate fibromyalgia pain.

Points to assess (see Special topic Fig. 10.1)

Seated

- mid-forehead (control point)

- occiput: suboccipital muscle insertions

- trapezius: midpoint of upper border

- supraspinatus: above medial border of scapular spine

- gluteal: upper outer quadrant of buttocks

- low cervical: anterior aspect of the intertransverse space of C5–C7

- 2nd rib: 2nd costochondral junction

- lateral epicondyle of elbow: 2 cm distal to epicondyle

- dorsum right forearm (control point): junction of proximal two thirds and distal one third

- left thumbnail (control point).

Side-lying

- greater trochanter: posterior to trochanteric prominences.

Supine, feet slightly apart

- knee: medial fat pad proximal to the joint line.

Special topic Exercise 10.1 *Fibromyalgia Tender Point Assessment*

Time suggested: 5–7 minutes

Perform the test (all 18 points as listed above plus the 3 control points) on someone with widespread pain (ideally already with an FMS diagnosis), as well as on someone with limited, or no, somatic pain.

- Compare the feel of these palpated sites.

- What differences do you note in respect to the responses of the two individuals to pressure on these areas – particularly when comparing "real" points and "control" points?

- Learn to ask for pain responses in terms of a scale out of 10 after each test point.

- Chart each point's pain response.

Note: In a study in New Zealand in 2007 it was found that, a number of participants "changed" their FMS diagnosis during the course of a menstrual cycle, fulfilling the diagnostic criteria during the menstrual or luteal phase, but never during the follicular phase (Dunnett et al. 2007). It is suggested that pain thresholds drop post-ovulation as progesterone levels rise, accelerating the breathing rate, potentially influencing pain thresholds via inducement of respiratory alkalosis – as discussed in Chapter 12.

References

Clayton E W (2015) Beyond myalgic encephalomyelitis/chronic fatigue syndrome: an IOM report on redefining an illness. JAMA 313.11: 1101-1102.

Dommerholt J and Issa T (2009) Differential diagnosis of fibromyalgia, in Chaitow L (ed) Fibromyalgia syndrome, 3rd edn. Edinburgh: Churchill Livingstone/Elsevier.

Dunnett A, Roy D, Stewart A and McPartland J (2007) The diagnosis of fibromyalgia in women may be influenced by menstrual cycle phase. Journal of Bodywork and Movement Therapies 11: 99–105.

Wolfe F, Smythe HA, Yunus MB et al. (1990) The American College of Rheumatology criteria for the classification of fibromyalgia: Report of the Multicenter Criteria Committee. Arthritis and Rheumatism 33: 160–172.

Chapter 11

The learning experience in acquiring palpation skills depends upon the development of an awareness of what "normal" feels like. Without that baseline for comparison it is hard to know what "abnormal" feels like. Remembering what normal feels like offers an instant sense of "this is not right."

In the 1950s and 1960s, research, most notably by Irvin Korr (1947), coincided with a resurgence of interest in what is known as "functional technique." This involved palpation of tissues that are being gently and sequentially taken, by means of passive positioning, towards a state of "comfort," "ease," "dynamic neutral."

The "ease" position is subjectively sensed by means of your palpation skills, rather than relying on feedback from the patient as to comfort, or reduction in pain, as fine-tuning repositioning progresses. This approach is in contrast to the method of Laurence Jones's strain/counterstrain (SCS), as discussed in Chapter 5, which also aims at identifying "comfort" positions, but that depends on verbal feedback from the patient regarding the sensitivity of the tissues being positioned (Jones 1981).

In this chapter we explore the theme of functional palpation, and it will be up to you to start to recognize, and imprint on your proprioceptive memory, what the tissue responses are to passive repositioning of joints and soft tissues – normal and abnormal – and ultimately, "maximal ease."

The following series of exercises includes reference to, and thoughts derived from, the research work of: Edward Stiles (Johnston et al. 1969), CA Bowles (1955), William Johnston (1966, 1988a, b, 1997), John Glover and Herbert Yates (1997), Philip Greenman (1989, 1996), as well as descriptive observations from British osteopath Laurie Hartman (1985). Also included later in this section (Exercises 11.3, 11.8) is a functional exercise based on the work of the developer of functional technique, H.V. Hoover (1969).

Hartman analyzes this "indirect palpation technique," saying that the practitioner's objective is to palpate the affected tissues, seeking "a state of ease and release, rather than looking for the point of bind and barrier" that characterizes so many other manipulative approaches (high-velocity thrust, articulation, muscle energy methods, and so on).

We have already experimented with an indirect form of assessment/palpation in Chapter 4, Box 4.4, where skin was moved on its underlying fascia in various directions, seeking a combined position of comfort/ease. That was an example of a purely "functional palpation" exercise.

Finding dynamic neutral

The term "functional technique" grew out of a series of study sessions organized by the Academy of Applied Osteopathy in the 1950s, under the general heading of "a functional approach to specific osteopathic manipulative problems."

An exercise will be described in this chapter (Exercise 11.9) in which a functional palpation for ease of a particular area will be compared with using SCS methodology in the same area. Theoretically (and commonly in practice), the palpated position of maximum ease (reduced tone) in the distressed tissues, located using functional palpation, should correspond with the position which would have been found were pain being used as a guide – as in SCS.

Bowles (1955) gives an example of functional palpation:

- *A patient has an acute low back and walks with a list.*

- *A structural diagnosis is made and the fingertips palpate the most distressed tissues, within the area of most distress. The practitioner begins tentative positioning of the patient, preferably sitting.*

- *The fingertips pick up a slight change toward a dynamic neutral response, a little is gained, a little, not much, but a little.*

- *little, but enough so the original segment is no longer the most distressed area within the area of general distress.*

- *The fingers then move to what is now the most acute segment.*

- *As much feeling of "dynamic neutral" (ease) is obtained here as possible.*

- *Being temporarily satisfied with slight improvements here and there, this procedure continues until no more improvement is detectable.*

- *That is the time to stop.*

- *Using [palpated] tissue response to guide the treatment, the practitioner has step by step eased the lesioning [dysfunction], and corrected the structural imbalance, to the extent that the patient is on the way to recovery.*

Functional objectives

Hoover (1957) summarizes the key elements of functional technique:

- Diagnosis of function involves passive evaluation as the part being palpated responds to physiological demands for activity made by the practitioner or the patient.

- Functional diagnosis determines the presence, or absence, of normal activity of a part that is required to respond to normal body activities (say, respiration, or the introduction of passive or active flexion or extension). If the participating part has free and "easy" motion, it is normal; however, if it responds to activity by demonstrating palpated restricted or "binding" motion, it is dysfunctional.

- The degree of ease and/or bind – present in a dysfunctional site when motion is demanded – is a fair guide to the severity of the dysfunction.

- The most severe areas of dysfunction are the ones to treat first.

- The directions of motion which induce ease in the dysfunctional tissues indicate precisely the most desirable pathways of movement.

- Use of these guidelines automatically prevents undesirable manipulative methods, since bind would result from any movement towards directions of stress for the tissues.

- Treatment using these methods is seldom, if ever, painful and is well received by patients.

- The application requires focused concentration on the part of the practitioner and may be mentally fatiguing. Functional methods are suitable for application to the very ill, the extremely acute and the most chronic situations.

The "listening" hand

Bowles (1955) offers advice to those attempting to use their palpating contacts in ways that will allow the application of functional methods:

- The palpating contact ("the listening hand") must not move.

- It must not initiate any movement.

- Its presence, in contact with the area under assessment/treatment, is simply to derive information from the tissue beneath the skin.

- It needs to be "tuned into" whatever action is taking place beneath the contact and must temporarily ignore all other sensations such as "superficial tissue texture, skin temperature, skin tension, thickening or doughiness of deep tissues, muscle and fascial tensions, relative positions of bones and range of motion.

- All these signs should be assessed and evaluated and recorded separately from the functional evaluation, which should be focused single-mindedly on tissue response to motion. "It is the deep segmental tissues, the ones that support and position the bones of a segment, and their reaction to normal motion demands, that are at the heart of functional technique specificity."

Terminology

Bowles explains the shorthand use of common descriptive words:

Normal somatic function is a well-organised complexity, and is accompanied by an easy action under the palpating fingers. The message from within the palpated tissue is dubbed a sense of "ease", for convenience of description. Somatic dysfunction could then be viewed as an organised dysfunction, and rec-

ognised under the quietly palpating fingers as tissues under stress, an action dubbed as having a sense of "bind".

In addition to the "listening hand" and the sensations it is seeking, of ease and bind, Bowles suggests we develop a "linguistic armament," which will allow us to pursue the subject of functional technique without "linguistic embarrassment" and without the need to impose quotation marks around the terms each time they are used.

He therefore asks us to become familiar with the additional terms "motive hand," which indicates the contact hand that directs motion (or fingers, or thumb, or even verbal commands for motion – active or assisted); and also "normal motion demand," which indicates what it is that the motive hand is asking of the body part. The motion could be any normal movement such as flexion, extension, side bending, rotation, or a combination of movements – the response to which will be somewhere in the spectrum of ease and bind, which will be picked up by the "listening hand" for evaluation.

At its simplest, functional technique sets up a "demand–response" sequence that allows for the identification of dysfunction – as bind is noted – and for therapeutic intervention, as the tissues are guided into ease. Functional technique, palpation or treatment (there is really no difference), seeks the loose, free, easy, comfortable directions of movement and avoids anything that produces feelings in the palpated tissues of increased tone, tension, restriction, bind, or pain.

Bowles's summary of functional methods

In summary, whatever region, joint or muscle is being evaluated by the listening hand, the following results might occur:

1. The motive hand makes a series (in any order) of motion demands (within normal range) that includes as many as possible physiological variations. If the response noted in the tissues by the listening hand is ease in all directions symmetrically, then the tissues are functioning normally.

2. The motive hand makes a series of motion demands that includes as many as possible variations; however, some of the directions of movement produce bind, although the demand is within normal physiological ranges. The tissues are responding dysfunctionally.

3. For therapy to be introduced, in response to an assessment of bind relating to particular motion demands, the listening hand's feedback is required, so that, as the motions which produced bind are reintroduced, movement is modified so that the maximum degree of possible ease is achieved.

Therapy is monitored by the listening hand, and fine-tuned information, as to what to do next, is then fed back to the motive hand. Motion demands are selected which give an increasing response of ease and compliance, under the quietly palpating fingers.

The results can be startling, as Bowles explains:

Once the ease response is elicited, it tends to be self-maintaining in response to all normal motion demands. In short, somatic dysfunctions are no longer dysfunctions. There has been a spontaneous release of the holding pattern.

The palpating contact

Some practitioners mold the hand, part of the hand, or palmar surface of the fingers to the tissues which are being evaluated for ease and bind, as the area is moved actively or passively. Others use a method (termed a "compression test") described by Johnston (1997) as follows:

The compression test is the application of pressure, through the finger(s), to sense any increased tissue tension, at one segment, compared with adjacent segments. Even at rest, a compression test of a dysfunctional segment will register the local increased resistance of that segment's deep musculature ... The segment's tissues change during motion testing. This provides a palpable measure of the degree of disturbed motor function ... During motion testing, palpatory cues of increasing resistance in one direction are sensed immediately, along with an immediate sense of decreasing resistance (increasing ease) in the opposite direction.

Exercise 11.1 Bowles's Self-Palpation Method

Time suggested   3–4 minutes

- Stand up and place your fingers on your own neck muscles, paraspinally, so that the fingers lie, very lightly, without pressing but constantly "in touch" with the tissues, approximately over the transverse processes.

- Start to walk for a few steps and try to ignore the skin and the bones under your fingers.

- Concentrate all your attention on the deep supporting and active tissues as you walk.

- After a few steps, stand still and then take a few steps backwards, all the while evaluating the subtle yet definite changes under your fingertips.

- Repeat the process several times, once while breathing normally and once while holding the breath in, and again, holding it out.

- Standing still, take one leg at a time backwards, extending the hip and then returning it to neutral, before doing the same with the other leg.

- What do you feel with your listening hands in all these different situations?

Comment

This exercise should help to emphasize the "listening" role of the palpating fingers and of their selectivity about what they wish to listen to. The listening hand contact should be "quiet, non-intrusive, non-perturbing," in order to register the compliance of the tissues and to evaluate whether there is a greater or lesser degree of ease or bind on alternating steps, and under different circumstances, as you walk, stand still, move your leg.

Exercise 11.2 Stiles and Johnston's Sensitivity Exercises

Time suggested   11.2A 3–4 minutes; 11.2B and 11.2C 7–10 minutes

11.2A

- Stand behind your seated palpation partner, resting your palms and fingers over their upper trapezius muscle, between the base of the neck and shoulder.

- The object is to evaluate what happens under your hands as your partner takes a deep breath.

Notes

> This is not a comparison between inhalation and exhalation, but is meant to help you assess how the areas being palpated respond to inhalation.

- Do the tissues under your hands stay easy – or do they bind?

You should specifically not try to define the underlying structures, or their status, in terms of tone or fibrosity. Simply assess the impact, if any, of inhalation on the tissues.

- Do the tissues resist, restrict, bind or do they stay relaxed on inhalation?

Compare what is happening under one hand with what is happening under the other, during inhalation only – specifically avoiding comparison of the feel of the tissues during inhalation and exhalation.

11.2B

Your palpation partner should be seated with you standing behind.

The objective this time is to "map" the various areas of "restriction" or bind in the thorax, anterior and/or posterior, during the time your partner is inhaling.

In this exercise, try not only to identify areas of bind but map the territory, by assigning what you find into large (several segments of near the spine) and small (single segment) categories.

Exercise 11.2 *continued*

- To commence, place a single hand, mainly fingers, on (say) the upper left thoracic area, over the scapula, and have your partner breathe deeply several times, first while seated comfortably hands on lap and then with the arms folded on the chest (exposing more the costovertebral articulation).

- After several breaths, with your hand in one position, resite it a little lower or more medially or laterally, as appropriate, until the entire back has been "mapped" in this way.

Most importantly for this exercise, remember that you are not comparing how the tissues "feel" on inhalation as compared with exhalation, but how different regions compare (in terms of ease and bind) with each other, in response to inhalation.

- Map the entire back and/or front of the thorax, in this way, for location of areas of bind and for the size of these areas.

- Return and repalpate any large areas of bind and, within them, see whether you can identify any small areas, using the same simple contact, with inhalation as the motion component.

- Individual spinal segments can also be mapped by sequentially assessing them, one at a time, as you evaluate their response to inhalations.

- How would you normally handle the information you have uncovered if this were a "patient"?

- Would you try in some way to mobilize what appears to be restricted? If so, how?

- Would your therapeutic focus be on the large areas of restriction or the small ones?

- Would you work on areas distant from or adjacent to the restricted areas?

- Would you attempt release of the perceived restriction by trying to move it mechanically towards and through its resistance barrier or would you rather be inclined to use some indirect approach, moving away from the restriction barrier?

- Or, would you try a variety of approaches, mixing and matching, until the region under attention was free or improved?

There are no correct or incorrect answers to these questions. However, the various exercises in this section should open up possibilities for a variety of treatment options to be considered, ways which do not impose a solution, but that allow one to emerge spontaneously.

11.2C

Your palpation partner should be seated, arms folded on the chest, with you standing behind, with your listening hand/fingertips placed on the upper left thorax, on or around the scapula area.

Your motive hand should be placed at the cervicodorsal junction, so that it can indicate to your partner your request that he move forward of the midline (dividing the body longitudinally in the coronal plane), not into flexion but in a manner which carries the head and upper torso anteriorly.

The movement will be more easily accomplished if your partner has arms folded, as suggested above.

The repetitive movement forward into the position described, and back to neutral, is initiated by the motive hand, while the listening hand evaluates the palpated tissues' response to the movements.

The comparison that is being evaluated is of one palpated area with another, in response to this normal motion demand.

As Johnston and his colleagues (1969) state, in relation to this exercise: "It is not anterior direction of motion, compared with posterior direction, but rather a testing of motion into the anterior compartment only, comparing one area with the ones below, and the ones above, and so on."

Your listening hand is asking the tissues whether they respond easily or with resistance to the motion demanded of the trunk. In this way, try to identify those areas, large and small, which bind as the movement forward is carried out.

Compare these areas with those identified when the breathing assessment was used.

Comment

The patterns elicited in Exercise 11.2C involve movement initiated by you as the practitioner, whereas the information derived from 11.2A and 11.2B involved intrinsic motion, initiated by exaggerated respiration.

Chapter 11

Johnston and his colleagues (1969) have, in these simple exercises, taken us through the initial stages of palpatory literacy, in relation to how tissues respond to motion, self-initiated or externally induced. You should, by these means, have become able to localize (map) areas of dysfunction (bind), large and small, and, within large areas, become able to identify small dysfunctional tissue localities. These localities can then be used as monitors in subsequent treatment, as the area is moved into positions which minimize the restrictions you are able to palpate in them.

Hoover's "experiments"

Hoover (1969) poses a number of questions in the following exercises ("experiments" he calls them), the answers to which should always be "yes." If your answers are indeed positive at the completion of the exercise, then you are probably sensitive enough in palpatory skills to be able to effectively utilize functional technique.

Exercise 11.3 *Hoover's Thoracic Experiment*

Time suggested   11.3A 7–10 minutes; 11.3B and 11.3C 3–4 minutes each

---

11.3A

You should stand behind your seated partner, whose arms are folded on their chest.

Having previously assessed by palpation, observation, and examination the thoracic or lumbar spine of your partner, lightly place your listening hand or finger pad contact on those segments you judge to be the most restricted (perhaps as assessed in Chapter 8?) or in which the tissues are most hypertonic.

● Wait, and do nothing as your hand "tunes in" to the tissues.

● Make no assessments as to structural status. Wait for at least 15 seconds.

Hoover says: "The longer you wait, the less structure you feel. The longer you keep the receiving fingers still, the more ready you are to pick up the first signals of segment response, when you proceed to induce a movement demand."

● With your other hand, and by voice, guide your partner into flexion and then extension.

● The motive hand should apply very light touch, just a suggestion, to indicate to your partner in which direction you want movement to take place.

● The listening hand does nothing but wait to feel the functional response of ease and bind, as the spinal segments move into flexion and then extension.

A wave-like movement should be noted as the segment being palpated is involved in the gross motion demanded of the spine.

A change in the tissue tension under palpation should be noted as the various phases of the movement are carried out.

Can you feel this?

● Practice the same assessment of tissue response at various segmental levels.

● Try to feel the different responses of the palpated tissues during the phases of the process, as bind starts and then becomes more intense as the first barrier approaches, then eases somewhat as the direction of movement reverses, becoming ever easier, before a hint of bind reappears, and then becomes intense again, as the opposite barrier is approached.

● Decide where the maximum bind is felt and where maximum ease occurs. These are the key pieces of information required for functional technique, as you assiduously avoid bind and home in on ease.

Can you feel this?

Can you locate the point where the distressed tissues are at their most comfortable in response to whatever movement you are using as the challenge?

Try also to distinguish between the bind response that is a normal physiological result of an area coming towards the end of its normal range of movement and the bind that is a response to dysfunctional restriction.

Can you feel this?

11.3B

● Return to the starting position as in 11.3A and, while palpating an area of restriction or hypertonicity, induce

Exercise 11.3 *continued*

straight side-flexion to one side and then the other, while assessing for ease and bind in exactly the same way as in 11.3A.

Can you locate the position of maximum ease during these movements?

11.3C

- Return to the starting position and, while palpating an area of restriction or hypertonicity, induce rotation to one side and then the other, while assessing for ease and bind, in exactly the same way as in 11.3A and 11.3B.

Can you locate the position of maximum ease during these movements?

Comment

Hoover (1969) describes variations in what might be felt as the response of the tissues palpated during these various positional demands.

1. *Dynamic neutral.* This response to motion is an indication of normal physiological activity. There is minimal signaling during a wide range of motions in all directions. Hoover states it in the following way: "This is the pure and unadulterated unlesioned (i.e. not dysfunctional) segment, exhibiting a wide range of easy motion demand-response transaction."

2. *Borderline response.* This is an area or segment which gives some signals of some bind fairly early in a few of the normal motion demands. The degree of bind will be minimal and much of the time ease, or dynamic neutral, will be noted. Hoover states that "most segments act a bit like this"; they are neither fully "well" nor fully "sick."

3. *The lesion response.* Note that the use of the word "lesion" predates the introduction of the term "somatic dysfunction" to describe abnormally restricted segments or joints. To update this term we should call this a "dysfunctional response." This is where bind is noted at the outset of almost all motion demands, with little indication of dynamic neutral.

Hoover suggests that you:

Try all directions of motion carefully. Try as hard as you can to find a motion demand that does not increase bind, but on the contrary, actually decreases bind, and introduces a little ease. This is an important characteristic of the lesion [dysfunction].

Indeed, he states that the more severe the restriction, the easier it will be to find one or more slight motion demands that produce a sense of ease, dynamic neutral, because the contrast between ease and bind will be so marked.

Hoover's summary

Practice is suggested with dysfunctional joints and segments, in order to become proficient. Three major ingredients are required for doing this successfully, according to Hoover.

1. A focused attention to the process of motion demand and motion response, while whatever is being noted is categorized as "normal," "slightly dysfunctional," "frankly or severely dysfunctional," and so on.

2. A constant evaluation of the changes in the palpated response to motion, in terms of ease and bind, with awareness that this represents increased and decreased levels of signaling and tissue response.

3. An awareness that, in order to thoroughly evaluate tissue responses, all possible variations in motion demand are required, which calls for a structured sequence of movement demands. Hoover suggests that these be verbalized (silently):

Mentally set up a goal of finding ease, induce tentative motion demands until the response of ease and increasing ease is felt, verbalise the motion-demand which gives the response of ease in terms of flexion, extension, side-bending and rotation. Practise this experiment until real skills are developed. You are learning to find the particular ease-response to which the dysfunction is limited.

In addition, depending upon the region being evaluated, the directions of abduction, adduction, translation forwards, translation backwards, translation laterally and medially, translation superiorly and inferiorly, etc., all need to be factored into this approach.

Bowles describes your goal

Bowles's (1955) words summarize succinctly what is being sought:

> *The activity used to test the segment (or joint) is largely endogenous, the observing instrument is highly non-perturbational, and the information gathered is about how well or how poorly our segment (being palpated) of structure is solving its problems.*

> *Should we find a sense of ease and non-distortion following examination of the structures we diagnose the segment as normal.*

> *If we find a sense of binding, tenseness, tissue distortion, a feeling of lagging and complaining in any direction of the action, then we know the segment is having difficulty properly solving its problems. The diagnosis would be of dysfunction.*

> *The treatment would be functional; by holding a segment, an area, in its position of ease, resolution of dysfunction begins (spontaneously).*

The whole key to successful normalization of dysfunction in this manner, lies in the finding of the position of dynamic neutral, of ease, and the degree of your palpatory sensitivity is what decides whether this will be achieved or not.

Spinal application of functional technique palpation

In order to practice functional evaluation (and ultimately) treatment of the spine or a joint, an area (of the spine, for example) needs to be identified as being dysfunctional, different or abnormal, as compared with the rest of the spine, using one of the many forms of assessment already described (see Chapter 8).

The identification of areas of muscle fullness during the seated and standing spinal flexion tests (see Chapter 8) or the neuromuscular assessment methods, or of "flat" spinal areas as described in the assessment sequence for tight muscles in Chapter 5, or the previous exercises in this chapter, could all direct you to such a "different" area, requiring further investigation or normalization.

Hartman (1985) suggests another possibility, after initial suspicion has been alerted: "Diagnosis of textural abnormality in the tissues is made in the normal way with palpation. A gradient of abnormality can be felt in a particular area and the centre of this area is made a focus." He suggests light tapping be introduced over the spinous processes and paravertebral musculature, to emphasize and localize the area of difference. There will be a variation in the resonance noted which, he suggests, will be subjectively picked up by the patient and can guide you to the most central portion of the dysfunctional tissues. (See Special topic 8, Percussion palpation and treatment.)

Johnston's views on the barrier

Johnston (1966) explains the terms "direct" and "indirect" as follows:

> *When the incremental aspects of these cues [directions of motion restriction] are appreciated as an immediately increasing resistance towards a sense of barrier in one direction, and an immediate increasing ease towards a sense of potential release, in the opposite direction, then the terms direct [towards the sense of resistance] and indirect [away from the sense of resistance] offer a classification of osteopathic manipulative procedures, based on diagnosed asymmetry, to be addressed.*

It is then easy to move from such a diagnostic assessment into active treatment.

Johnston's protocol

Johnston's summary of the planning and criteria involved in a functional approach to assessment and treatment can be expressed as follows:

- It is necessary to introduce motion in any one direction at a time which involves minimal force.

- Motion direction is towards a sense of increasing ease, which is manifested by a lessening in the sense of resistance to pressure from the palpating fingers.

- Different direction elements are combined, such as rotation and translation, producing variations in torsion.

- Active respiration is also monitored for its influence on ease.

- The examiner follows the continuous flow of information, signaling increasing ease/decreasing resistance during all procedures.

Exercise 11.4 *Functional Spinal Palpation*

Time suggested   **10–15 minutes**

Evaluate the spine of your seated palpation partner, assessing areas of flatness or fullness, as you observe the flexed spine from the side or from in front.

Palpate the area and seek out the central site of tissue dysfunction, greatest hypertonia or sensitivity, using one of the previous exercises such as Exercise 11.3A. Using the flexed fingertips of one hand, tap lightly and steadily on the tissues identified, as well as on those surrounding the area. (See Special topic Fig. 10.1.)

Can you identify a different sound in the most affected tissues?

Once a suitably "different" (from adjacent segments) sound has been identified, one hand (the listening hand) should be placed on these tissues. The other hand is used to introduce motion into the region, passively or with some active cooperation, but only if directed to do so by you.

A sequence of normal physiological motions should be introduced to the region and in each instance (in each direction) the palpating hand, on the tense dysfunctional tissues, should be feeling for greater ease or greater bind, trying to find a point where a combination of the greatest directions of ease (see below) are summated, in order to achieve maximal relaxation of the tissues.

This, says Hartman, is a form of inhibition for the tense tissues, "in that areas of irritability are quieted, the practitioner constantly looking for the state of ease and release."

The movements introduced (sequence is irrelevant) for assessment of ease and bind should include:

- flexion and extension
- side-flexion, left and right
- rotation, left and right
- translation, anterior and posterior
- translation (shift), left and right
- translation, cephalad and caudad (involving traction and compression); followed by
- respiration, involving both inhalation and exhalation.

Greenman describes the process of achieving the point of ease, involving the first six motions, as "stacking" (the order in which these are applied is not significant; simply it is useful to apply them sequentially so that none is forgotten).

This should be followed by the final respiratory screening, seeking the phase of the cycle that produces maximum ease. Johnston (1997) has described this:

- *The final component step of the functional procedure involves a request for a specific direction of active respiration, whichever direction (inhalation or exhalation) contributes further to the increasing ease. For example, if inhalation, the request is for the subject to take a deep breath slowly, and to hold briefly.*

- *After a position of greatest ease has been established using one of the planes of movement (say, flexion and extension), that position of ease is used as the starting point for the next direction (say, rotation left and right) or plane (say, side-flexion left and right) to be assessed for its position of greatest ease.*

- *When this is discovered you will have found a combined position of ease for the first two directions of movement tested, say extension and side-flexion or rotation.*

- *You will have "stacked" the second onto the first and from that combined position of ease you would then introduce the next direction for assessment, say translation right and left ... and so on, until all directions have been evaluated and their positions of ease "stacked", one onto the other.*

- *Then the respiratory assessment is introduced and the final position of ease held for 60–90 seconds or so, before complete reevaluation of previously identified restrictions.*

- *A sense of a wider range of normal (greater ease) should be felt by the practitioner as these releases occur [Fig. 11.1].*

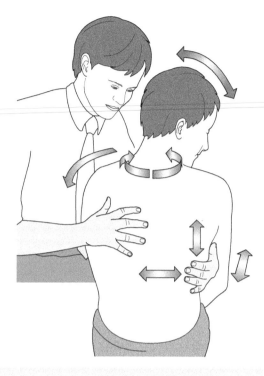

Figure 11.1
Arrows show directions of movement, as ease and bind are
assessed by the "listening" hand on the spinal tissues during
functional evaluation of spinal segments. Movements are:
flexion–extension, rotation left and right, side-bending left and
right, translation to each side, translation forward and back,
translation up and down (traction and compression).

Exercise 11.5 *Greenman's Functional Literacy Palpation*

Time suggested 15–20 minutes for the three phases of the exercise

Greenman describes a sequence of exercises for achievement
of "functional literacy." The following is a modified summary
of his sequence.

11.5A

- Stand behind and to the side of your seated palpation
  partner, whose arms should be folded, so that the hands
  are holding the opposite shoulders.

- Place a "listening" hand, or finger pads, onto the upper
  thoracic spine, where tissue tightness or fullness has
  been identified.

- Allow the hand to be very still. Wait until it feels "nothing"
  (no movement).

- Your other hand ("motive" hand) should be placed on
  your partner's head, in order to lead it through specific
  motions, such as flexion or extension (very slowly performed, without jerking).

- The palpating hand tries to identify tissue changes, in
  terms of increased ease or increased bind.

- Keep repeating a single movement of the head into slow
  flexion, back to neutral, into flexion, back to neutral …
  noting where the point of *maximum ease* is located in
  this plane of movement.

- Then introduce slow repetitive backward bending of the
  head as you palpate for ease. Extend slowly, return to
  neutral, extend, back to neutral.

Is the ease greater with the head in a flexed or extended
direction?

11.5B

- Return to neutral and introduce side bending right and
  rotation to the left of the head and neck on the trunk,
  several times (back to neutral after each excursion).

- Then introduce side bending left and rotation to the
  right of the neck and head on the trunk, all the while
  palpating the area being assessed for alterations in their
  ease and bind characteristics.

- In which parts of this compound series of movements do
  the tissues relax most or become most tense?

- Is there a symmetrical range of ease and bind in both
  directions?

Identify the point – somewhere between extreme side
bending left, rotation right, and side bending right, rotation
left – in which the palpated tissues feel at their most relaxed.

Exercise 11.5 *continued*

11.5C

Return the neck and head to neutral and introduce, and try to combine, the following movements, as you palpate for ease and bind:

- Small amount of forward bending, accompanied by right side bending and right rotation of the head and neck on the trunk.

- Follow this with slight flexion, left side bending and left rotation of the head and neck on the trunk.

- Palpate constantly for ease in the thoracic segment under your listening hand.

- Evaluate the symmetry of the findings.

Was ease/bind found at the same place moving the head and neck to the left and to the right?

Comment

Greeman (1996) suggests that similar palpation exercises be performed in various regions of the spine.

- In each case what you are looking for in normal tissue, or where there is only minimal dysfunction, is a wide range of motion accompanied by minimal signaling (i.e., most of the tissue being palpated is in relative ease and feels relaxed).

- Where a significant degree of dysfunction exists, there will be narrow ranges which produce signals of ease – and increased evidence of bind.

- Experience is the only teacher as to what is and what is not significant clinically in this information.

Exercise 11.6 *Greenman's Functional Spinal Palpation*

Time suggested **20 minutes**

Note

This is more or less the same exercise as Exercise 11.5, with the difference that you should first practice it on a dysfunctional segment and then a normal one.

11.6A

Your palpation partner should be seated. You stand behind and to one side, palpating a previously identified area of dysfunction in the thoracic spine.

Adopt a contact where the patient has their arms folded and you embrace the shoulder furthest from you with one hand, drawing the opposite shoulder into your axilla, so that you can control the various directions of motion.

- Sequentially introduce the elements of:

—forward bending, followed by backward bending

—left side bending, right side bending

—rotation left, rotation right

—a combination of side bending in one direction, with rotation to the same side, during flexion and then extension.

- Then introduce side bending in the other direction, with rotation to the opposite side during flexion and then extension.

- Add to a combination of positions of ease, discovered during these assessments, elements such as translation anterior and posterior, translation from side to side and translation cephalad and caudad, in order to discover where the maximum point of ease occurs.

Can you sense ease positions in any of these motions?

Exercise 11.6 *continued*

Can you find a "most easy" position, by combining elements of these motions?

Maintain the final position of ease and after a minute return the area to neutral.

Re-evaluate the positions of ease. Have they changed?

11.6B

Perform exactly the same sequence on a segment lower down the spine which does not display evidence of dysfunction.

Compare your findings of range, and positions of ease and bind, with those discovered during the previous exercise.

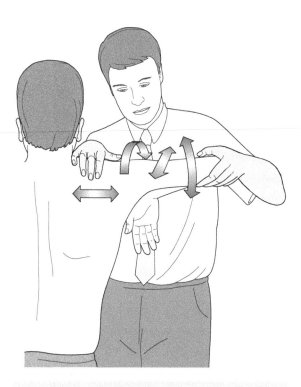

Figure 11.2
Assessing positions of the arm which induce ease or bind at the acromioclavicular joint. (After Hoover 1969.)

Exercise 11.7 *Greenman's Functional Spinal Palpation, with Breathing Assistance*

Time suggested **20 minutes**

Repeat all the components of Exercise 11.6A but now introduce a held breath (only for as long as is comfortable to the person), in both inhalation and exhalation, in each of those positions in which maximum ease was previously palpated.

Is there any additional release (or increase) of resistance during or after either phases of held breath?

The secret of this approach is learning to apply *all suitable directions of motion which enhance ease, together with the respiratory component which produces maximal ease.*

Hoover's clavicle "experiment"

The developer of functional technique, H.V. Hoover, explained the essence of this approach in the words of the founder of osteopathy, Andrew Taylor Still: "I am doing what the body tells me to do."

Hoover (1969) asks the beginner to perform the following three "experiments," grouped together in Exercise 11.8. In each case a question is posed, the answer to each being "yes." Your answers will tell you whether you are ready to use this method – whether you have achieved palpatory literacy.

Exercise 11.8 *Hoover's Clavicle Palpation*

Time suggested **20–30 minutes**

11.8A

Question 1: Does the clavicle move in a definite and predictable manner when demands are made upon it by definite movements of an adjacent part?

● Stand facing your seated palpation partner and place the pads of the (relaxed) fingers of your right hand lightly over the right clavicle, just feeling the skin overlying it (Fig. 11.2). This hand is the listening hand. It is there to evaluate what happens.

Exercise 11.8 *continued*

- With your left hand, hold the right arm close to the elbow (this is your motive or moving hand).

- Your partner must be relaxed, passive, and cooperative, not helping or hindering the introduction of movements by your motive hand.

- The listening hand should barely touch the skin, no pressure at all being applied to the clavicle.

- Raise and lower the arm slowly, several times, until you are certain that it is relaxed, that you have the weight of the arm without assistance. The exercise can now begin.

- Slowly take the arm backwards from the midline, introducing shoulder extension, just far enough to sense a change in the tissues under the palpating hand. Then return the arm to its starting position.

- Do not move quickly or jerk the arm, so ensuring that the sensations being picked up by both the motive and the listening hand are accurate.

- Repeat this several times, slowly, so that you become aware of the effect of a single, simple, movement (*remember the question you are asking your partner's body*).

- Now take the arm forward of the midline (shoulder flexion) and again assess the effect on the palpated tissues (clavicle and surrounding tissue).

- Subsequently, in no particular sequence, abduct and then adduct the arm; rotate the arm externally and subsequently internally, each time slowly and if necessary repeatedly, each time noting the tissue response to a single direction of movement.

- What response was noted to each of these single physiological movements?

- Remember this was not an exercise in which you were meant to compare the effect of one movement with another (that comes next), but a time to evaluate what effect single movements produced, as perceived by your palpating hand and also by the motive hand.

- Revisit Exercises 5.16A and B, where you evaluated the feeling of resistance as you moved the leg into abduc-

tion, as well as the palpated feeling of "bind" in the medial hamstrings and other adductors.

11.8B

Question 2: Are there differences in ease of motion, and feeling of ease and bind in the tissues associated with this clavicle when it is caused to move in different physiological motions?

- Follow the same starting procedure until the exercise proper begins (i.e., ensure a relaxed, supported arm, with your palpating contact in place).

- Move the arm backwards into extension very slowly as you palpate the changes in the tissues around the clavicle.

- Compare the feeling of the tissues when this is done with what happens as you take the arm into flexion, bringing it forwards.

- Now compare the feelings in the listening hand as you abduct and then adduct the arm, slowly, deliberately, gently.

- Compare the tissue changes (ease/bind) as you first internally and then externally rotate the arm.

- Did there appear to be directions of motion which produced enhanced feelings of ease in the tissues? If so, what were they?

11.8C

Question 3: Can the differences of ease of motion, and tissue texture, be altered by moving the clavicle in certain ways?

- Repeat the introductory steps up until the exercise proper begins.

- Flex the patient's arm, bringing it forward of the midline, slowly and gently, until you note the clavicle moving or the tissue texture under your palpating hand changing. Stop at that point.

- Now extend the arm backwards from the midline, slowly and gently, until you note the clavicle moving or the tissue texture under the palpating hand changing. Stop at that point.

- Find a point of balance between these two states, a point of balance from which movement, in any direction,

Exercise 11.8 *continued*

causes the clavicle to move, along with a change in tissue texture.

- Hold this point of physiological balance, which Hoover called "dynamic neutral."

- Starting from this first position of ease, you should next find the point of balance between adduction and abduction.

- Once this has been established you will have found a combined position of ease between flexion and extension, as well as adduction and abduction.

- Starting from this combined ease position you should then move on to find the point of balance between internal and external rotation.

- You will then have achieved a state of reciprocal balance between the arm and the clavicle.

Were you able to identify this point of balance?

If so, from here Hoover leads you to another important finding.

11.8D

- Holding the arm and clavicle in dynamic neutral, as at the end of Exercise 11.8C above, test to see whether any of the six physiological motions (flexion/extension/adduction/abduction/internal and external rotation, as in 11.8B), on its own, gives a sensation of improved tissue texture, compared with the other physiological motions.

- One of the directions may be found which does not increase bind, or which increases ease more than the others.

- Having found this motion, slowly and gently continue to repeat it for as long as the sensory hand continues to report that tissue conditions, motion of the clavicle, are gaining in ease.

- Should bind begin to be noted as this is done, Hoover suggests that the various directions of motion should all be rechecked, to find that which introduces the most ease.

- If none do, then stop at this point, noting what it is that you have been feeling.

- If a further direction of motion producing ease is found, this is repeated until bind seems to occur again.

- Repeat the retesting procedure of all the directions of motion.

Hoover says:

This process of finding the easy physiological motion, and following it until bind starts, and then rechecking, may go on through two or more processes, until a state of equilibrium is found from which tissue texture indicates ease in all [directions of] physiological motion.

Exercise 11.9 *Combined Functional and SCS Palpation of Atlanto-Occipital Joint*

Time suggested 10–15 minutes

11.9A

A final functional exercise in this chapter introduces many of the methods "tested" in the exercises above, and involves their application to the atlanto-occipital joint.

- Your palpation partner is supine. You sit at the head of the table, slightly to one side, so that you are facing the corner.

- One hand (your caudal hand) cradles the occiput, with opposed index finger and thumb palpating the soft tissues adjacent to the atlas.

- The other hand is placed on the forehead or the crown of the head.

- The caudal hand assesses for feelings of "ease," "comfort," or "release" in the tissues surrounding the atlas, as the hand on the head directs it into a compound series of motions, one at a time.

- As each motion is "tested," a position is identified where the tissues feel at their most relaxed or easy. This position of the head is used as the starting point for the next element in the sequence of assessment.

Exercise 11.9 *continued*

In no particular order (apart from the first movements into flexion and extension), the following directions of motion are tested, seeking always the position of the head and neck that elicits the greatest degree of ease in the tissues around the atlas, to "stack" onto the previously identified positions of ease:

- flexion/extension (suggested as the first directions of the sequence)

- side bending left and right

- rotation left and right

- anteroposterior translation (shunt, shift)

- side-to-side translation

- compression/distraction.

Notes

To repeat, each of these functional assessments of the tissues surrounding the atlanto-occiptal joint commences from the combined positions of ease of all previous assessments, apart from the initial assessment which starts from neutral.

One "position of ease" is therefore being stacked onto previously identified positions of ease.

- Once three-dimensional equilibrium has been ascertained (known as dynamic neutral), in which a compound series of ease positions have been "stacked," the person is asked to inhale and exhale fully, to identify which stage of the breathing cycle enhances the sense of palpated "ease," and then to hold the breath in that phase of the cycle for as long as is comfortable (Fig. 11.3).

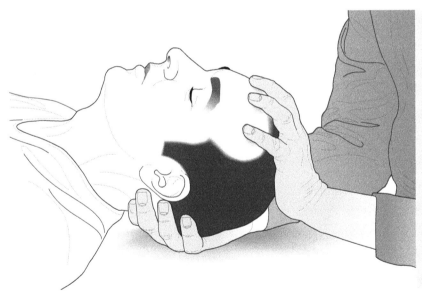

Figure 11.3
Hand positions for application of functional assessment and/or treatment of the atlanto-occipital joint and surrounding tissues.

Exercise 11.9 *continued*

- The final combined position of ease is then held for not less than 90 seconds – or until a profound sense of changes is palpated – before slowly returning to neutral.

Note

> The sequence in which directions of movements are assessed is not relevant, providing as many variables as possible are employed in seeking the combined position of ease.

This held position of ease is thought to allow neural resetting to occur, reducing muscular tension, and also to encourage improved circulation and drainage through previously tense and possibly ischemic or congested tissues.

11.9B: Counterstrain exercise for atlanto-occipital area

- With your palpation partner lying supine and with you seated at the head of the table, palpate the tissues around the atlanto-occipital joint, using drag palpation, and locate what you consider to be the area of greatest sensitivity/tenderness.

- Apply a single-digit pressure to this sensitive area, sufficient to evoke a reported score of 10 on the pain scale (where 10 = marked discomfort and 0 = no pain).

- Maintain this pressure as you carefully reposition (fine-tune) the head and neck, in order to reduce the reported pain score to 3 or less.

- The most likely position to ease reported pain of this sort is slight extension, followed by slight side bending toward, and slight rotation away from, the painful point.

- If such a combination is not effective, fine-tune until you identify the head/neck position that reduces the score most.

Once you have established this position of ease, hold it for 90 seconds and then, on release, repalpate to see whether the tissues are less sensitive.

Pay particular attention to the final position of ease and decide whether it is in any way similar to the final position

achieved when you sequentially stacked positions of ease, in Exercise 11.9A.

This exercise offers you the chance to explore the two major methods of positional release technique, and also gives you a very useful method for easing distressed tissues in this sensitive and vulnerable area.

Conclusion

The exercises in this chapter are extremely important. They are elegant in their objectives (to locate comfort/ease/balance), apparently simple – and yet demanding of intense focus. They also represent, as clearly as is possible, the objective of a seamless transition from assessment to treatment. This is so because once the point of optimal ease has been identified, for as long as this is held, self-generated, homeostatic normalization processes are operating.

The tissues appear to take advantage of being held in a state of ease, to commence normalization, of circulation, neural status, and tone. Everything negative that is taking place when tissues are tense and contracted (increased pain perception, ischemia, drainage impairment, mechanical and chemical irritation, etc.) is put into reverse.

So finding the point of "ease" by palpation is the task of the practitioner, while using that position advantageously is the prerogative of the body itself.

If these concepts excite you then you are urged to investigate further by studying the practice of positional release (D'Ambrogio & Roth 1997; Chaitow 2014; Deig 2001).

References

Bowles C (1955) Functional orientation for technic. Newark, OH: Yearbook of the Academy of Applied Osteopathy.

Chaitow L (2014) Positional release techniques, 4th edn. Edinburgh: Churchill Livingstone.

D'Ambrogio K and Roth G (1997) Positional release therapy. St Louis, MI: Mosby.

Deig D (2001) Positional release technique. Boston: Butterworth Heinemann.

Glover J and Yates H (1997) Strain and counterstrain techniques, in Ward R (ed) Foundations for Osteopathic Medicine. Baltimore: Williams and Wilkins.

Greenman P (1989) Principles of manual medicine. Baltimore: Williams and Wilkins.

Greenman P (1996) Principles of manual medicine, 2nd edn. Baltimore: Williams and Wilkins.

Hartman L (1985) Handbook of osteopathic technique. London: Hutchinson.

Hoover H (1957) Functional technique. Newark, OH: Yearbook of the Academy of Applied Osteopathy.

Hoover H (1969) A method for teaching functional technique. Newark, OH: Yearbook of the Academy of Applied Osteopathy.

Johnston WL (1966) Manipulative skills. Journal of the American Osteopathic Association 66 (4): 389–407.

Johnston W (1988a) Segmental definition, Part I. A focal point for diagnosis of somatic dysfunction. Journal of the American Osteopathic Association 88 (1): 99–105.

Johnston W (1988b) Segmental definition, Part II. Application of an indirect method in osteopathic manipulative. Journal of the American Osteopathic Association 88 (2): 211–217.

Johnston W (1997) Functional technique, in Ward R (ed) Foundations for Osteopathic Medicine. Baltimore: Williams and Wilkins.

Johnston W, Robertson A and Stiles E (1969) Finding a common denominator. Newark, OH: Yearbook of the American Academy of Applied Osteopathy.

Jones L (1981) Strain and counterstrain. Colorado Springs: Academy of Applied Osteopathy.

Korr I (1947) The neural basis for the osteopathic lesion. Journal of the American Osteopathic Association 47: 191.

Special topic 11

About hyperventilation
Leon Chaitow

The effect of overbreathing is to rapidly reduce the levels of carbon dioxide in the blood, altering the acid–alkaline balance (increasing alkalinity), increasing nociceptor sensitivity and a sense of apprehension and anxiety, resulting in a variety of unpleasant symptoms.

Many studies have concentrated on the widespread problem of overbreathing and much of this has related to its connection with anxiety states, panic attacks of an incapacitating nature, and, all too often, phobic behavior (Chaitow et al. 2002, 2014; Timmons 1994).

The symptoms most often associated with hyperventilation include: giddiness, dizziness, faintness, numbness in the upper limbs, face or trunk, loss of consciousness (fainting), visual disturbances in which blurring or even temporary loss of vision is experienced, headaches of a general nature often accompanied by nausea and frequently diagnosed as migraine, inability to walk properly (ataxia) as well as trembling and tinnitus.

A number of symptoms often associated with cardiac function ("pseudo-angina") can become apparent during or after hyperventilation, including: palpitation, chest discomfort, difficulty in taking a deep breath, feelings of pressure in the throat, insomnia, fatigue, weakness in the limbs, and much more (Ajani 2007).

Of patients diagnosed with hyperventilation, more than half are found to be undergoing stress, related to marriage, work, or finance. Hyperventilation is not, however, always associated with psychiatric stress and this is made clear by Lum (1987): "The underlying disorder (of hyperventilation) may be psychiatric, organic, a habit disorder or a combination of these." However Lum (1981) also observed that:

> *Neurological considerations can leave little doubt that the habitually unstable breathing is the prime cause of symptoms. Why they breathe in this way must be a matter for speculation, but manifestly the salient characteristics are pure habit.*

Lum has also summarized some of the confusion surrounding the phenomenon:

> *Although Kerr et al. (1937) had pointed out that the clinical manifestations of anxiety were produced by hyperventilation, it was Rice who turned this concept upside down by stating that the anxiety was produced by the symptoms and, furthermore, that patients could be cured by eliminating faulty breathing habits. Lewis identified the role of anxiety as a trigger, rather than the prime cause. Given habitual hyperventilation, a variety of triggers, psychic or somatic, can initiate the vicious cycle of increased breathing, symptoms, anxiety arising from symptoms exacerbating hyperventilation and thus generating more symptoms and more anxiety.*

Despite the literature providing evidence of various symptom patterns being linked to hyperventilation, the concept of selecting patients for treatment and breathing retraining on the basis of symptoms alone might be flawed according to some. Bass and Gardner (1985) point out:

> *Diagnostic criteria for the hyperventilation syndrome [HVS] are imprecise. The practice of basing diagnosis on symptom checklists is unreliable and equivalent to diagnosing diabetes on the basis of symptoms without measuring blood glucose concentrations.*

When Bass and Gardner examined 21 patients with unequivocal hyperventilation and a host of unexplained symptoms they found that all but one complained of "inability to take a satisfying breath" but that there was enormous variety when a host of different physical and psychological markers and signs were evaluated. They concluded: "Severe hyperventilation can occur in the absence of formal psychiatric or detectable respiratory or other organic abnormalities." Not everyone agrees with Bass's view that symptoms cannot provide a clue as to whether HVS exists.

A symptom questionnaire, the Nijmegen Questionnaire (Special topic Table 11.1), was evaluated by Van Dixhoorn and Duivenvoorden (1985). They compared the results of the questionnaire when completed by 75 confirmed HVS patients and 80 non-HVS individuals (health workers).

Special topic Table 11.1

The Nijmegen Questionnaire	Never 0	Rare 1	Sometimes 2	Often 3	Very often 4
Chest pain					
Feeling tense					
Blurred vision					
Dizzy spells					
Feeling confused					
Faster or deeper breathing					
Short of breath					
Tight feelings in chest					
Bloated feeling in stomach					
Tingling fingers					
Unable to breathe properly					
Stiff fingers or arms					
Tight feelings round mouth					
Cold hands or feet					
Palpitations					
Feelings of anxiety					
Total:	/64				

©2010 Elsevier Ltd. Leon Chaitow, Palpation and Assessment Skills, 3rd edn.

A score of 19 or more, out of 64, offers a strong indication of hyperventilation.

Note: Never = never; rare = less than monthly; sometimes = at least monthly but not weekly; often = weekly but not daily; very often = daily.

Three dimensions were measured in the questionnaire:

- shortness of breath
- peripheral tetany
- central tetany.

All three components had an unequivocally high ability to differentiate between HVS and non-HVS individuals.

- Together they provided a 93% correct classification.
- Statistical double cross validation resulted in 90–94% correct classifications.
- The sensitivity of the Nijmegen Questionnaire in relation to diagnosis was 91% and the specificity 95%.

More recent refinement of the questionnaire suggests that a cut-off point of a score of 19 or more (out of a possible 64 – see Special topic Table 11.1) strongly suggests a tendency to hyperventilation (Grammatopoulou et al. 2014; Courtney et al. 2011).

How to deal with hyperventilation

In most instances of hyperventilation a combination exists of a learned pattern of breathing coming into operation in response to real or assumed stressful situations. This is usually found to coexist alongside severely contracted muscles relating to the ribcage, spinal regions, and the diaphragm area that are readily palpable or observable. Such changes are a common feature amongst people who are chronically fatigued, since the combination of energy wastage through long-held tension and reduced oxygenation due to impaired respiratory function can produce profound fatigue.

Muscles that are chronically hypertonic, shortened, or contracted cannot function normally and this is usually the case in people who hyperven-

tilate who, it seems, have learned to overbreathe excessively in response to both stressful events and non-stressful ones. (See Chapter 12 for more detail on structural changes associated with breathing dysfunction.)

It is perfectly normal to hyperventilate when excessive demands are required of the body, for example, on physical exertion or in situations of increased acidosis (advanced pregnancy or liver disease as examples). If, however, this response occurs inappropriately, in the face of a perceived but unreal crisis, such as exists when we are abnormally anxious about something, then the sequence of overbreathing would lead to imbalanced blood gas levels, changes in acidity/alkalinity, and the whole sequence of hyperventilation symptoms previously listed.

This may become a habitual method of responding to all minor stress situations, leading to the complete misery of phobic states compounded by panic attacks and virtual incapacity and inability to function. People affected in this way often respond well to breathing retraining. By recognizing that it is possible to learn to use more appropriate patterns of breathing in the face of a stressful (real or imagined) situation, they may be able to control the symptoms, because they simply will not hyperventilate.

Ample research evidence exists to indicate that arousal levels (how rapidly and severely an individual responds to stressful situations) can be markedly reduced via the habitual use of specific patterns of calming breathing. Thomas et al. (2003), Hagman et al. (2011), McLaughlin et al. (2011), among many others, have shown that breathing retraining is a valid and highly successful approach.

Pranayama breathing

Cappo and Holmes (1984) in particular have incorporated into their methodology a form of traditional yoga breathing that produces specific benefits that have gone largely unrecognized in the protocols of most other workers. The pattern calls for a ratio of inhalation to exhalation of 1:4 if possible, but in any case, for exhalation to take appreciably longer than inhalation. Research indicates that this pattern markedly lowers arousal.

Conclusion

There is a clear link between abnormal breathing patterns, excessive use of the accessory breathing muscles, upper chest breathing, etc. and increased muscle tone, which is itself a major cause of fatigue, over and above the impact on the economy of the body of reduced oxygenation and the unbalanced, malcoordinated patterns of use that stem from the structural and functional changes, as detailed by Garland (see Chapter 12).

These patients will be fatigued, plagued by head, neck, shoulder and chest discomfort and a host of minor musculoskeletal problems as well as feeling apprehensive or frankly anxious. Many will have digestive symptoms (bloating, belching, and possibly hiatal hernia symptoms, etc.) associated with aerophagia, which commonly accompanies this pattern of breathing, as well as a catalog of symptoms.

And yet none of the major medical researchers into hyperventilation seem to have examined the structural machinery of respiration! There is scant attention in the quoted literature to the status of the muscles that perform the task of breathing.

And none of them seem to have considered that modifying the structural component (muscles, rib cage, spinal attachments, etc.) could encourage more normal function, despite evidence from manual medicine that this is possible (Lewit 1991).

Nor is there any seeming concern for those many patients whose condition does not fit the strict criteria for a diagnosis of hyperventilation, those whose breathing is demonstrably out of balance but who fail to display evidence of arterial hypocapnia.

There is always a spectrum in such cases, with some being patent and obvious, others being borderline, and many being somewhere on their way towards a point where they will indeed show evidence of arterial hypocapnia and thus achieve the status of "real" hyperventilators.

The fact that before someone displays frank symptoms they are possibly progressing towards that state should be our concern in breathing dysfunction, to recognize people who are borderline hyperventilators and to prevent that progression, as well of course as trying to help those already entrenched in this pattern of dysfunction.

References

Ajani A (2007) The mystery of coronary artery spasm. Heart, Lung and Circulation 16: 10–15.

Bass C and Gardner W (1985) Respiratory and psychiatric abnormalities in chronic symptomatic hyperventilation. British Medical Journal (Clinical Research Edition) 290 (6479): 1387–1390.

Cappo B and Holmes D (1984) Utility of prolonged respiratory exhalation for reducing physiological and psychological arousal in non-threatening and threatening situations. Journal of Psychosomatic Research 28 (4): 265–273.

Chaitow L, Bradley D and Gilbert C (2002) Multidisciplinary approaches to breathing pattern disorders. Edinburgh: Churchill Livingstone.

Chaitow L, Bradley D and Gilbert C (2014) Recognizing and treating breathing disorders. Edinburgh: Churchill Livingstone.

Courtney R, Van Dixhoorn J, Greenwood KM and Anthonissen EL (2011) Medically unexplained dyspnea: Partly moderated by dysfunctional (thoracic dominant) breathing pattern. Journal of Asthma 48 (3): 259–265.

Grammatopoulou EP, Skordilis EK, Georgoudis G et al. (2014) Hyperventilation in asthma: A validation study of the Nijmegen Questionnaire–NQ. Journal of Asthma 51 (8): 839–846.

Hagman C, Janson C and Emtner M (2011) Breathing retraining – a five-year follow-up of patients with dysfunctional breathing. Respiratory Medicine 105 (8): 1153–1159.

Kerr WJ, Dalton JW and Gliebe P (1937) Some physical phenomena associated with the anxiety states and their relation to hyperventilation. Annals of Internal Medicine 11: 961–992.

Lewit K (1991) Manipulative therapy in rehabilitation of the locomotor system. London: Butterworths.

Lum L (1981) Hyperventilation and anxiety state. Journal of the Royal Society of Medicine 74 (1): 1–4.

Lum L (1987) Hyperventilation syndromes in medicine and psychiatry: A review. Journal of the Royal Society of Medicine 80 (4): 229–231.

McLaughlin L, Goldsmith CH and Coleman K (2011) Breathing evaluation and retraining as an adjunct to manual therapy. Manual Therapy 16 (1): 51–52.

Thomas M, McKinley RK, Freeman E, Foy C, Prodger P and Price D (2003) Breathing retraining for dysfunctional breathing in asthma: A randomised controlled trial. Thorax 58 (2): 110–115.

Timmons B (1994) Behavioral and psychological approaches to breathing disorders. New York: Plenum Press.

Van Dixhoorn J and Duivenvoorden H (1985) Efficacy of Nijmegen Questionnaire in recognition of hyperventilation syndrome. Journal of Psychosomatic Research 29 (2): 199–206.

Accurate visceral palpation requires a high degree of palpatory literacy and that can only be accomplished by practice, practice, practice. And there is much to practice on.

Goldthwaite and his colleagues (1945), in their classic text, described the changes that are commonly found in association with a slumped posture leading to loss of diaphragmatic efficiency and abdominal ptosis (see Chapter 5).

- Breathing dysfunction and restrictions develop.

- There is drag on the fascia supporting the heart, displacing this organ and resulting in traction on the aorta. Nerve structures supplying the heart are similarly stressed mechanically.

- The cervical fascia is stretched (recall that this can lead to distortion anywhere from the cranium to the feet, as the fascia is continuous throughout the body).

- Venous stasis develops below the diaphragm (pelvic organs and so on) as its pumping action is inhibited and diminished, leading to varicose veins and hemorrhoids.

- The stomach becomes depressed and tilted, affecting its efficiency mechanically.

- The esophagus becomes stretched, as does the celiac artery. Symptoms ranging from hiatus hernia to dyspepsia and constipation become more likely.

- The pancreas is mechanically affected, interfering with its circulation.

- The liver is tilted backwards, there is inversion of the bladder, the support of the kidneys is altered and the colon and intestines generally become mechanically crowded and depressed (as does the bladder). None of these can therefore function well.

- The prostate becomes affected due to circulatory dysfunction and increased pressure, making hypertrophy more likely. Similarly, menstrual irregularities become more likely.

- Increased muscular tension becomes a drain on energy, leading to fatigue which is aggravated by inefficient oxygen intake and poor elimination of wastes.

- Spinal and rib restrictions become chronic, making this problem worse.

- Postural joints become stressed, leading to spinal, hip, knee, and foot dysfunction, increasing wear and tear.

All these changes are palpable and all may be correctable, if caught early enough.

A more precise examination of the biomechanical aspects of visceral dysfunction is now available through texts such as the highly recommended *Visceral Manipulation* (Barral & Mercier 2006), which gives a host of directions, instructions and useful hints for anyone interested in this area of palpation and treatment. These British-trained French osteopaths have developed the art of visceral palpation and manipulation to a very high level of expertise. Additional exploration of this topic is to be found in *Visceral and Obstetric Osteopathy* (Stone 2007).

In their opening chapter, Barral and Mercier (2006) outline what we need to know about visceral motility and mobility:

> There is an inherent axis of rotation in each of these motions (mobility and motility). In healthy organs, the axes of mobility and motility are generally the same. With disease, they are often at variance with one another, as certain restrictions affect one motion more than another. What a surprise it was for us to discover that the axes of motion reproduce exactly those of embryological development! Neither preconceived ideas nor hypotheses directed this research. The discovery of this phenomenon was purely empirical, and tends to confirm the idea that "cells do not forget".

Chapter 12

Additionally, visceral motion is influenced by:

1. the somatic nervous system (body movement, muscular tone and activity, posture). An example mentioned by Barral and Mercier is the motion of the liver during flexion, as it slides forwards over the duodenum and the hepatic flexure of the colon below. Similar motions occur in all viscera, determined by the particular support they have and their anatomical relationships.

2. the autonomic nervous system. This includes diaphragmatic motion, cardiac pulsation and motion as well as peristaltic activity. Clearly these automatic motions influence other closely associated organs, as well as some at a distance (for example, diaphragmatic motion, 24,000 times daily, influences and to some extent moves or vibrates all organs).

3. craniosacral rhythm. As we will see in Chapter 14, this is believed to involve palpable movement throughout the body, including the viscera.

Embryological influences

These three influences produce visceral mobility and there is also inherent organ motility which Barral and Mercier have indicated relates very much to the embryological development phases. As an example, they describe how, during the development of the fetus, the stomach rotates to the right in the transverse plane and clockwise in the frontal plane. The transverse rotation therefore orients the anterior lesser curve of the stomach to the right, and the greater posterior curvature to the left. The pylorus is therefore rotated superiorly and the cardia inferiorly.

Barral and Mercier found that these directions "remain inscribed in the visceral tissues," with motion occurring around an axis, a point of balance, as it moves further into the direction of embryological motion and then returns to neutral (very similar to what is thought to take place in the craniosacral mechanisms during flexion and extension of the structures of the skull).

Inspir and expir

The motility cycle is divided by Barral and Mercier (2006) into two phases, termed *inspir* and *expir*. These are unrelated to the breathing cycle, being similar to the descriptions used in cranial osteopathy for cranial motion, flexion, and extension.

Inspir describes the inherent motion and *expir* the return to neutral afterwards (7–8 cycles per minute). An example of this is that the liver's inherent *inspir* phase involves rotation posterosuperiorly (its mobility, as influenced by inhalation's diaphragmatic movement, is almost exactly opposite, anteroinferior).

In palpation, it is often easier to feel the *expir* phase (although *inspir* is more "active" as there is less resistance to it), being a return to neutral.

Visceral articulation

Just as joints have articulations, so do viscera. These are made of sliding surfaces (meninges in the CNS, pleura in the lungs, peritoneum in the abdominal cavity, and pericardium in the heart), as well as a system of attachments (including ligaments, intercavity pressure, various folds of peritoneal structures forming containment and supportive elements). Unlike most joints, few muscular forces directly move organs.

Stone (2007) describes the movement of organs:

Visceral biomechanics relate to the movements that the organs make against each other, and against the walls of the body cavities that contain them. The viscera "articulate" by utilizing sliding surfaces formed by the peritoneal (and pleural or pericardial) membranes that surround the organs and line the body cavities. [Due to normal body movement including bending and locomotion, as well as body processes such as micturition] ... as the body cavities distort and change their shape, so the individual organs must adapt to those changes, and they do so by slightly sliding over each other, given the constraints of their attachments and surrounds.

By moving in these ways organs adapt to mechanical pressures and as they do so, they impart "internal massage" and assist in fluid motion. Restrictions to normal visceral motion can derive from externally applied changes (restrictions, shortened soft tissue structures, etc.) involving the musculoskeletal system while conversely, local visceral scarring or adhesions can impact on the musculoskeletal system via adverse tensions involving the suspensory ligaments that attach to, for example, the spine (Fig. 12.1).

Figure 12.1 shows the way in which mesenteric attachments to the thoracic and lumbar spine support intestinal structures. Spinal changes (restrictions, positional modifications, increased or decreased spinal curves, etc.) could affect organ position and function, while conversely, internal changes to the mesenteric ligaments (in a case of visceroptosis, for example) could affect the spinal structures to which they attach.

Three visceral palpation elements

Barral and Mercier (2006) suggest that there are three elements involved in evaluation of visceral function and these are the traditional ones of:

- palpation (which informs as to tone of the walls of the visceral cavity)

- percussion (which informs about the position and size of the organ in question; see Special topic 8 and later in this chapter)

- auscultation (which informs as to factors such as circulation of air, blood, and secretions such as bile).

Muscular influences

Barral and Mercier stress the importance of the influence on visceral function of muscular activity and suggest mobility tests to identify dysfunction in the musculoskeletal system. However, they state: "We believe that visceral restrictions are the causative lesions much more frequently than are musculoskeletal restrictions."

Mobility and motility

Mobility describes the potential for movement at an articulation or interface. The movement associated with mobility would be produced by external forces, such as active muscular contractions or passive movements.

Motility, on the other hand, describes the inherent movement, such as pulsation, of an area, organ, or specific tissues: for example, the rhythmic motions that may be palpated in the cranium, as described in Chapter 14.

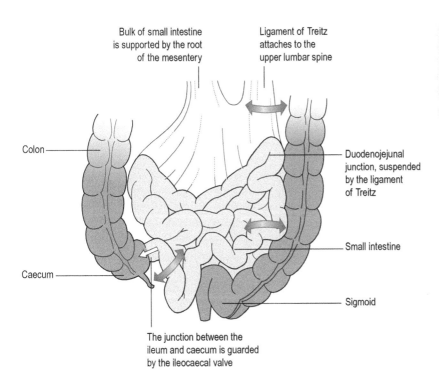

Bulk of small intestine is supported by the root of the mesentery

Ligament of Treitz attaches to the upper lumbar spine

Colon

Caecum

Duodenojejunal junction, suspended by the ligament of Treitz

Small intestine

Sigmoid

The junction between the ileum and caecum is guarded by the ileocaecal valve

Figure 12.1
Suspensory mesenteric ligaments supporting the small intestine attach to the spine. (After Stone 1999.)

How do you palpate an organ for mobility?

By means of precise movements, say Barral and Mercier. In order to do this, though, you need to know the normal movements of the organ in question. They give an example of the liver, which "you literally lift up to appreciate the elasticity of its supporting structures and the extent of its movement."

Mobility assessment (which provides information as to elasticity, laxity/ptosis, spasm and structural injury of muscular or ligamentous supports) requires less skill than does finer evaluation of inherent motility and variations in it from the norm.

How do you palpate organs for motility?

The most effective method for evaluating motility, according to Barral and Mercier, is that described by Rollin Becker (see Chapter 14) in which the hand "listens" for information. This is how they describe application of Becker's work to this task.

Place your hand over the organ to be tested, with a pressure of 20–100 g, depending on the depth of the organ. In some cases the hand can adapt itself to the form of the organ. The hand is totally passive, but there is an extension of the sense of touch used during this examination. Let the hand passively follow what it feels – a slow movement of feeble amplitude which will show itself, stop and then begin again (7–8 per minute in health). This is visceral motility.

It is then desirable, after a few cycles, to estimate elements such as frequency, amplitude and direction of the motility.

The advice is very much as that offered by Becker, Upledger, Smith, and others (see Chapter 14). Do not have preconceived ideas as to what will be felt. Trust what you feel. Empty the mind and let the hand listen. (Both organs of a pair should be assessed and compared.)

One visceral palpation exercise for motility (based on the work of Barral & Mercier) is suggested below. Those exercises, relating to Becker's work, as outlined in Chapter 14, should be performed satisfactorily before performing this exercise – so you might want to move ahead to review that chapter and its exercises before continuing with this chapter.

Study of visceral manipulation and attendance at seminars and workshops covering this subject is suggested for those keen to explore this subtle and rewarding field.

Exercise 12.1 *Palpation for Liver Motility*

Time suggested **10 minutes**

The person to be palpated should be supine. You should be seated or standing on the right, facing the person.

Place your right hand over the lower ribs, molding to their curve, covering the outer aspect of the liver. Your left hand should be laid over the right hand. Your mind should be stilled as you visualize the liver.

You are trying to assess the return to neutral (the *expir* phase of the motility cycle), which means that the direction of active motion would be the opposite of that palpated during this phase.

Barral and Mercier (2006) suggest that the *expir* phase is the easiest for the beginner to palpate. During this phase, three simultaneous motions may be noted.

- In the frontal plane, a counter-clockwise motion, from right to left, around the sagittal axis (of your hand and therefore the liver). This takes the palm of the hand towards the umbilicus (Fig. 12.2).

- In the sagittal plane the superior part of the hand should rotate anteroinferiorly around a transverse axis through the middle of your hand.

- In the transverse plane, the hand rotates to the left around a vertical axis, bringing the palm off the body as the fingers seem to press more closely.

Each of these planes of movement can be assessed separately before they are assessed simultaneously, providing a clear picture of liver motility in the *expir* phase of the cycle (*inspir* is the exact opposite).

This palpation exercise should be performed with eyes closed.

Periodically the person should be asked to hold the breath for a 20-second period to see whether this provides a less confused feeling of motion.

It may be useful to review Becker's method of assessment (Chapter 14), in which elbows or forearm are used as a fulcrum, to enhance palpatory sensitivity and perception.

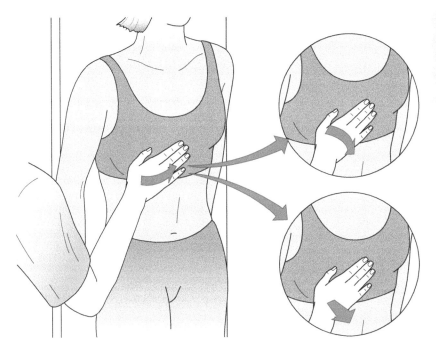

Figure 12.2
Palpation of the liver (after Barral & Mercier 2006) in which frontal, sagittal, and transverse planes of motion are sequentially assessed.

Palpation and observation for respiratory dysfunction

(See also Chapter 8, rib assessment, breathing wave, etc.)

Lewit (2009) has synthesized much of the current knowledge about respiratory influence on body mechanics and describes useful methods for assessing its efficiency and coordination.

> *Thinking of breathing, one naturally has in mind the respiratory system. Yet it is the locomotor system that makes the lungs work, and the locomotor system that has to coordinate the specific respiratory movements with the rest of the body's locomotor activity. This task is so complex that it would be a miracle if disturbances did not occur.*

It is important to distinguish between respiratory problems that relate to habitual use patterns and those that derive from pathology.

- Breathing pattern disorders (such as a tendency toward hyperventilation) are extremely common dysfunctional patterns that are often remediable through a combination of breathing retraining and bodywork (Chaitow et al. 2002, 2013).

- Respiratory diseases (such as emphysema or asthma) are also common and usually require expert medical attention (Pryor & Prasad 2002), even though the methods used to manage breathing dysfunction may also enhance respiration where pathology exists.

Structural considerations

Garland (1994) has summarized the structural modifications that are likely to inhibit successful breathing retraining, as well as psychological intervention, until they are at least in part normalized. He describes a series of changes including:

> *Visceral stasis/pelvic floor weakness, abdominal and erector spinae muscle imbalance, fascial restrictions from the central tendon via the pericardial fascia to the basi-occiput, upper rib elevation with increased costal cartilage tension, thoracic spine dysfunction and possible sympathetic disturbance, accessory breathing muscle hypertonia and fibrosis, promotion of rigidity in the cervical spine with pro-*

motion of fixed lordosis, reduction in mobility of 2nd cervical segment and disturbance of vagal outflow … and more.

These changes, he states, "run physically and physiologically against biologically sustainable patterns, and in a vicious circle, promote abnormal function which alters structure which then disallows a return to normal function."

In simple terms, until there is some degree of normalization of the breathing mechanism, it cannot be used normally, whatever instructions the individual gives it. However:

If assistance can be given to an individual who hyperventilates, by minimising the effect of somatic changes, and if these structural changes can be provided with an ability to modify, therapeutic interventions via breath retraining and counselling will be more effective.

Garland concludes: "In hyperventilation, where psychology overwhelms physiology, the role of [manual therapy] can be very beneficial."

Lewit (1980, 2009) has given due attention to structure and function as it relates to respiration, and states that: "The most important disturbance of breathing is overstrain of the upper auxiliary muscles by lifting of the thorax during quiet respiration." The implications of this have been described by Garland, as detailed above.

Other researchers have examined the relationship between respiration and the function of the musculoskeletal system. For example, Cummings and Howell (1990) have looked at the influence of respiration on myofascial tension, and have clearly demonstrated that there is a mechanical effect of respiration on resting myofascial tissue (using the elbow flexors as the tissue being evaluated).

They also quote the work of Kisselkova and Georgiev (1979), who reported that resting EMG activity of the biceps brachii, quadriceps femoris and gastrocnemius muscles "cycled with respiration following bicycle ergonometer exercise, thus demonstrating that nonrespiratory muscles receive input from the respiratory centres." The conclusion was that:

These studies document both a mechanically and a neurologically mediated influence on the tension produced by myofascial tissues, which gives objective verification of the clinically observed influence of respiration on the musculoskeletal system and validation of its potential role in manipulative therapy.

Recent research by Bradley and Esformes (2014) has clearly illustrated the practical implications of such changes. The study on which they report demonstrated that "Inefficient breathing could result in muscular imbalance, motor control alterations, and physiological adaptations that are capable of modifying movement."

They found that functional movements were less efficiently performed by individuals with breathing pattern disorders (BPD), that is, not pathology, just "poor breathing" habits: "Individuals who exhibited signs of BPD were likely to demonstrate greater movement dysfunction as represented by lower scores on the Functional Movement Screen." These findings provide evidence for incorporating breathing evaluations into clinical practice by clinicians and trainers, as they could be contributing to problems with motor control and movement.

Breathing and muscle pain

Pellegrino (1993, 1994, 1995, 1997) has studied fibromyalgia syndrome (FMS) and its link with chest pain. He notes that: "FMS patients are more prone to getting anxiety or panic attacks, especially when placed in a stressful situation."

Breathing irregularities often have a connection with the symptoms of anxiety. Hyperventilation and anxiety also have an intimate link with poor stress-coping abilities. At its simplest, the connections can look as follows (Chaitow et al. 2013; Timmons & Ley 1994):

- A person responds habitually to what they find to be a stressful situation by breathing shallowly, using the upper chest and not the diaphragm.

- This breathing pattern becomes a habit, so that it continues even when whatever they see as stress is not present (even when sleeping), although it tends to be much more obvious when they are stressed.

- With such a pattern of breathing the accessory breathing muscles become overactive and tense, and often develop painful local areas (e.g., trigger points).

- Irritation of local nerve structures in these muscles and/or interference with circulation to, and drainage from, the head can occur – with lightheadedness, dizziness, and possibly headaches resulting.

- The overbreathing pattern leads to excess carbon dioxide being exhaled (in relation to current metabolic requirements), causing carbonic acid levels in the blood to be lowered, leading to the bloodstream becoming too alkaline (respiratory alkalosis).

- Alkalization leads automatically to a feeling of apprehension/anxiety and the abnormal breathing pattern becoming worse. Panic attacks and even phobic behavior are not uncommon following this.

- Alkalization also leads to nerve endings becoming increasingly sensitive, so that the individual is more likely to report pain when previously only discomfort would have been reported.

- Respiratory alkalosis results in smooth muscle constriction leading to vasoconstriction of all blood vessels, including those in the head, further reducing oxygenation of the region.

- Along with heightened arousal/anxiety and cerebral oxygen lack, there is also a tendency for what oxygen there is in the bloodstream to become more tightly bound to its hemoglobin carrier molecule, leading to decreased oxygenation of tissues and easy fatigability.

- Inadequate oxygenation and retention of acid wastes in overused muscles takes place and these become painful and stiff.

- The muscles being overused in the inappropriate breathing pattern are mainly postural stabilizing muscles (scalenes, sternocleidomastoid, trapezius, pectoral, levator scapulae) and these will, with the repetitive stress involved in overbreathing, become short, tight and painful and will develop trigger points. Remember that the most common sites for tender points of fibromyalgia – and trigger points – lie in just these muscles of the neck, shoulder, and chest.

- The increased tension in these muscles adds to feelings of fatigue, since the muscles are constantly using energy in a non-productive way, even during sleep.

- The poor breathing pattern leads to a restriction of the spinal joints that attach to the ribs which, because their movement is reduced due to shallow breathing, are deprived of regular (each breath) motion, leading to stiffness and discomfort.

- The rib attachments to the sternum are also restricted, leading to pain.

- A similar lack of movement of the diaphragm leads to digestive organs missing out on a regular (each breath) rhythmic "massage" as the diaphragm rises and falls.

- Shallow breathing restricts the pumping mechanism between the chest and the abdomen, which normally assists in the return of blood from the legs to the heart. Cold feet and legs could be caused, or at least be aggravated, by this.

- The intercostal muscles become tense and tight with the likelihood of chest pain and a feeling of inability to get a full and deep breath.

The consequences of respiratory dysfunction that falls short of actual hyperventilation should not be underestimated since although the impact on health may well be less dramatic than the sequence indicated above, the same tendencies will be apparent (see Special topic 11, on hyperventilation).

Breathing and muscle and joint activity

In general, muscular activity is enhanced by inspiration and inhibited by expiration. There are exceptions to this, such as the abdominal muscles, which are facilitated by forced exhalation (Lewit 1999).

Flexion of the cervical and lumbar spines is enhanced by maximum exhalation, whereas flexion of the thoracic spine is enhanced by maximum inspiration, and these phases of respiration can be usefully employed in mobilization (and assessment, including palpation) of this region.

A further influence on spinal mechanics of respiration is described by Lewit (1999).

The most surprising effect of inspiration and expiration is the alternating facilitation and inhibition of individual segments of the spinal column during side-bending, discovered by Gaymans (1980). It can be regularly shown that during side-bending, resistance increases in the cervical as well as the thoracic regions, in the even segments (occiput–atlas, C2, etc. and again T2, T4, etc.) during inspiration; during expiration we gain the mobilising effect in these segments. Conversely, resistance increases in the odd segments during expiration (C1, C3, etc., T3, T5, etc.). There is a neutral zone between C7 and T1.

Inspiration increases resistance to movement in the atlas–occiput region in all directions, while expiration eases its motion in all directions, a most useful piece of information, of value during manipulation or assessment/palpation of motion.

Where maximum muscular effort is required we tend to neither inhale nor exhale, but to hold the inhaled breath (Valsalva maneuver). This achieves postural stability (no facilitation of spinal motion in any segments) at the cost of momentary loss of respiratory function. The diaphragm has therefore been described (according to Lewit (1999)) as "a respiratory muscle with postural function," while the abdominal muscles are "postural muscles with respiratory function."

These comments highlight the role of the diaphragm in supporting the spine. As Lewit explains, the abdominal cavity is a fluid-filled space which is not compressible as long as the abdominal muscles and the perineum are contracted (the shout of the judo wrestler, ski jumper, and weight lifter all attest to this enhanced stability being used).

A further stabilizing feature is the fact that, as we rise on our toes, the diaphragm contracts (at the start of a race or when jumping, for example), this being interpreted as a postural reaction. Lewit sees inspiration as largely dependent on contraction of the diaphragm which lifts the lower ribs as long as the central tendon is supported by counter-pressure from sound abdominal muscles. This, he says, is the only explanation for the widening of the thorax from below (see also Latey's discussion of this function in Chapter 15).

The thorax must be widened from below to achieve postural stability during respiration, never raised from above.

Therefore the shoulders, clavicles and upper ribs are not lifted, but rotate slightly to accommodate the movement from below as the thorax widens. This does not happen when supine or on all-fours, where no postural stabilizing effect is needed and pure abdominal respiration becomes physiologically normal, with the abdomen bulging while its wall remains relaxed.

Assessing breathing function

These preliminary explanations are necessary to understand what we should look for in the presence of respiratory dysfunction. What then should we observe and palpate?

- Inactive abdominal muscles are clearly undesirable for respiratory and postural normality, for the spine then loses its diaphragmatic support. Abdominal tone can be assessed with the patient seated and relaxed. There should be no flabbiness on palpation. On stooping from the standing position the abdominals should be felt to contract. Recall that Janda (1983) has shown (Chapter 5) that over-tight erector spinae muscles will effectively reciprocally inhibit the abdominal musculature, and that no amount of toning exercise can restore normality until the erector spinae group is stretched and normalized.

- The test for abdominal muscle efficiency involves having the patient sit up from the supine position while knees and hips are flexed. In order to have coordinated action from the glutei (maximus) in this action, the heels may press backwards against a firm cushion or support. If this is difficult, then lying backwards from a seated position will train the abdominals. The spine is flexed first and one segment at a time is laid on the table/floor without raising the feet from the floor. If the feet start to leave the floor, stop the move backwards at this point and slowly return to the upright seated position. Keep repeating the lie back, trying to increase the distance travelled before the feet start to rise.

- The thorax must be seen to widen from below on inhalation. Also, when sitting flexed or lying prone, there must be a visible ability to breathe "into" the posterior thoracic wall. This is evidenced by the respiratory "wave" described previously (see Chapter 8). Where this wave is limited, failing to start in the low lumbar spine and progressing throughout inhalation up to the cervicodorsal junction, there will be palpable restrictions in the thoracic spine due to the absence of the mobilizing effect of the breathing function.

- The most obvious evidence of poor respiratory function is the raising of the upper chest structures by means of contraction of the upper fixators of the shoulder and the auxiliary and obligatory cervical muscles (upper trapezius, levator scapulae, scalenes, sternomastoid). This is both inefficient as a means of breathing and the cause of stress and overuse to the cervical structures. It is clearly evident (see below) when severe but may require a deep inhalation to show itself if only slight.

Exercise 12.2 *Assessing Respiratory Function*

Time suggested **25 minutes**

12.2A

You and the person you are observing should be seated, facing each other.

- Ask the person opposite you to relax and to try to think pleasant thoughts – walking in a garden or lying on a grassy river bank, for example.

- Observe the shoulders and clavicles during this relaxed stage, and again when the person is speaking in reply to a question.

- Observable clues to a possible upper chest/ non-diaphragmatic breathing pattern might include all or any of the following: rapid speech, sighing, yawning, and prominent "air-hunger" (like a fish-out-of-water, a gasp for air), mouth breathing.

- Look for evidence of any of the following visible signs that are suggestive of breathing pattern dysfunction: visible cord-like and palpable hypertonicity of the accessory and obligatory respiratory muscles: scalenes, sternomastoid, upper trapezius (see discussion of postural muscles Chapter 5).

- Is the head held forward of its center of gravity ("chin-poke") – something often accompanied by mouth-breathing?

- Are the shoulders protracted, commonly associated with altered scapula control (see Exercise 5.14, the scapulohumeral rhythm test, in Chapter 5).

- The HiLo assessment involves the person placing one hand on the upper sternum, and the other on the upper abdomen (Fig. 12.3). As you observe – does the upper hand move before the one on the abdomen, suggesting that thoracic breathing is dominant?

- If, in addition, the lower hand also moves posteriorly during inhalation, paradoxical breathing is being observed.

Pryor & Prasad (2002) report: "Paradoxical breathing is where some or all of the chest wall moves inward on inspiration

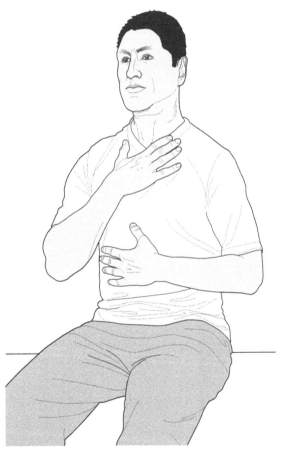

Figure 12.3
HiLo test.

and outward on expiration … localized paradox occurs when the integrity of the chest wall is disrupted."

Paradoxical breathing can also be habitual.

Lum (1987) discussed the reasons for people overbreathing: "Neurological considerations leave little doubt that habitually unstable breathing is the prime cause of symptoms."

While the person being tested continues to breathe slowly and deeply you should try to evaluate "continuity of motion" in the inhalation /exhalation phases.

- Is there any sign of starting and stopping, asymmetry, or apparent malcoordination, or any unexpected departures from smooth mobility?

- You should then palpate the abdomen, with the person still seated and inhaling deeply and slowly. Does the abdomen (slightly) bulge on inhalation? This is normal. In some instances, breathing is so faulty that the abdomen is drawn in on inhalation and pushed outwards on exhalation – further evidence of a paradoxical pattern.

- Is there obvious retraction of the epigastric area, or excessively tense intercostal spaces (see neuromuscular technique assessment methods in Chapter 5 and Fig. 5.3 in particular).

- Or does the person not quite get the end of the exhalation, before commencing the next inhalation? If so, this leads to retention of excessive levels of tidal air and carbon dioxide, preventing a full inhalation and leading to respiratory alkalosis.

- Inhalation efficiency can be said to depend on the completeness of the exhalation.

- Now ask the person to take as long as possible to breathe in completely. How long did it take? If less than 5 seconds, there is probably dysfunction.

- Next, after a complete inhalation, ask the person to take as long as possible to exhale, breathing out slowly all the time. This should also take not less than 5 seconds, although people with dysfunctional breathing status or who hyperventilate, and those in states of anxiety, often fail to take even as long as 3 seconds to inhale or exhale.

- Now time the complete cycle of breathing (inhalation plus exhalation). This should take not less than 10 seconds if function is good.

12.2B

Now stand behind the person and place your hands over their lower ribs, fingers facing forwards, thumbs touching on the midline posteriorly (Fig. 12.4).

- The person then exhales to their comfortable limit (i.e., not a forced exhalation) and then inhales slowly and fully.

- Is there a lateral widening and if so, to what degree? Pryor and Prasad (2002) report that normal total excursion is between 3 and 5 cm.

- Or do your hands seem to be move cephalad? The hands should move apart but they will rise if inappropriate breathing is being performed involving the accessory breathing muscles and upper fixators of the shoulders (Courteney 2013).

- Does one side seem to move more than the other? If so, in which directions? If so, local restrictions or muscle tensions are probably involved.

- Is there evidence of paradoxical breathing?

- Now rest your hands over the upper shoulder area, fingers facing forwards, fingertips lightly touching the superior surface of the clavicles.

- On inhalation, do the hands rise?

- Does either clavicle rise on inhalation – and if so is this symmetrical? Neither the clavicles, nor your hands should rise, except on maximal inhalation.

- Assess whether one side moves more than the other. If so, local restrictions or muscle hypertonicity (scalenes, sternomastoid) may be implicated.

- Observe the upper trapezius muscles as they curve towards the neck. Are they convex (bowing outwards)? If so, these so-called "gothic" shoulders are very taut, and probably accompanied by inappropriate breathing, lifting the upper ribs (along with scalenes, sternomastoid, and levator scapulae).

- Palpate these muscles and test them for shortness (see Chapter 5 and Exercise 12.3 below).

Exercise 12.2 *continued*

12.2C

The person should now lie supine, knees flexed.

Rest a hand, lightly, just above the umbilicus, and have the person inhale deeply.

- Does your hand move towards the ceiling (ideally "yes")?

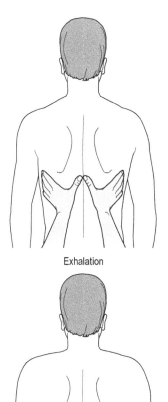

Exhalation

Inhalation

Figure 12.4

Palpation of thoracic expansion on inhalation. (After Pryor & Prasad 2002.)

- Are the abdominal muscles relaxed (ideally "yes")?
- Or did your hand actually move toward the floor on inhalation (ideally "no")?
- If the abdomen rises, was this the first part of the respiratory mechanism to move, or did it inappropriately follow an initial movement of the upper or lower chest?

Paradoxical breathing such as this involves the mechanism being used in just such an uncoordinated manner.

- Now lightly palpate underneath the subcostal margins for excessive tissue tension, suggestive of excessive tone in the attachments of the diaphragm, or the oblique abdominal muscles, or rectus abdominis, possibly accompanied by an abnormal xiphicostal angle (see above).
- Is there a reduced, or increased xiphicostal angle? (considered "normal" at about 90º; Fig. 12.5). This is best observed in the supine position. If excessively narrow, suggestive of thoracic cage rigidity and hypertonic abdominal and intercostal muscles and dysfunctional diaphragm, the angle commonly normalizes as breathing function improves (Clifton-Smith 2013).
- With the person still lying supine, observe and/or palpate the xiphoid process and the umbilicus during respiration. Do they rise cranially, rather than the norm, which is to move in a slightly anterior direction, on inhalation?

12.2D

Ask the person to lie prone.

Observe the wave as inhalation occurs, moving upwards in a fan-like manner from the lumbars to the base of the neck (see breathing wave discussion in Chapter 8, Exercise 8.19 and Fig. 8.12).

This wave can be observed by watching the spinous processes or the paraspinal musculature or palpated by a feather-light touch on the spine or paraspinal structures.

Cross-referral to other palpatory findings

Whatever restrictions or uncoordinated movements you observe or palpate during this exercise can now usefully be related to findings of spinal joint and rib restrictions (see Chapter 8), respiratory and postural muscular shortening, as well as trigger point activity, especially in the intercostal muscles (Chapter 5), postural imbalance, pelvic

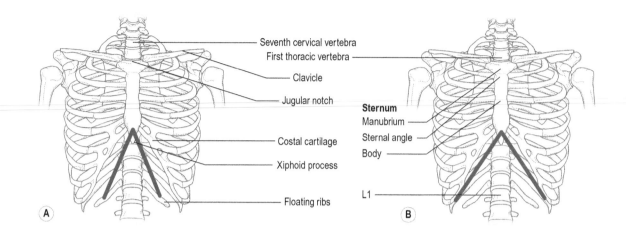

Figure 12.5
Xiphicostal angle: (A) very narrow; (B) normal.

dysfunction and other anomalies (Chapter 8), and emotional involvement (Chapter 15).

Integrating the various components of palpation, as described throughout this book, enhances clinical thinking, as evidence from one source is supported or contradicted by additional (palpation and other) findings.

Charting results

Boxes 12.1 and 12.2 offer examples of the kind of forms you can create to record breathing dysfunction in individual cases.

Observation

Bradley (Chaitow et al. 2002, 2013) describes those features which should be observed when breathing function is being evaluated, whether in the presence of pathology or a habitual breathing pattern disorder.

- Resting respiratory rate? (Normal adult range 10–14 per minute; West 2000)

- Nose or mouth breather?

- Resting breathing pattern:

Box 12.1 Primary and accessory respiratory muscle assessment for shortness (see previous chapters for guidance on individual muscle assessments)

E = Equally short (circle if both are short)

L and R (circle if left or right is short)

1. Psoas	E	L	R
2. Quadratus lumborum	E	L	R
3. Pectoralis major	E	L	R
4. Latissimus dorsi	E	L	R
5. Upper trapezius	E	L	R
6. Scalenes	E	L	R
7. Sternocleidomastoid	E	L	R
8. Levator scapulae	E	L	R
9. Spinal flattening when slumping*		LowL LD LowT MidT UpperT	
10. Cervical spine extensors short?		Yes	No

* LowL, low lumbar; LD, low dorsal; LowT, low thoracic; MidT, mid thoracic; UpperT, upper thoracic.

—effortless upper chest/hyperinflation

—accessory muscle use

—frequent sighs/yawns

—breath-holding ('statue breathing')

—abdominal splinting

● Combinations of the above

● Repeated throat clearing/air gulping.

Observe:

● Jaw, facial and general postural tension, tremor, tics, twitches, bitten nails

● Chest wall abnormalities, for example:

—pectus carinatum (anterior sternal protrusion)

—pectus excavatum (depression or hollowing of the sternum)

Box 12.2 Respiratory function assessment

Seated

a. Is lateral rib expansion symmetrical?   YES   NO

Specify differences:

b. Measure range of unforced expansion:*
EXHALED   INHALED

From: … cm to … cm

c. Measure range of full expansion:*
EXHALED   INHALED

From: … cm to … cm

d. Does inhalation start before
exhalation complete?   YES   NO

e. Does clavicle rise on inhalation?   YES   NO

f. If there is movement, is it
symmetrical?   YES   NO

Specify differences:

g. Does abdomen draw inwards
on inhalation?   YES   NO

h. Timed breathing elements:

Does inhalation last at least 3 seconds?   YES   NO

Record inhalation in seconds:

Does exhalation last at least 5 seconds?   YES   NO

Record exhalation in seconds:

Does full cycle last at least 10 seconds?   YES   NO

Record cycle in seconds:

i. Evaluate thoracic spinal restrictions (see Chapter 8).

j. List and chart findings.

* To measure the amount of expansion taking place, sit or stand facing your patient/model and place your thumbs, with their tips touching, on the anterior or posterior midline, with the index fingers resting along the shafts of a pair of ribs. As your palpation partner inhales, either fully or normally, your thumbs will separate. Judging the degree and equality of expansion by this means is rapid and accurate (Bockenhauer et al. 2004). Alternatively, use a flexible tape measure to record the unexpanded circumference and the expanded circumference in order to measure the range of expansion.

Prone

k. Observe "breathing wave" of prone patient as he/she takes full breath.

Is there a wave-like movement from the base of the sacrum to the base of the neck?
(see Exercise 8.19)   YES   NO

l. Where does the wave start and stop?

LowL   LD   LowT   MidT   UpperT

Supine

m. Evaluate for elevated or depressed rib restrictions (see Exercises 8.20 and 8.21).

n. Note any asymmetry in breathing function (e.g., lateral expansion).

- Kyphosis (abnormal forward anteroposterior spinal curvature)

- Scoliosis (lateral spinal curvature)

- Kyphoscoliosis, a combination of the former two

- Adaptive upper thoracic and shoulder girdle muscle changes, e.g., raised shoulders, protracted scapulae (see Chapter 5). See Exercise 5.14, the scapulohumeral rhythm test, in Chapter 5.

Exercise 12.3 *Comprehensive Respiratory Assessment*

Time suggested **10 minutes**

12.3A

- Look at the list of muscles below, in Box 12.1. How many of these can you assess for shortness?

- If guidelines for doing so are not contained in this book (Chapter 5 mainly), identify sources that will allow you to acquire such information and practice evaluating the muscles on this list for shortness.

Having identified asymmetrical differences in any of these postural muscles – what would your clinical approach be toward restoring balance?

The evidence of the research by Janda (1983) strongly suggests that primary attention should be towards reducing hypertonicity in overused postural muscles, before starting on rehabilitating (toning) their inhibited antagonists. This approach is supported by Lewit (2009) and others.

12.3B

- Look at the list of assessments below, in Box 12.2.

- Do your best to fulfill these observations, tests, and assessments, and circle the appropriate result.

Assessing for pathology

This book cannot cover detailed palpation for pathology but several evaluations involving palpation can be usefully practiced to enhance clinical skills.

Palpation of vocal fremitus

- When speaking, vibrations pass through the entire thoracic cavity and these can be palpated on the chest wall by placing the flat hands bilaterally and comparing the sensation as the person being evaluated repetitively speaks the words "ninety nine." Pryor and Prasad (2002) note:

- The hands are moved from the apices to bases, anteriorly and posteriorly, comparing the vibration being felt. Vocal fremitus is increased when the lung underneath is relatively solid (consolidated), as this transmits sound better.

- As sound transmission is decreased through any interface between lung and air or fluid, vocal fremitus is decreased in patients with pneumothorax or pleural effusion.

Exercise 12.4 *Percussion and Vocal Fremitus Palpation*

Time suggested **3–4 minutes**

Perform the vocal fremitus and the percussion evaluation as described above and relate this to the body type of the person.

If possible perform these exercises on a variety of different body types.

Percussion

See Special topic 8 on the subject of percussion. Percussion of the chest is a useful means of evaluating areas of consolidation. Pryor and Prasad explain:

> *Resonance is generated by the chest wall vibrating over the underlying tissues. Normal resonance is heard over aerated lungs, while consolidated lung sounds dull, and a pleural effusion sounds "stony dull". Increased resonance is heard when the chest wall is free to vibrate over an air-filled space, such as pneumothorax or bulla. In … obese patients the percussion note may sound dull even if the underlying lung is normal.*

Conclusion and discussion

If all the exercises in this chapter have been successfully attempted, ideally more than once, you should have gained an appreciation of the importance and subtlety of these methods.

While not everyone will be drawn to or feel comfortable regarding visceral palpation as such, the evaluation of breathing function is one of the skills that simply "have to" be acquired, if a comprehensive understanding of the patient/client is to be gained.

Awareness of breathing pattern disorders leads naturally to a need to uncover structural modifications (short tight muscles, restricted ribs, etc.) which might be impacting on this vital function. Reviewing the notes in Special

topic 11 (on hyperventilation) and the chapters that cover muscle and joint evaluation (Chapters 5 and 8) will provide a solid foundation for clinical interventions.

References

Barral J and Mercier P (2006) Visceral manipulation. Seattle: Eastland Press.

Bockenhauer S et al. (2004) Reliability of a measure of thoracic excursion. Journal of Osteopathic Medicine 7: 104.

Bradley H and Esformes J (2014) Breathing pattern disorders and functional movement. International Journal of Sports Physical Therapy 9 (1): 28.

Chaitow L, Bradley D and Gilbert C (2002) Multidisciplinary approaches to breathing pattern disorders. Edinburgh: Churchill Livingstone.

Chaitow L, Bradley D and Gilbert C (eds) (2013) Recognizing and treating breathing disorders. Edinburgh: Churchill Livingstone.

Clifton-Smith T (2013) Breathing pattern disorders and the athlete, in Chaitow L, Bradley D and Gilbert C (eds) Recognizing and Treating Breathing Disorders. Edinburgh: Churchill Livingstone, ch 7.7.

Courteney R (2013) Questionnaires and manual methods for assessing breathing dysfunction, in Chaitow L, Bradley D and Gilbert C (eds) Recognizing and Treating Breathing Disorders. Edinburgh: Churchill Livingstone, ch 6.5.

Cummings J and Howell J (1990) The role of respiration in the tension production of myofascial tissues. Journal of the American Osteopathic Association 90 (9): 842.

Garland W (1994) Somatic changes in hyperventilating subject – an osteopathic perspective Presentation to Paris Symposium.

Gaymans F (1980) Die Bedeutung der Atemtypen für Mobilisation der Wirbelsäule. Manuelle Medizin 18: 96–101.

Goldthwaite J, Brown LT, Swaim LT and Kuhns JG (1945) Body mechanics in health and disease. Philadelphia, PA: JB Lippincott.

Kisselkova H and Georgiev V (1979) Effects of training on postexercise limb muscle EMG synchronous to respiration. Journal of Applied Physiology 46 (6): 1093–1095.

Janda V (1983) Muscle function testing. London: Butterworths.

Lewit K (1980) Relation of faulty respiration to posture. Journal of the American Osteopathic Association 79 (8): 525–529.

Lewit K (1999) Manipulation in rehabilitation of the motor system, 3rd edn. London: Butterworths.

Lewit K (2009) Manipulative therapy. Edinburgh: Churchill Livingstone.

Lum LC (1987) Hyperventilation syndromes in medicine and psychiatry: A review. Journal of the Royal Society of Medicine 80: 229–231.

Pellegrino M (1993/1994) Fibromyalgia Network Newsletters, Tucson, AZ.

Pellegrino M (1995) The fibromyalgia survivor. Columbus, OH: Anadem Publishing.

Pellegrino M (1997) Fibromyalgia, managing the pain, 2nd edn. Columbus, OH: Anadem Publishing.

Pryor J and Prasad S (2002) Physiotherapy for respiratory and cardiac problems. Edinburgh: Churchill Livingstone.

Stone C (1999) The science and art of osteopathy. Cheltenham: Stanley Thornes.

Stone C (2007) Visceral and obstetric osteopathy. Edinburgh: Churchill Livingstone.

Timmons B and Ley R (1994) Behavioral and psychological approaches to breathing disorders. New York: Plenum Press.

West J (2000) Respiratory physiology. Philadelphia: Williams and Wilkins.

Special topic 12

Synesthesia
Sasha Chaitow

Have you ever seen letters and numbers as having colors? Does your favorite song smell of roses? Do you remember people's names according to their color?

Oddly enough, a number of individuals live permanently in such a polychrome world, in some cases with a perpetual orchestra playing in the background. Far from being a step away from disturbing hallucinations, this crossover between senses and perception is in fact a recognized condition – or rather gift – which strengthens memory, enriches perception, and offers a distinctly different view of the world to that experienced by non-synesthetes.

Deriving its name from the Greek *syn* + *aestheses*, meaning "combined sensation," synesthesia is a sensory phenomenon in which increased brain connectivity causes a perceptual overlap. In practical terms, synesthetes perceive one kind of stimulus by means of two or more senses, so for instance they can taste, as well as see, colors or shapes, or they may perceive a word or texture via an olfactory or even auditory response, in combination with the reaction of the primary sense.

The number "3" may be perceived as "red," or as having a "fluffy" texture or "sour" taste, for example, and the synesthete may experience a separate set of responses when encountering the written word "three," if the sensory pairing is such that letters of the alphabet evoke alternative responses.

The synesthetic perception is often perceived as being either in the mind's eye, or in an undefined but nearby locus (Dixon & Smilek 2002) and characterizes the primary sensation (the number or letter for instance) as strongly as the actual and relevant attributes of the stimulus itself. It is for this reason that synesthetic responses enhance the memory; a synesthete may not immediately recall someone's name, but they may first recall that the name/person is "turquoise," this association often being connected with the "strongest" color in the person's name. Then the leap is made to the name itself (Cytowic 1995).

There are as many types of synesthesia as there are sensory-modality pairings, where modalities are broad groups of sensory stimuli (color–graphemic, color–auditory and so on). According to research thus far (Day 2005; Rich et al. 2005), the most common type of synesthesia is color–graphemic, the association of written, or spoken letters and numbers, with colors.

A close second is color–auditory; the association of a sound with a color which is "seen" in the mind's eye, or even a series of colors corresponding to the tones in a melody. "True" or "strong" synesthesia is classified by the lifelong presence of the phenomenon, in addition to the fact that the associations between given stimuli and perceptions remain unchanged. For instance, for a particular individual, the number "3" will always be red; a flute sound will taste salty, or sound blue, and so forth. Stability of association displaying accuracy upon repetition is the main criterion for identifying true synesthesia, strengthening the case for an internal causative mechanism and debunking the suggestion that it could be caused by conditioned responses, learned unconsciously in childhood, such as through the use of colored alphabets.

Synesthesia is termed "weak," or "pseudo-synesthesia," when the accuracy rate decreases, or when an individual produces a synesthetic response with diminished or irregular frequency.

Synesthesia research is a very young field, perhaps only really spanning the last 20 years, and it has to a large extent been treated as a "curiosity condition" by the scientific community (Cytowic 1995), although greater efforts are now being made to isolate and explore its precise provenance and stages of development, with large-scale experiments being implemented at a number of research centers.

Although it was first tentatively identified in the 1880s (Galton 1883), and in the past there have been isolated cases of artists and poets, Charles Baudelaire, Richard Wagner and Wassily Kandinsky among them, proclaiming their synesthetic abilities, and actively utilizing them in their respective arts, these were frequently written off as products of an overactive artistic imagination or the effects of too much absinthe. However, more recently, the serious examination of synesthesia has become more widespread, particularly in the fields of cognitive neuroscience and consciousness research, although there is still a tendency to emphasize its status as a curiosity, or as part of an innate artistic ability (Heyrman 2005, 2007), though this is rapidly fading as new studies emerge (Smilek & Dixon 2002; Hochel & Milan 2008).

Researchers are still unsure as to whether it is a pre- or postnatal developmental anomaly, one theory (Baron-Cohen, 1996, Maurer & Mondlach 2005) suggesting that while normally the senses differentiate in infancy, in synesthetes the neural pathways retain an overlap. Statistics also seem to indicate that there is a tendency for synesthesia to run in families, particularly in the maternal line, and between twins (Cytowic 1989, 2002; Baron-Cohen et al, 1993). Further research difficulties include a demographic bias in statistics gathered, as few people recognize synesthesia for what it is. Certain individuals may not realize that it is actually a rare ability; others have thought it was an abnormality and spent years hiding it in the belief that they had some kind of mental illness (Cytowic 1989, 2002; Day 2005). The statistics gathered so far are mainly from volunteers who generally originate from a Western, middle-class, reasonably literate background, which may be the reason for the relative commonality of color-graphemic synesthesia, and so the findings cannot as yet provide a clear indication as to the prevalence and distribution of synesthesia and its subtypes.

What has also not been established is the extent to which synesthesia can actually be "learned" or developed by non-synesthetes, or for synesthetes displaying one sensory-modality pairing to be able to develop others. Ongoing research into this continues, such as that by Baron-Cohen into developmental aspects of synesthesia, and whether it is a faculty that we are all born with but some lose, or that we all have but is simply dominant in some and latent in others (Cytowic 2003).

Possible bodywork implications

Although one might wonder what practical application this may have, from a phenomenological viewpoint, its potential applications – beyond the artistic fields – are of considerable interest to the area of manual assessment and therapy.

A synesthete, born or made – if research indicates the latter possibility – might be able to perceive and interpret tensions and subfascial disparities via touch, but with the added advantage of picking up subtleties and deeper tissue anomalies. To a synesthete's perceptual framework, this would be directly differentiated to a further extent than normal, and with more clarity, thus increasing accuracy and sensitivity during assessment.

When palpating for fluid continuity in initial evaluation, it may be possible to categorize and interpret the subtle levels of rhythm and pulsation being sought to the effect that these variations can be traced more clearly and offer a greater understanding of the associated dysfunctions.

Natural synesthetes also display an above-average mnemonic ability (Cytowic 1995), and in conjunction with a deeper understanding of the intuitive mechanisms and techniques as described in Chapter 13, these faculties may be of great value in numerous applications, once their inner workings are better understood.

One such case of synesthesia applied to bodywork (Bishop 2000) utilizes a tactile-olfactory pairing via which the practitioner is able to tap into cellular memory (see Chapter 14), communicated via the synesthetic link, and through communication with the patient, track the trauma and its effects by interpreting the "smells" generated by the tactile stimuli during palpation.

An extension of this is what has been termed mirror-touch synesthesia, in which a synesthete watching another person being touched, on the head or neck, for example, can feel the tactile sensation as if they themselves are being touched. Neuroimaging studies (Banissey & Ward 2007; Blakemore et al. 2005) have indicated that the somatosensory cortex is hyperactivated in mirror-touch synesthetes, when observing another person being touched, and participants reported back with a high degree of accuracy when describing the sensation. They also perceived the "mirrored" sensation as being stronger than when they themselves were being touched on a different part of their body, indicating a high degree of empathy overriding their own sensory messages. Such an ability could well be useful when a therapist is seeking to understand the nature of a given problem, its causes and influences within the body. It is equally useful if one considers that in order to understand the condition of the patient, it is also important to enhance our understanding of our own bodies. The visceral, or downright physical, reaction we may feel when identifying with a character in a film or book, particularly in disturbing scenes, is an extreme example of how mirror-touch synesthesia may work. This new research does suggest that there is a far more sensitive faculty underlying such empathetic reactions, and with encouragement, it may be possible for it to be developed and utilized to an extent where the therapist can sense – in their own body – how the patient's body is responding, and so fine-tune their actions accordingly.

As with the ability to visualize, the ability to synesthetically perceive what the fingers are feeling offers a tool which, with training, might forge new paths in terms of the therapist–patient relationship, on both a practical level and a theoretical one. The earlier example relating to memory, and recalling of a name through synesthetic association, could work equally well in terms of committing to memory, and then intuitively (see Chapter 13) working with the types of tissue texture and sensation when palpating.

If you know, or suspect, that you are synesthetic, it may well be worth paying closer attention to how your synesthesia works and where, as described in Bishop's work, as you may be able to use it in your assessment and evaluation techniques. If you are not synesthetic it may nevertheless be useful to retain an awareness of this capacity, as feedback from occasionally synesthetic patients will be easier to work with. Also, by understanding the empathetic perception involved in mirror-touch synesthesia, you may find ways to develop your rapport with the patient on a more subtle level.

Synesthesia research in the field of cognitive neuroscience in particular is continually evolving, and it will be of great interest to see what findings are reached regarding the prevalence and evolution of synesthesia, particularly whether it is after all a latent faculty that can be awoken in non-synesthetes and its relationship to consciousness. Artists were using it before it had a name; now scientists are seeking to place and understand it and already it is demonstrating its uses in bodywork. It may be worth following these developments given that the more we understand about *how* we understand, the more likely we are to be able to help both the bodies and the minds of others regain their equilibrium.

References

Banissy MJ and Ward J (2007) Mirror-touch synesthesia is linked with empathy. Nature Neuroscientist 10: 815–816.

Baron-Cohen S (1996) Is there a normal phase of synesthesia in development? Psyche 2 (27). Online. Available at: http://hstrial-tridenttechnical.homestead.com/BaronCohen1996.pdf

Baron-Cohen S, Harrison J, Goldstein JH and Wyke M (1993) Coloured speech perception: Is synaesthesia what happens when modularity breaks down? Perception 22: 419–426.

Bishop R (2000) Synesthesia and its relevance to bodywork. Rolf Lines 28 (3): 40–42.

Blakemore SJ, Bristow D, Bird G, Frith C and Ward J (2005) Somatosensory activations during the observation of touch and a case of vision-touch synaesthesia. Brain 128: 1571–1583.

Cytowic RE (1989) Synesthesia: A union of the senses. Cambridge MA: MIT Press.

Cytowic RE (1995) Synesthesia: Phenomenology and neuropsychology; a review of current knowledge. Psyche 2 (10).

Cytowic RE (2002) Synesthesia: A union of the senses, 2nd edn. Cambridge MA: MIT Press.

Cytowic RE (2003) The man who tasted shapes. Exeter: Imprint Academic.

Day SA (2005) Some demographic and socio-cultural aspects of synesthesia, in Robertson L and Sagiv N (eds) Synesthesia: Perspectives from cognitive neuroscience. Oxford: Oxford University Press, pp 11–33.

Galton F (1883) Inquiries into human faculty and its development. London: Macmillan.

Heyrman H (2005) Art and synesthesia: In search of the synesthetic experience. Lecture presented at the First International Conference of Art and Synesthesia, 25–28 July 2005, Universidad de Almeria, Spain. Online. Available at: http://www.doctorhugo.org/synaesthesia/art/index.html

Heyrman H (2007) Extending the synesthetic code: Connecting synesthesia, memory and art. Online. Available at: http://www.doctorhugo.org/synaesthesia/art2/index.html

Hochel M and Milan EG (2008) Synaesthesia: The existing state of affairs. Cognitive Neuropsychology 25 (1): 93–117.

Maurer D and Mondlach CJ (2005) Neonatal synesthesia: A reevaluation, in Robertson LC and Sagiv S (eds) Synesthesia: Perspectives from cognitive neuroscience. New York: Oxford University Press, pp 193–213.

Rich AN, Bradshaw JL and Mattingley J B (2005) A systematic, large scale study of synaesthesia: Implications for the role of early experience in lexical-colour associations. Cognition 98 (1): 53–84.

Smilek D and Dixon M (2002) Towards a synergistic understanding of synaesthesia: Combining current experimental findings with synaesthetes' subjective descriptions. Psyche 8 (01). Online. Available at: http://journalpsyche.org/files/0xaa9d.pdf

Sasha Chaitow

Intuition is an intellectual capacity that is frequently surrounded by an aura of mystery. In truth it is intuition that is responsible for those sudden insights that are often difficult to explain in concrete terms. Despite its somewhat mysterious reputation, it is in fact a skill inherent in the intellectual makeup of each of us. And just as it has been suggested that "we are all athletes, but only some of us are in training," so can this latent intuitive skill be developed and enhanced. A well trained intuitive faculty can therefore, together with your subtle sensory memory, exploit your embedded theoretical and empirical knowledge, in both therapeutic and assessment settings. An example might involve awareness of the way in which your senses, including your memory, can help to construct in your "mind's eye" a picture of a particular tissue or a joint, involving its structure and function, and how to approach its treatment or rehabilitation. While it is vital to have a solid theoretical and clinical knowledge base – for otherwise assessment and diagnosis would become guesswork – the use of intuition in its various subtle manifestations offers you an amplified ability to view and treat a given dysfunction from a holistic viewpoint.

Intuition can be seen as a way of "superior knowing" of the essence of things, without resorting to empirical intellectual analysis of a situation. Hippocrates, the father of medicine (5th century BC), considered that three faculties were necessary for accurate diagnosis and treatment: the senses, the intellect, and intuition (Antoniou et al. 2012). As Hippocrates states, "judgment is difficult" – when it comes to diagnosis and appropriate therapeutic approaches, intuition is the faculty that draws together the others in order to reach a solid conclusion (Antoniou et al. 2012).

In modern times, the theoretical exploration of intuition has been defined by, and based on, the philosophical method of the influential philosopher Henri Bergson (1859–1941). It involves an approach by means of which the mind can come to know a thing in itself as more than the sum of its parts. This *knowing* occurs outside a logical analytic framework, so rationalizing it requires something of a quantum leap in thinking, as it places the essence of

material objects outside of time. Where motion through space, measured in time, is the traditional scientific method of comprehending material attributes, the intuitive method places the essence of objects in a perpetual *now*, whereby the significance for intuiting their fundamental nature is related to memory, with prediction being seen to represent same thing.

The roots of intuition research are found in existentialist theory; but its presence and usefulness in a number of fields are undeniable. These range from the more obviously relevant humanities, to quantum physics and abstract mathematics. In these fields – where extreme abstractions can only be intuited at first, and then set down as formulae – it has become the subject of much exploration by neuroscientists and consciousness researchers. These explorations of intuitive function are based on conceptual models borrowed from semiotics (the theory and study of meaning, and how our intellect approaches and processes it) and linguistic studies, in conjunction with neurophenomenology and genetic epistemology (Winkelman 1996), which is the study of how knowledge originates and develops, based mainly on the work of clinical psychologist Jean Piaget (1896–1980).

In plain terms, the sensory perceptions that we gather from our environment, or from a situation, or an object, are committed to a part of our memory. When we find ourselves in a similar situation, or approach a similar object, we do not enter into a process of full recall – one or two stimuli are enough for the rest of the experience to be intuited, and for us to then form a judgment about the new stimulus and react to it. Intuition is also differentiated from instinct on the basis that instinctual responses are inherited and related to survival; intuited responses are rooted in a constant process of synthesizing our sensory perceptions deriving from our environment and our place within it. When reactions and learning processes are "hard-wired" into the brain, so as to have become second nature, they are naturally embedded into the unconscious, and our responses, actions, and what we perceive as independent intuitive insights are in fact based on these unconscious learned patterns.

The essential difference between comprehending something via intuition and via analytic method can be compared to the difference between describing an archetypal experience – the vision of a sunset, or reading a line of poetry, as compared with reams of commentary and description of either of these. The latter communicates and describes around the sum of parts of the experience, the former instantaneously presents to consciousness *the thing as it is,* and one of the hallmarks of intuition is that flash of realization, as opposed to labored analytical reasoning.

According to one aspect of communication theory, the essential formula by which we communicate consists of a pattern of "encoding–transmission–decoding" (Hall 1973):

- Person A formulates a thought and encodes it in what they consider appropriate language.

- Person A then transmits the thought through speech, writing, or non-verbal signals.

- The message is then decoded by person B, according to the common codes of communication they share.

- Miscommunication occurs when the recipient misinterprets the encoding used by the transmitter.

The more experienced we are in the use of language, and the more proficient in understanding appropriate modes of encoding and decoding, the more astute we become at understanding the actual message being transmitted, although rarely do we even momentarily stop to think about the process that we all participate in many times a day. The process of "decoding" the more subtle elements present in the encoding of a message, such as body language, or vocal nuance, is a more familiar example of intuition. Precisely the same idea applies to our responses and comprehension of sensory perceptions from environmental stimuli – as when palpating tissues.

In more commonplace situations, therefore, we use intuition on a daily basis without being aware of it. In the context of palpation it can be explained as the inexplicable "knowing" of the nature of a given dysfunction, usually gained through long experience and hands-on practice, as opposed to simply theoretical – and so analytical – knowledge, without the added dimension of being able to simply feel and simultaneously know what is wrong. In this way intuition is connected to memory, though, it must be clarified, not the kind of linear memory we are more familiar with, such as being able to remember the theoretical underpinnings of why and how a given trauma affects tissue in the way it does.

Modern neuroscience places the understanding of intuition in a trans-disciplinary framework where biology, psychology, physics, and philosophy respectively reveal empirical, structural, cognitive, systematic, and conceptual aspects of its form, function, and phenomenology (Freeman 1997). From a biophysical perspective, we are able to perceive stimuli well beyond the frequencies to which our senses are tuned; even if our hearing only allows us to consciously discern sound within a given set of wavelengths, nonetheless our brain can pick up and perceive sounds outside that wavelength, albeit on a subconscious level (von Arx 2001).

A similar process occurs with our perception of light and color, so that although our eyes do not, and cannot, consciously analyze a given color into its component wavelengths of light, with experience we can begin to separate it into shades and constituent parts, as most artists can attest. This occurs by way of indirect perception based on recall whereby the neural system "fills the gaps" between what is seen and what can be perceived (von Arx 2001). Research and analysis of this phenomenon has often fallen into a dualistic bind consisting of the separation between sensory data and perceived data, because our brains are seen to be in a continuous process of perceiving and processing two sets of data. This paradox is reconciled by what is termed *whole systems theory*: the brain is seen as a closed nonlinear system with the capacity to create and continually self-determine its perceptions (Freeman 1997). These processes do not occur at a conscious level, but consciousness is necessary for them to occur (Marcel 1983; von Arx 2001) because only then does the perception acquire meaning which is then embedded as part of the learning process. The more aware we become of these processes, by observing our own reactions to them, the more able we are to utilize them in whichever capacity we choose.

Inherent in the process of intuition is the ability to visualize; and although this is based on prior experience and the hard-wiring within the neural pathways of our brains, it is sparked by the active imagination. This should in no way be confused with the imagination of storybooks and fantasy (Voss 2004): it is an intellectual faculty which recreates neural processes, not due to an external sensory stimulus, but based on inner conceptual models and the will or intention to do so (Perlovsky 2006). Just as an artist can visualize a body and transfer that image onto canvas without a model – the more experienced the artist, the more accurate the representation – similarly a manual therapist can learn to enhance their awareness of their own tactile perceptions of the human body, and so recreate the sensations and perceptions acquired while palpating. It is thus possible to build up a mental touch-image of tissue layers when in a normal state, and, through experience, to recall that image for comparison when meeting dysfunctions, which will gradually become equally familiar. We learn to intuit from the outside in; firstly by internalizing the perceptions we gather from outside ourselves using our senses, and secondly, on a smaller scale and in the context of manual therapy, from the skin inwards. The ability to visualize at will from the inside out (whether this visualization is in the mind's eye or the fingertips) demonstrates our developing ability to work with this skill, and to learn to discern what it is we are sensing at ever more subtle levels.

By understanding the theoretical underpinnings of intuitive knowledge, we are in a position to not only enhance our own sensory perceptions but, in a therapeutic context, also to approach the patient with a heightened awareness of what it is to view the organism holistically. In order to enhance our own intuitive skills for the purpose of therapeutic application, we might first conceive of our own mind and the knowledge it contains. We should also conceive of ways in which we can use our senses, as a unified whole, with the capability to reach outside ourselves, both to discover and to extend the limits of our perceptions. When palpating tissue, we observe and process the sensory input on a number of levels, all of which are needed to make a satisfactory assessment. That sense of sudden and meaningful inner knowledge of what is being palpated and what therapeutic input it may need, when correlated against and confirmed by your clinical knowledge, is the synthesis and integration of these diverse mental processes and a valuable tool for hands-on therapy in particular.

Exercise 13.1A *Developing Intuition via Sensory Awareness Part 1*

Some individuals may find spatial and tactile visualization reasonably easy, others not so easy. However recall-based visualization is not so challenging; for example, closing one's eyes and visualizing the layout of one's home, or a familiar object such as an apple or orange.

The following exercise is intended to:

- exercise your awareness of sensory input
- help develop your visualization skills
- teach you to use those skills to recreate and recognize a variety of individual sensory stimuli.

These skills can then be applied in a variety of evaluation and clinical contexts.

If you find visualization quite easy, then after familiarizing yourself with the procedure you may wish to progress to the development of the other senses, although it is useful to begin by treating them individually and gradually building up the sensory image the exercise requires. This is mainly so that you sharpen your own awareness of how you perceive each kind of sensory input. It may be useful to keep notes of any insights or reactions you have as you repeat the exercise: which senses you find easier to recall, which harder, what changes in awareness you may note. This will give you a roadmap to your own particular sensory abilities and guide you as to which senses you may work best with.

As with all exercises that deal with subtle and minute sensations, it is important that you relax and center yourself before you begin. You are trying to observe very slight sensations and so a steady focus is needed. If at any point your concentration is broken or you find your mind wandering, take a few moments to clear your mind and begin again.

- Close your eyes and visualize an apple. It can be as simple as a black silhouette on a contrasting white background. Focus on the outline, complete with stalk and leaf.
- Concentrate on holding the image firmly in your mind's eye, without interfering thoughts. After a minute or so, open your eyes, clear your visual field, and then close them again and repeat the exercise.

Exercise 13.1A *continued*

- After a few daily repetitions of a minute at a time, begin to fill the apple out, making it three-dimensional. It may help to first observe a real apple in front of you for 10 seconds or so and then close your eyes and try to hold the image firmly in your mind's eye.

- Once you are comfortable with visualizing the apple, begin to work with the other senses to manifest your perception of the apple as much as possible.

- Hold the apple in your hand with your eyes closed. Focus on its texture and weight.

- Put it down, keeping your hand outstretched and hold the visualization again. Can you add its texture and weight to the visualization?

- As with the image, look, then close your eyes and visualize. Hold it, and draw out the sensation of how it feels. Add smell as well, and then taste.

- After a number of gradual repetitions, you should begin to be able to visualize the apple strongly enough, to the point where you can recreate the apple in the palm of your hand, first by building the image, then by giving it texture, weight, and all the other qualities that you recognize and that impact directly on your senses.

- Once you are reasonably comfortable with this exercise, at least to the extent where you can hold the visualization and recall tactile sensation, try to repeat it with a different fruit, or other inanimate object.

- Begin to observe differences in weight and texture.

- What are the differences between an apple and a pear? Can you recall their textures on your fingertips without picking them up? How does the difference in shape affect the pressure you feel on your palm? When you put the fruit down, can you bring back the sense of how they felt in your hand?

- When familiar with at least two different kinds of fruit in the manner described above, begin to try to "extend" your sensory perception of them below the surface of the skin. It is best to work with two quite different fruits, such as an apple and an orange, for example. Use the real fruit at first, with your eyes closed, and as you palpate each fruit, begin to "feel" for the textures below the surface. An apple is crisp while an orange is juicy, its surface springier. Can you sense these differences?

- Now move to the visualization, drawing in each sense at a time to enhance it, and "build" the fruit in your mind's eye and hand. This is perhaps the hardest stage; you should, however, slowly be able to recreate the sense of holding an entirely solid fruit in the palm of your hand, while seeing it in your mind's eye and even smelling it and sensing its texture under the skin.

Exercise 13.1B *Developing Intuition via Sensory Awareness Part 2*

It is suggested that you refer back to Exercises 3.10–3.14 to see how those exercises can usefully incorporate the ideas expressed in this chapter.

- Once you are comfortable with building your awareness of sensory perception, begin combining it with your knowledge of anatomy and physiology. In the same way that you visualized the apple and gradually added its other qualities, visualize the human body, or a portion of it – a limb perhaps. You can use your own arm or leg for reference, as well as anatomical drawings.

- With closed eyes, begin to build up an image of an arm or joint; add muscle, ligaments, fascia, and skin.

- As you add layers, observe each of them using as many textural sensations as possible, focusing particularly on the differentiation between tissue types.

- Which are more elastic and which less so?

- Which are springier and which tougher?

- Concentrate on the sensations that are most meaningful to you in order to differentiate between the various tissue types. With time the subtleties will become easier to observe.

- Building from the inside out in this case will give you a stronger awareness of the complexity of the limb and the behavior and connections between the substrata of its anatomy.

- At this stage use as much of your anatomical knowledge as you can, to quite literally "flesh out" the visual and textural mental picture you are working with.

Exercise 13.1B *continued*

- As you become more proficient with the exercise, approach the fibrous, and then cellular level. Once again, use as many of your inner senses as you can to recreate your mental image of the elements you are observing.

- Try to sense the rhythm and motions within the tissue. As you repeat the exercise, you should be able to "zoom in" quite quickly to whichever level of tissue you wish. You should also notice that the mental image that you acquire is the same each time, and that you can begin to sense and recall the differences in feeling between tissue types (muscle, skin, joint, etc.).

- In extension, these skills can then be applied to the location and assessment of dysfunction. If developed sufficiently, in combination with other palpation skills and a sound training, the depth and quality of dysfunction should become more clearly discernible via palpatory examination. Just as you should become able to discern between a "bruised" apple and a withered or rotten one, and learn to recall, build and recognize the sense of each, so subcutaneous dysfunctions such as trigger points, strains, or fascial tension, should become easier to differentiate and their sources easier to locate.

- Some individuals may detect changes in temperature between healthy and dysfunctional tissue, or their visualization may change color depending on the problem. It is at this point that the intuitive faculty has begun to bridge the actual sensory information with the "deeper" knowledge of what the nature of the problem is, leading to a more accurate assessment.

Do note that as you progress with this exercise, you should not be analyzing what it is you are feeling, so much as seeking to recognize it for what it is. Even when zooming in to a muscle fiber, for example, you should be focusing on the feeling of what it is in relation to the whole and to your fingertips or mental picture, not thinking about it in an anatomical sense – just as when looking at a painting you would not analyze the individual brushstrokes or the composition of a particular color; you would observe that color in relation to what it represents in terms of the whole painting.

This should become second nature after a while. A good way to add to your proficiency would be to try to observe the sensory impressions you gain from everyday objects; different fabrics you wear, or shaking someone's hand. Gradually you should be able to recall a number of sensations or mental pictures at will, and so apply this heightened sensory awareness to your palpatory practice.

With reference to the process of building a mental touch-image "from the inside out," as previously discussed, when in the process of healing we necessarily approach from the "outside in," beginning from our own center and gradually feeling our way into whichever part of the body we are working with. One way to use some of the concepts described above, particularly the visualization skill (as discussed in Chapter 14), would be in conjunction with energy and non-touch palpation to which the value of practitioner intuition is indispensable.

The skills developed in those exercises can be combined and applied as an adjunct to any kind of manual therapy, and depending on the situation, you may choose for it to be a secondary or primary element of whichever other type of treatment you decide to work with. It can also be very useful in guiding your hands and you may build up a particular style of rhythm which helps you both to synchronize with the patient and approach to the problem.

Exercise 13.2A *Energy Fields and Healing Part 1*

- Before attempting this exercise, and although out of sequence, it is suggested that you skip forward to Exercise 14.6 in the next chapter.

- When/if you are able to sense what is described as an 'energy field' in that exercise, return to this one.

- Hold your hands at a comfortable distance apart and close your eyes.

- Visualize the energy field that you can feel as colored light.

- White, gold, or pale blue are best as these colors are associated with calming and healing influences and will also be conducive to your own state of mind.

- Observe the flow and rhythm that you feel. Begin to "translate" this into a visual image.

- As with the previous exercise, after a few repetitions this should settle into a particular preferred color and visualization which you are comfortable with. These may resemble wave patterns or even fractals.

Chapter 13

Exercise 13.2B *Energy Fields and Healing Part 2*

- When you are comfortable with Exercise 13.2A, above, place your hands at a comfortable distance, as before, with a plain white surface behind them. Focus on the space between your hands.

- Can you see anything? If not, close your eyes, repeat part 1, and then open them. Try to hold the visualization with your eyes open.

- After some repetitions, you should observe a shimmering or blurring between your hands where you sense the tingling of the energy field. With some practice you should be able to hold the visualization you had with your eyes closed when you open them.

- Now begin to practice without "creating" the energy field. Close your eyes, and place the one hand above the other, with the fingertips of the uppermost hand just touching the lower.

- Visualize the same light as before flowing out from the fingertips or the palm of the uppermost hand into the lower. You may experience a tingling sensation where the hands meet, possibly accompanied by a change in temperature.

- Gradually lift the uppermost hand a few millimeters while holding the visualization. The sensation should remain the same.

- Increase the distance again. Continue doing this by small increments and observe when, or if, the tingling sensation starts to fade. Does the visualization weaken as you increase the distance?

- Repeat this as many times as you need to until you are able to hold the visualization steady as you increase the distance. Repeat with your eyes open as well as closed.

- You should eventually find that you can hold the visualization even when looking at something entirely different, if you have learned to focus your mind on the particular activity.

You should then be able to develop this skill to the point where you can direct the light as an "invisible finger" as you palpate or treat. Used together with the method learned in Exercise 13.1, this should heighten your awareness when treating or evaluating a patient, by any given manual therapy method, in order to enhance your perception and assessment ability as well as your treatment applications on very subtle levels.

Energy fields are related to the type of sensory perception that is on the edge of consciousness, as previously described in the discussion of light frequencies perceptible to the human eye. Intuition is the stepping stone, or tool, with which we can raise our awareness of them and draw them into our conscious perception and so learn to utilize them, just as with any other latent faculty. In a number of places in this book, for example in Chapter 3, involving Frymann's (1963) series of palpation exercises (Exercises 3.10–3.12, 3.14), what you are essentially learning to do with these techniques is to perceive and trust non-material and non-visible signals.

Since antiquity and until the Enlightenment, which began in the mid-17th century, the perception and understanding of medicine and healing was very different and was arguably more holistic than in modern times. The homeostatic functions of body, mind, and soul were considered to be vital to well-being, and the idea of correspondences between Nature and Man, microcosm and macrocosm, were taken as fact, so concepts such as invisible energy fields acting on a body were entirely acceptable within a worldview characterized by anagogical and symbolic perception, where anagogical thinking is the process of finding meaning and knowledge by observing natural processes and viewing them as metaphors for other levels of reality (Voss 2004).

Holism is a modern term, yet the separation of mind and body, reason and intuition were unheard of until the Age of Reason dictated that anything that was not proven according to the scientific method and empirical data was worthless, in a reaction stemming from social and religious factors. The philosopher and physician Paracelsus (1493–1541) is not only considered the true precursor of homeopathy via his work on toxicology, but also emphasized the importance of hands-on practice and evidence-based medicine, and broke new ground in the use of chemicals and minerals to effect cures against what he recognized as externally engendered diseases. So far-reaching was his influence that where "holistic" ideas survived after the Enlightenment, Paracelsianism is credited. It is only in our time that this way of thinking has become scientifically accredited and is beginning to find a new framework within which to promote healing and harmony within the human organism, and by extension with nature.

Concepts such as intuition and subtle energies within the healing profession are therefore part of a much longer tradition and are gradually being reinstated through work in the fields of energy medicine, neuroscience and quantum coherence. Research still has a long way to go in many of these areas, but the most useful message to be gleaned from these developments is the fact that the stigma attached to what may have seemed to be arcane and esoteric ideas, is fading as their re-examination within the scientific establishment allows them to enrich and complement holistic treatment methods.

References

Antoniou GA, Antoniou SA, Georgiadis GS and Antoniou AI (2012) A contemporary perspective of the first aphorism of Hippocrates. Journal of Vascular Surgery 56 (3): 866–868.

Freeman WJ (1997) Three centuries of category errors in studies of the neural basis of consciousness and intentionality. Neural Networks 10 (7): 1175–1183.

Frymann V (1963) Palpation – its study in the workshop. Newark, OH: Yearbook of the American Academy of Osteopathy, pp 16–30.

Hall S (1973) Encoding/decoding, in Centre for Contemporary Cultural Studies, Culture, Media, Language: Working Papers in Cultural Studies, 1972–79. London: Hutchinson.

Marcel AJ (1983) Conscious and unconscious perception: An approach to the relations between phenomenal experience and perceptual processes. Cognitive Psychology 15 (2): 238–300.

Perlovsky LI (2006) Towards physics of the mind: Concepts, emotions, consciousness, and symbols. Physics of Life Reviews 3: 23–55.

von Arx WS (2001) On the biophysics of consciousness and thought and characteristics of the human mind and intellect. Medical Hypotheses 68 (3): 302–313.

Voss A (2004) From allegory to anagoge: The question of symbolic perception in a literal world, in Campion N, Curry P and Yorke M (eds) Astrology and the Academy. Bristol: Cinnabar Books, pp 1–9.

Winkelman M (1996) Neurophenomenology and genetic epistemology as a basis for the study of consciousness. Journal of Social and Evolutionary Systems 19 (3): 217–236.

Further reading

Bergson H (1903) The creative mind: An introduction to metaphysics.

Biley F (1992) The science of unitary human beings: A contemporary literature review. Nursing Practice 5 (4): 23–26.

Debus AJ (2002) The chemical philosophy. New York: Dover.

Debus AJ (ed) (2004) Alchemy and early modern chemistry: Papers from Ambix. Huddersfield: Jeremy Mills.

De Saussure F [1916] (1983) Course in general linguistics (trans Roy Harris). London: Duckworth.

Engebretson J and Wind DW (2007) Energy based modalities. Nursing Clinics of North America 42: 243–259.

Goodrick-Clarke N (ed) (1999) Paracelsus: Essential readings. Western Esoteric Masters Series. Berkeley: North Atlantic.

Heidegger M [1927] (1962) Being and time (trans J Macquarrie and E Robinson). New York: Harper.

Jakobson R and Halle M (1956) Fundamentals of language. The Hague: Mouton.

Jakobson R (1971) Language in relation to other communication systems, in Selected Writings, vol 2. The Hague: Mouton.

Koffka K (1935) Principles of gestalt psychology. New York: Harcourt Brace.

Krieger D (1993) Accepting your power to heal. Rochester, VT: Bear and Company.

Oschman JL (1997) Polarity, therapeutic touch, magnet therapy and related methods. Journal of Bodywork and Movement Therapies 1 (2): 123–128.

Oschman JL (2002) Clinical aspects of biological fields: An introduction for healthcare professionals. Journal of Bodywork and Movement Therapies 6 (2): 117–125.

Piaget J (1972) Psychology and epistemology: Towards a theory of knowledge. Harmondsworth: Penguin.

Prigogine I (1980) From being to becoming: Time and complexity in the physical sciences. San Fransisco: WH Freeman.

Special topic 13

Palpating the traditional Chinese pulses
Leon Chaitow

A method of diagnosis that has existed and been refined over a period of 5000 years deserves to be taken seriously, even if its precepts and conclusions seem to fly in the face of current Western medical thinking.

Not surprisingly, there are different versions and interpretations of pulse diagnosis; however, the basic methodology is similar in all schools.

As an exercise in palpation the methods of pulse diagnosis have much to commend them, even if the interpretations of what is being palpated are not generally accepted by Western medicine or if the language in which these findings are expressed is difficult to follow in the West.

Precisely the same can be said for cranial palpation, in which there is little dispute that "something" is being felt when "cranial impulses" are being palpated, although there is a great deal of debate as to what "it" is, and what "it" may mean, in health terms (see Chapter 14).

It should be remembered that the TCM practitioner who is using pulse diagnosis incorporates the impressions gained in this way with other methods of assessment, including the presenting signs, symptoms, and history, as well as methods such as tongue diagnosis (where descriptors such as "pale," "fat," "moist," "dry," "yellow," and so on, are used to discriminate one pathophysiological state of the tongue from another, each indicating an imbalance of one sort or another) (Ryan & Shattuck 1994).

History

Austin (1974) pointed out that in Western medicine, taking the pulse is an important part of the diagnostic process:

- How many beats to each breath?

- Is the pulse strong or weak, even or irregular?

- Is blood flow full or thin, strong or weak, hard or soft, regular or intermittent, etc.?

TCM pulses

The Chinese pulse is, however, quite a different story. In TCM it is considered that through the pulse it is possible to read not merely the health of the organism as a whole, but that of each inner organ separately:

- whether it has too much or too little *energy*

- whether it is congested, over-full, or deficient

- whether it is hyper- or hypoactive

- whether the polarity predominance and polarity changes are in proper order

… and so on (Austin 1974).

The Chinese identified 12 (some say 14) positions on the radial pulse that could be used to indicate the status of specific organs and functions. How is this possible? Austin explains:

If you have fluid flowing through a resilient tube, a rubber or plastic tube attached to a water tap, and very lightly touch the tube with a finger, the flow of water can be felt. The tube need hardly be compressed at all for us to feel the flow quite distinctly. Let the finger tip linger a while, so that the kind of sensation of flow registers in you; now steadily compress the tube by increasing the pressure until you have stopped the flow, then lift ever so slightly – maintain this pressure and note what you are feeling. The kind of sensation you now experience in your finger tip is different from that of the first light touch. You may, for example, be more aware of the resilience of the tube itself, at one pressure level rather than another; or of volume, water pressure, speed of flow, etc. *Continue your experiment by varying the surface on which the tube rests. A tube resting on a hard surface will feel different from when it is resting upon a soft surface (folded towel, for example). This will apply to both levels of palpation. There will also be a difference if one places a layer of material between finger and tube.*

If, instead of the tube described by Austin, we think of an artery, and of the hard surface as an underlying bone, and of the gauze as soft tissues, we can see that it may indeed be quite possible for palpation to detect variations in flow, depending upon what lies between the palpating finger and the artery, and what lies below the artery.

Some of the many descriptors used in TCM to describe the different sensations imparted by the various pulses include, "wiry," "bounding," "full," "rapid," "empty," "thin," "thready." Each of these descriptors is thought to represent the current state of energy balance relative to the organ and its functions that are being assessed in this way. When you attempt this exercise (see Exercise 13.2 below) see how many different descriptors you can contrive (Ryan & Shattuck 1994).

For a more recent evolution of this method of palpation see the paper by Shu and Sun (2007), who describe a quantitative approach that complements the qualitative nature of traditional pulse diagnosis. They note:

Chinese pulses can be recognized quantitatively by the newly-developed four classification indices, that is, the wave length, the relative phase difference, the rate parameter, and the peak ratio. The new quantitative classification not only reduces the dependency of pulse diagnosis on Chinese physician's experience, but also is able to interpret pathological wrist-pulse waveforms more precisely.

Special topic Exercise 13.1 *Palpating Water Flow Through a Tube*

Time suggested: 2–3 minutes

Connect a plastic or rubber tube to a bath or kitchen tap and conduct the experiment as described by Austin.

● Can you sense differences depending upon the surface the tube rests on and materials between your finger and the tube?

Special topic Exercise 13.2 *Pulse Palpation on Self and Others*

Time suggested: 3–5 minutes

Learn to assess your own pulses and those of patients, friends or volunteers (Special topic Figs 13.1 and 13.2). Oshawa (1973) states that:

The extreme end of the finger, the pulp, which is the most sensitive part, should be used to evaluate the pulses.

The last phalanges should be perpendicular to the plane of the wrist. The nails must be cut short.

The superficial yin pulse corresponds to the hollow organs; the deep yang pulse corresponds to the full yang organs.

You judge the superficial pulse by feeling the position lightly and then gradually increasing the pressure of the finger. To determine the deep pulse, one compresses the artery completely at the beginning and then releases it little by little.

The deep pulse corresponds to the blood pressure, to the fundamental composition of blood; the superficial pulse to the variable blood pressure.

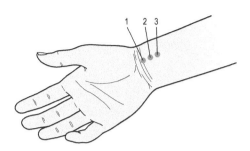

Figure ST 13.1
Location of pulses (right hand only illustrated) for assessment in Traditional Chinese Medicine.

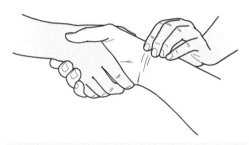

Figure ST 13.2
Taking the pulse in Traditional Chinese Medicine. One finger at a time would apply suitable degrees of pressure to make an assessment, superficially or at depth.

Method

- Sit in a relaxed manner and with your right hand feel the (TCM) pulses of the left wrist.

- Resting the back of your, or your patient's, left hand on the palm of your right hand, curl your fingers so that they rest on the radial artery.

- Place the middle finger at the level of the styloid prominence, just below the wrist crease. Your forefinger will then rest naturally on the crease, near the thenar eminence, and the ring finger will fall naturally onto the third pulse position.

- Position 1 is where your index finger rests, position 2 is where the middle finger rests, and position 3 is where the ring finger rests.

- Adopt the palpation position as described, right hand palpating the left radial pulse.

Left wrist: TCM interpretations

- Position 1 light pressure (superficial) is said to relate to the Small Intestine meridian and deep pressure detects the Heart meridian status.

- Position 2 light pressure (superficial) relates to Gall Bladder and deep pressure detects Liver meridian status.

- Position 3 light pressure (superficial) relates to Bladder meridian and deep detects the Kidney meridian.

Right wrist: TCM interpretations

- Position 1 light pressure (superficial) is for Large Intestine and deep is for Lungs.

- Position 2 light pressure (superficial) is for Stomach and deep is for Spleen.

- Position 3 light pressure (superficial) is Triple Heater and deep is Circulation.

Notes

It is suggested in relation to these exercises, that you revisit Chapter 3, particularly Exercise 3.15

Notes

Oshawa states that the allocation of organs to pulses on the right and left hand, as described above, relates to men only. The pulse allocations are said by him to be reversed in women. This sort of controversial statement helps to explain why so many Western-trained therapists find difficulty in accepting the conclusions drawn from TCM pulse diagnosis.

A simpler view

Stiefvater (1956) gives the following simplified breakdown of what pulse readings may indicate:

- Small, thin, and fine indicates insufficiency.

- Full and hard indicates hypertension and hyperfunction.

- Soft and strong indicates inflammation.

- Small, hard and pointed indicates spasticity, contracture, and the associated organ will usually be painful.

- Overflowing and large indicates excess, usually with inflammation and pain.

- Very weak, scarcely perceptible indicates energy depletion.

Giving a numerical value to the palpated pulse

As you palpate, try to gain a sense of normal (score of 4), excess (score of 5–8) or deficiency (score of 0–3).

Lawson-Wood (1965) states that a score of 0 is applicable to someone who is "almost dead" and a score of 8 represents a patient "*in extremis.*"

When feeling the pulses the practitioner "listens" to them much as one listens to an orchestra – each pulse representing one of the instrumentalists. Taken together the "melody" should be a happy and harmonious one. If the melody is not joyous and harmonious at least one of the players is out of tune. You need to locate which is the discordant player. You must be relaxed and receptive and when you palpate each level quite deliberately say to yourself, "I am now listening to the pulse of (name of meridian) to hear and understand what it has to say to me."

The exercises in this segment should help you to sense the difference in what you feel in the various indicated pulse positions. You are not meant to make a diagnosis on this basis or to necessarily accept the interpretations of TCM offered above, merely to gain an awareness of what is being suggested by TCM.

References

Austin M (1974) Acupuncture therapy. London: Turnstone Books.

Lawson-Wood D (1965) Five elements of acupuncture and Chinese massage. Rustington, Sussex: Health Science Press.

Oshawa G (1973) Acupuncture and the philosophy of the Far East. Boston, MA: Tao Publications.

Ryan M and Shattuck A (1994) Treating AIDS with Chinese medicine. Berkeley, CA: Pacific View Press.

Shu JJ and Sun Y (2007) Developing classification indices for Chinese pulse diagnosis. Complementary Therapies in Medicine 15 (3): 190–198.

Stiefvater A (1956) Akupunktur als Neuraltherapie. Heidelberg: Hang.

Subtle palpation

Leon Chaitow

It is suggested that both Special topic 12 (Synesthesia) and Chapter 13 (Understanding and using intuitive faculties) should be read with care, before this chapter and its exercises are approached.

There are probably few areas of palpation that can be labelled "subtle" with more accuracy than that involving cranial palpation, and the start of this chapter will incorporate palpation exercises relating to that topic. Irrespective of the validity of the explanations of the different models associated with cranial, and craniosacral therapy (biomechanical, biodynamic, etc.), there is no doubt that palpable rhythms can commonly be sensed when the hands are appropriately molded to cranial structures.

What these subtle fluctuating pulsations and rhythms represent is another matter – although it should be acknowledged that the perceived sensations may possibly be self-generated, rather than deriving from what is being palpated.

It is also important to acknowledge that we can often *describe* what we feel, even when we cannot *explain* what it is that we are palpating. That lack of explanation may represent a barrier for some individuals exploring the potential usefulness of palpating the rhythmic sensations associated with cranial methodology.

In Chapter 13 the phenomenon of intuition was discussed, and it is suggested that as you work your way through the exercises in this chapter, involving subtle palpation, you should allow the non-intellectual, non-cognitive aspects of your mind to operate, free from the shackles of critical judgement. The advice is to "trust what you feel" and to "suspend disbelief." In other words, allow yourself to be intuitive.

This does not mean that you should necessarily accept the theories and concepts that surround some of these subtle palpation approaches, only that you are open to what "might" be being sensed.

Questions we need to ask ourselves as we explore cranial concepts include:

- What might we be feeling during cranial palpation?

There are numerous suggestions, but one that seems most plausible relates to fluid dynamics – relating to the recent identification of a cranial lymphatic ("glymphatic") system (Iliff et al. 2013).

Cerebrospinal fluid and glymphatic motion: possible explanation for cranial sensations?

Meert (2012) has explained that:

> The CSF shows three flow patterns: a ventricular flow, a subarachnoidal flow and a transmural flow. The transmural flow represents the transport of CSF along paravascular spaces, whereby CSF enters the brain parenchyma and exchanges with the interstitial fluid of the brain, facilitating an efficient removal of waste and solutes (Iliff et al. 2012–2013). This transmural pathway is also termed the "glymphatic system", as it is formed by a combination of the glia cells of the brain and the cervical lymphatic system. (Johanson et al. 2008)

Palpating inherent motion

In seeking methods for evaluation of subtle movement in the body we can once again turn to Viola Frymann (1963), as she describes what we should expect when we begin to palpate tissues for anything other than their mechanical status (see Chapter 1):

> If the hand is laid on a healthy muscle mass, of a resting limb, it is often possible, in the space of a few seconds, to "tune in" to the inherent motion within. A state of rapport, of fluid continuity, between the examiner and the examined may be established, leading to a whole new realm of palpatory exploration of fluid motion within the body – possibly including intra and extra-cellular fluid, lymph, cerebrospinal fluid – in a constant state of rhythmic, fluctuant motion.

Frymann maintains that the vitality of tissue can be judged by the *strength* of such motions, with a wide variety of grades of tissue vitality being apparent. The example is given of the difference in the "feel" noted when a previously paralysed limb and a presently paralysed limb are palpated. In the first a mere "murmur" of motion will be felt, whereas in the latter there will be no detectable rhythmic motion at all.

These thoughts are expanded on in the work of Fritz Smith (1986) and his methods, known as Zero Balancing, which are described later in this chapter.

However, nowhere is subtle palpation more controversial or difficult to explain, than in palpation of cranial rhythms.

Nelson et al. (2006) acknowledge that cranial palpation is often criticized as inaccurate, when the so-called cranial rhythmic impulse (CRI) is assessed:

> *The sensitivity of palpation necessary to perform cranial diagnosis and manipulation, and the failure of its practitioners to demonstrate interrater reliability (Hartman & Norton 2002), has led many to question its validity. Yet, the topic is taught in all colleges of osteopathic medicine, and the American Osteopathic Association's textbook, "Foundations for Osteopathic Medicine", devotes an entire chapter to it.*

So what is being palpated?

Nelson et al. explain:

> *Many low-frequency oscillations in the 6 to 9 cpm (0.1–0.15 Hz) range are found in the human body, such as blood pressure, blood flow velocity (TH), heart rate (R-to-R interval) variability, sympathetic tone in muscle, and intracranial fluid oscillations. These phenomena can be directly or indirectly linked to oscillations in the autonomic nervous system, particularly the sympathetic nervous system.*
>
> *The cranial rhythmic impulse (CRI), with reported rates ranging from 4 to 14 cpm (0.06–0.23 Hz), shares the spectral frequency band with these physiologic oscillations. The CRI has been shown to correspond to the low-frequency TH in blood flow velocity (Nelson et al 2001). In addition, it has been demonstrated that manual cranial techniques affect TH (Sergueef et al 2002), and similar low-frequency oscillations in intracranial fluid (Moskalenko & Kravchenko 2004). It is naive, however, to therefore draw the conclusion*

that these measurable phenomena are expressions of the primary respiratory mechanism or even the CRI. Rather, these phenomena offer points of access through which researchers may study the elusive aspects of cranial osteopathy.

These words, and those of Meert above, should help to establish what *might* be being palpated. They do not, however, do more than that – and the objective of the exercises below are to take us to the point where we feel something subtle, the explanations for which remain to be explored elsewhere.

Palpation hint

It is suggested that in all early exercises in which cranial motion or craniosacral rhythms are being assessed, you should think in terms of a slight "surging" sensation, sometimes described as feeling "as though the tide is coming in" or a feeling of "fullness" under the palpating hand, rather than expecting to feel movement of a grosser nature. After a few seconds this "surge" will be felt to recede; the tide goes out again. This is a subtle sensation but once you have tuned into it, it is unmistakable and very real indeed.

Exercise 14.1 Cranial Rhythmic Impulse (CRI) Palpation

Time suggested not less than 10 minutes

The rate of the "normal" cranial rhythm remains a matter for debate, and it is suggested that you try to perform this exercise with no preconceptions as to what you might sense or feel.

You need to be relaxed, focused and centered.

The amount of contact pressure required to accomplish CRI palpation is around 5 grams.

CRI is said to best be felt at the parietotemporal squama, using what is known as the vault hold (Fig. 14.1). This is achieved with the palms centered on the posterior surface of the parietal bones. The fingers are usually placed so that:

- the small finger rests on the occipital bone
- the ring and middle finger are resting one behind and one in front of the ear
- the index finger is on the great wings of the sphenoid

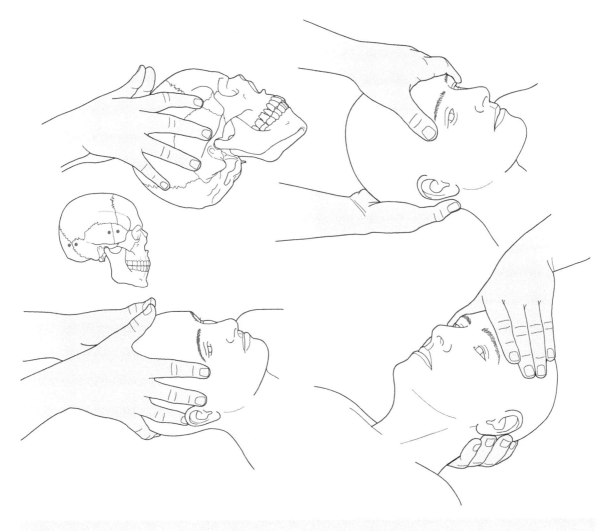

Figure 14.1
Vault hold hand positions and finger placements, for cranial palpation.

- thumbs are crossed and supporting each other, but not in contact with the head.

It is important that your forearms are supported on the table, your feet flat on the floor, eyes closed, with all tension in the shoulders, arms, and hands eliminated.

- Spend the first 2–3 minutes noting the various pulsations and subtle motions under your hands, both cardiovascular and respiratory and possibly others.

- After several minutes bring the focus of your attention to the motions of the head in relation to respiration only.

- Have your patient/partner breathe normally as well as, at times, with increased emphasis on inhalation and/or exhalation.

- Compare what you feel as the breathing pattern alters.

Exercise 14.1 *continued*

- Have the person hold the breath for 10–15 seconds and again see whether you notice any difference in the motions under your hands.

- Then for a minute or two screen out respiratory motion and try to pick up subtle cardiovascular pulsations.

- Now screen out and temporarily ignore both cardiovascular and respiratory motions and see what else you can feel in the background.

Imagine that your hands are totally molded to the head, with only a few grams of pressure, and with this whole hand contact shift your focus to the proprioceptors in your wrists and lower arms. Sense what these, rather than the neural receptors in your hands, are feeling.

Magnify in this way the very small amount of actual cranial motion available for palpation and you might gradually begin to feel as though quite a considerable degree of motion is taking place, as though the entire head were expanding and contracting laterally to a very slow rhythm, unrelated to cardiovascular or respiratory function, anything from 4 to 10 times per minute (or more?).

A faint, wave-like "pushing" might be noted.

At this stage trust what you feel uncritically.

- Can you sense a rhythm?

- Can you describe what you feel in words?

- Is there a periodic "prickling" or pressure sensation in the palms of the hand?

- Does it feel like a "tide" coming in and then receding?

- What words would you use to describe what you feel?

Once you are sensing a rhythmic impulse start to time it by counting silently to yourself as each impulse begins ("one hundred," "two hundred," etc. counts roughly a second at a time).

Remember what the count was as the sensation appeared and as it receded and later, after the exercise, count at the same rate and check the number of seconds it takes from the start of one cranial impulse to the start of the next. Work out the rate per minute.

See also what happens when your patient/partner holds his/her breath as you continue to assess the CRI.

- Does it change?

As time goes by and you palpate more heads, become aware of not just the rate of any rhythmic pulsation you may sense but also the amplitude of these pulsations.

Does the impulse feel sluggish and labored or energetic and brisk or something else?

And are the feelings symmetrical or is there a difference felt by one hand or the other?

Record all your findings in a journal or onto tape.

Variation: It is possible to palpate the CRI on your own head if you are seated, elbows on a table and hands resting on the head, fingers interlaced, or with a palm on each asterion.

The feeling you are seeking, in your own or anyone else's head, is of a "fullness" in your palms, a warmth, a wave-like pushing, a sensation rather than an actual osseous movement.

The craniosacral connection

The physical connection between the occiput and the sacrum involves the dural membrane, which is itself continuous with the meningeal membranes. Therefore, *if* the occiput moves (albeit minutely) anteriorly, as the flexion phase of the cranial cycle commences, a synchronous movement should occur at the sacral base (Fig. 14.2), which would move posteriorly during this phase (taking the sacral apex and coccyx anteriorly). Remarkable video evidence of this synchrony of motion has been made as a result of the clinical and research work of Dr Marc Pick (2001).

What should we be trying to learn from our palpation of these rhythms and cycles? Upledger (1987) summarizes:

> From the diagnostic, prognostic and therapeutic points of view, we are interested in a qualitative estimate of the strength of the inherent energy which is driving the physiological motion, the symmetry of the body motion response (both of the craniosacral system and of the extrinsic body connective tissues), and in the range and quality of each cyclical motion. Is it fighting against a resistance barrier?

Not only is there useful information available when palpating the cranial and sacral components of this complex but it is possible to feel the cycle in any tissues of the body, even in patients who are in a vegetative state.

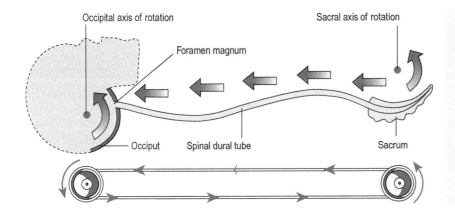

Figure 14.2
Schematic representation of synchrony of motion between the sacrum and the occiput.

Exercise 14.2 *Palpation of Synchrony Between Occiput and Sacrum*

Time suggested **approximately 5 minutes for each of Exercises 3.12, 3.13, 3.14, which should be repeated, plus 5–8 minutes for Exercise 14.2**

Go back to Chapter 3 and repeat Exercises 3.12, 3.13, 3.14, which focused your attention on inherent motion of tissues. Then continue with the following exercise.

Your partner lies on her side, pillow under the head in order to avoid any side bending of the neck. You are seated behind and place one hand on the occiput (fingers going over the crown) and the other on the sacrum, fingers towards the coccyx.

Take some minutes to "tune in to" the motions of the occiput and the sacrum.

Are they synchronous?

When you have satisfied yourself (5 minutes should be ample), have the model remove the pillow so that the neck is side bent (Fig. 14.3).

Repalpate and compare the results.

- Can you feel the synchronous motions under your hands?

- What changes occur when the neck is not supported on the cushion?

Exercise 14.3 *Palpating Cranial Motion from the Legs*

Time suggested **3–5 minutes**

Have your palpation partner lie supine.

You stand at the foot of the table, cradling one foot (heel) in each hand.

Close your eyes and feel for external rotation of the leg during the flexion phase of the craniosacral cycle and internal rotation as it returns to neutral, during the extension phase (Fig. 14.4).

- Does holding the breath change this?

Once you have become keenly aware of this motion, compare the ease of motion in the intrinsic rotation of the two legs.

- Does there seem to be an easier feel to the external or the internal rotation, symmetrically or in one leg or the other?

Exercise 14.4 *Sphenoidal Decompression "Layer" Palpation*

Time suggested **5–7 minutes**

In this palpation you should attempt to evaluate sensations which partly involve mechanical/structural cranial features, as well as more subtle sensations.

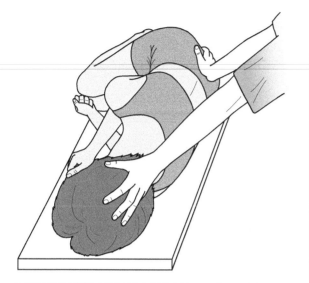

Figure 14.3
Palpation for the synchrony of motion between the sacrum and the occiput.

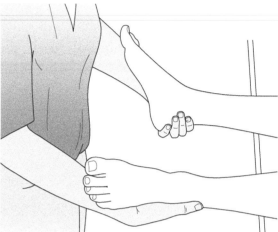

Figure 14.4
Palpating craniosacral rhythmic motion via the feet.

The patient's head is cradled in your hands so that the fingers enfold the occiput and the thumbs rest lightly on the great wings of the sphenoid.

First take out all the skin slack under your thumbs, so that you have a firm contact over the wings themselves, *not on the supraorbital ridges or the orbital portions of the zygomae*. Milne (1995) suggests fifth of an ounce contact pressure, which is approximately 5.5 grams, which is much the same as recommended by Upledger and Vredevoogd (1983).

By lightly drawing your thumbs toward your hands, the sphenoid is "crowded toward the occiput." This crowding is held for several seconds, after which the thumbs should alter their direction of effort, as they are lightly drawn directly toward the ceiling, so (theoretically) decompressing the sphenobasilar junction and applying traction to the tentorium cerebelli (one of the reciprocal tension membranes within the skull) as the weight of the cranium drags onto your palms and fingers.

Milne (1995) suggests that it is possible to distinguish six levels of tissue separation, from first contact to final completion, during this exquisite palpation exercise:

1. skin, scalp and fascia

2. slow release of the occipitofrontalis and temporalis muscles (mainly)

3. sutural separation ("akin to prising apart a magnet from a piece of metal")

4. dural release (like "elastic bands reluctantly giving way")

5. freeing of the cerebrospinal fluid circulation ("the whole head suddenly feels oceanic, tidal, expansive. This is the domain of optimized cerebrospinal fluid")

6. finally energetic release ("a tactile sensation of chemical electrical fire unrolling and spreading outwards in waves under your fingers").

In this poetic language we can sense the nature of the debate between those who wish to understand what is happening in orthopedic terms, and those who embrace "fluid/electric" and energetic concepts.

Creating a still point

Upledger's writings are a rich source of information for anyone who wishes to add craniosacral work to their repetoire. Instruction in workshop or seminar settings is, however, essential before this is applied therapeutically.

It is both possible and desirable during palpatory training for the student to learn to briefly interrupt the cranial cycles, a process known as inducing a "still" point. This can be done from many places in the body, for example from the feet, as in Exercise 14.3, or from the sacrum or occiput.

What is required is that the palpating hands follow the palpated part as it goes to the limit of the flexion or extension phase and to then "lock" (restrain) the part(s) at this limit of motion, not by applying pressure but by means of restraining the tendency to go into the next phase of the cycle, the return to neutral.

This attempt to halt normal motion is repeated after subsequent cycles, until the rhythm stops completely, for some seconds or even minutes. This is the "still" point (see Exercise 14.5).

After a while, the palpating (restraining) hand(s) will begin to sense the movement trying to start again. The normal motion is then allowed and a general improvement is usually noted in the amplitude and symmetry of the motion. Therapeutically this has the effect of enhancing fluid motion, restoring flexibility and reducing congestion.

Exercise 14.5 *Creating a Still Point*

Time suggested **10–12 minutes**

To start the exercise in establishing a "still" point, go back to Exercise 14.3.

When you have established that you can clearly sense a rhythm of external and internal rotation of the legs, during the flexion and extension phases of the craniosacral movement cycle, start to follow the external rotation, while preventing any return to internal rotation of the legs, when this phase is perceived.

Do not forcibly rotate the legs, simply go with the external rotation each time it occurs, taking up additional slack to its limit, and then prevent any return to the neutral position.

After a number of cycles (Upledger says anywhere from five to 20 repetitions), during which slight increases in external rotation will be noted, the impulses should cease.

There may be sensations of tremor, slight shuddering or pulling, noted through your contact hands, possibly arising

from elsewhere in the system (as the cranial impulses try to respond to the restriction), but eventually this too should cease and the "still" point will have been reached.

During this phase the person acting as your model will relax deeply, breathing may alter, and corrections may occur spontaneously within the musculoskeletal system.

CAUTION: The "still" point may easily be initiated via cranial and sacral structures, but practicing of this approach on such structures is not recommended without guidance and training, as it is all too easy to traumatize the craniosacral mechanisms. Working on the same mechanism from the feet is safe.

Discussion regarding Exercises 14.1–14.5

From a palpation point of view this is as far as we can go with our exercises in assessment and manipulation of cranial fluid fluctuations and rhythms. By practicing the exercises as described, you should have become sensitive to the subtle, yet powerful phenomenon that has been described as the primary respiratory mechanism, and which forms a major information source and therapeutic tool in cranial treatment.

Just how this is integrated into your work depends on the degree of interest this avenue excites in you, and how much cranial study/training you undertake. The heightened awareness of subtle rhythms which these palpation exercises should have produced is, however, of value whether or not your work ultimately involves cranial manipulative methods.

Energy

Our focus now moves from fluid/electric fluctuations and cranial rhythms to an area which can best be described as the palpation of energy flow, or energy fields. This is a topic which many find difficult to deal with, either intellectually or practically. The best advice is that you temporarily suspend disbelief and attempt the various exercises outlined below, based on the work of Becker, Smith, Oschman, and Upledger, amongst others, and see what you feel. Whether or not you accept the explanations that these respected researchers and clinicians give for "their" approach to reading and manipulating what they conceive as energy fluctuations in the body is quite another matter.

Chapter 14

If you have patience, you will undoubtedly feel movements and rhythms as you follow the exercises given below – and for the purpose of learning to "feel", you are asked to accept that these represent, in one form or another, "energy." In this chapter we will be looking at very subtle approaches, as used in methods such as "Therapeutic Touch", for we are entering an area which is ill-defined, where function and concepts of energy interactions are mixed and blurred.

That something palpable exists that is called energy by numerous researchers and practitioners is not in question. What remains controversial is its nature and function. Before exploring the work of clinicians, a major researcher into energy phenomena offers a glimpse of what may be happening as we enter this twilight zone of current understanding.

Oschman (2001) has researched this topic deeply and these are some of his observations:

- Over half a century ago Burr (1957, 1972) and his colleagues published evidence that early stages of pathology, including cancer, can be diagnosed as disturbances in the body's electrical field and that re-establishing a normal field will halt the progress of disease.

- In 1962 Baule & McFee (1963) used a pair of 2 million-turn coils on the chest to pick up the magnetic field produced by the electrical activity of the heart muscle.

- Also in 1962 Josephson (1965) developed the concept of quantum tunnelling which found many important applications, including the development of a magnetometer of unprecedented sensitivity, known as the SQUID (Superconducting Quantum Interference Device).

- By 1967 the SQUID was able to record the heart's biomagnetic field clearly (Cohen 1967). Magnetocardiograms produced in this way were clearer than electrocardiograms, because electrical fields are distorted as they pass through the various layers of tissue between the source and the skin surface, however these tissues are transparent to magnetic fields.

- By 1972 the biomagnetic field of the brain could be recorded (magnetoencephalogram). The field of the brain has been found to be hundreds of times weaker than the heart's field (Cohen 1972).

- In the 1970s Bassett and colleagues developed pulsing electromagnetic field therapy (PEMF) that stimulates repair of fracture non-unions. By 1979 the FDA approved this method and by 1995 more than 300,000 non-union fractures, world wide, had been treated this way. The PEMF method has since been modified for treating soft tissues, such as nerves, ligaments, skin, and capillaries (Bassett 1978, MacGinitie 1995).

- Using the SQUID magnetometer, Zimmerman (1990) has been able to demonstrate that a signal can be measured emanating from the hands of practitioners using Therapeutic Touch, as well as non-practitioners, in the range of 7–8Hz.

- Similar studies in Japan showed the hands of martial arts practitioners (QiGong, yoga, etc.) emitting pulsed biomagnetic pulses centered around 8–10 Hz, precisely the range used by biomedical researchers to "jump-start" the healing of soft and hard tissues (Seto et al 1992) [Fig. 14.5].

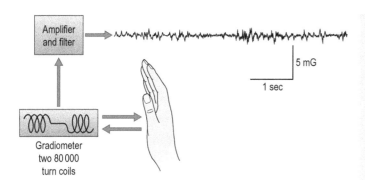

Figure 14.5
Biomagnetic field measurement during "chi emission" from the hand of a female subject in Tokyo. The double-coil magnetometer recorded a pulsating magnetic field that averaged 2 mGauss, peak to peak, with frequency of 8–10 Hz. (After Seto et al. 1992, with permission from Oschman 2001.)

You must make of this information what you will; however, the evidence is that forms of electromagnetic energy emerge from the human hand which, when generated by machines, may have a healing potential. And, as the SQUID evidence shows, large, measureable electromagnetic energy fields exist around the heart (and other organs), and particularly the brain.

Whether we can sense, feel, palpate these energies, and whether we can consciously activate the forces which our hands emit, is a matter for debate. Some of the ideas of different practitioners outlined later in this chapter seem clearly to impinge on this area of *energy medicine*.

Exercise 14.6 *Learning to Palpate Energy*

Time suggested 5–10 minutes

Center yourself and sit comfortably, both feet on the floor, and place your hands so that the palms face each other.

Your elbows should be held away from your trunk, the lower arms unsupported by anything.

Bring the palms as close together as you can without actually allowing them to touch (perhaps as close as under 0.5 cm (just under a quarter of an inch)).

Slowly separate your hands to a gap of around 5 cm (2 inches) and then return them to the first position (0.5 cm gap).

Next take them 10 cm (4 inches) apart and then slowly return them to the first position.

Now go to a 15 cm (6 inches) gap (always very slowly) and come again to the first position (Fig. 14.6).

- Do you feel anything as the hands come close together?
- A build-up of "pressure" in that small space, perhaps?
- Or do you feel any other sensation, such as a tingling or vibration?

Now take your palms 20 cm (8 inches) apart, and this time do not bring them together again immediately but rather do so in 5 cm (2 inch) increments; first to 15 cm (6 inches) apart, then 10 cm (4 inches), 5 cm (2 inches), and finally, the starting position.

At each position stop, sense and "test" what you can feel between your hands (Fig. 14.7).

- Do you sense a "compression" of *something* between your hands?
- A "bouncy" feeling?
- If so, at what distance did this become apparent?

Take a minute or more each time to practice this exercise over and over again.

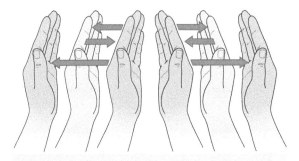

Figure 14.6
Bring hands as close together as you can without the palms touching each other. Then bring hands apart about 5 cm (2 inches). Return hands slowly to original position. Repeat and on each repetition, separate the palms by an additional 5 cm, until they are finally 20 cm (8 inches) apart.

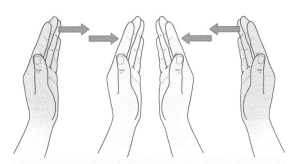

Figure 14.7
When the hands are about 20 cm (8 inches) apart, slowly bring them together. Every 5 cm (2 inches) test the field between your hands for a sense of bounciness or elasticity.

Chapter 14

Exercise 14.6 *continued*

Try to experience what you are feeling, and – hopefully – note the characteristics of the elastic, bouncy, energy field between your hands.

- Do you feel heat, cold, tingling, pulsation, or something else altogether?
- Try to put into words the sensations you feel.

Layers of energy?

Dr Fritz Smith (1986), developer of Zero Balancing (of which more later in this chapter), outlines his model of energy patterns within and around the body. Smith proposes that there is a non-differentiated field that pervades the body and extends some distance beyond the limits of the physical body, and suggests that the energy currents that move within us are organized into:

1. a deep layer that flows through the skeletal system
2. a middle layer that flows through the soft tissues (neurovascular bundles, fascia, muscle cleavages, and so on) as described in Traditional Chinese Medicine
3. a superficial layer that is found just below the skin.

These energy patterns are capable of disruption if the physical medium through which they pass (bone, muscle, fascia, skin) is traumatized or stressed. Smith also suggests that the non-differentiated field may carry "imprints" of imbalances caused by physical, toxic, or emotional insults and traumas, especially if these have not been absorbed by specific tissues or systems.

Chakras

Before examining the work of Smith and of Rollin Becker in relation to such energy patterns, we will also need to become familiar with Upledger's concept of the "energy cyst," and in order to do so we need to look at the chakra system, as described in Ayurvedic medicine.

One of the palpable phenomena of the energy system is said to be the chakras, or energy centers, that are described as being situated at specific sites on the body, and which – it is claimed – can be palpated on the surface, or just off the surface.

It is not necessary to accept the existence of chakras as such in order to palpate them, as they can simply be conceived of as areas where circulating energy is more organized, or dense, or where neurological activity creates increased rhythmic patterns of subtle movement.

The original concept of chakras was Ayurvedic (Indian), as was the word *prana* (energy), used to describe the vital "substance" with which they are associated. The chakras are described as involving a clockwise circulation of energy (prana, or chi, to use the equivalent Chinese word) at seven specific sites, said to range in size from about 3 cm to 15 cm (just over 1 inch to 6 inches) in diameter.

1. The *root chakra* is palpated just above the pubis, Upledger suggests, with one hand under the sacrum and the other resting on the lower abdomen. It is said to relate to sexual function.

2. The *navel chakra* is best palpated similarly, one hand under the lumbar spine, the other just below the navel (no hand pressure, just a touch). This is said to relate to emotions and sensitivity.

3. The *spleen chakra* is best palpated, says Upledger, with one hand over the lumbodorsal junction and the other over the epigastrium, and is said to relate to energy assimilation and immunity.

4. The *heart chakra* requires one hand under the midthoracic spine and the other touching the central sternal area and is said to relate to emotions connected with love as well as "hurt" feelings.

5. The *throat chakra* should be palpated with one hand behind the neck and the other over the center of the throat. It may be felt as two centers of spinning energy and is said to relate to personal communication and relationships.

6. The *brow chakra* may be palpated with a hand under the occiput and three fingers over the glabella. It has an intense energy "feel" relating, it is said, to intuitive perception.

7. The *crown chakra* is palpated at the crown of the head where it may be felt as an energy outflow rather than a spinning energy center, related, it is said, to the pineal gland and to spiritual factors.

Once again: "suspend disbelief"

For the purposes of the following three palpation exercises you should assume that there are indeed "energy dense" areas that can be subtly sensed by the non-touching hand, that can be termed chakras. If you are a skeptic, it is suggested that, for the moment at least, you might suspend disbelief in order to discover whether your palpation skills allow you to feel "something". What that "something" is can be left for another time.

Exercise 14.7 Scanning Someone's Energy Field

Time suggested 10–15 minutes

Having hopefully developed your skills in energy palpation with the earlier exercise, and having centered yourself (a calm, rested state of mind and body), practice the following assessment of someone else's energy field.

Have a "model," or a real patient, who is sitting comfortably.

Place your hands 5–8 cm (2–3 inches) from their skin surface, perhaps starting at the head.

"Test" the area to the left of the head for any sensations similar to those noted when doing Exercise 14.6, and compare this with the right side.

Scan from the top of the head, over the face to the chin, taking about 10 seconds to cover that area.

Be aware of whatever you feel: changes in sensation, temperature, and so on, but do not dwell on questions such as "Did I or did I not feel something?" Simply sense what comes through your hands. Gradually move over the entire front of the trunk, and then move to the back. Speed of movement is slow but steady.

When the complete scan is finished, recheck any areas that seemed unusual (especially those which seemed "hot" or "cold" or "dense"), and recheck your first impressions.

It may be that where there are significant variations in the energy field you will note temperature fluctuations through your hands. Or you may feel pressure changes, tingling, vibration, minute electric shock type sensations, or pulsations instead. All may be significant.

Note and record what you sense.

Exercise 14.8 Chakra Scanning

Time suggested 3–5 minutes per person

Relax and center yourself, then scan the body of a seated partner to see whether you feel any variations or changes in the texture and nature of the energy field in the regions of the chakras, as illustrated in Figure 14.8 (see also Figure 15.1 representing Ford's identical "cross-restriction" areas in the next chapter; Ford 1989).

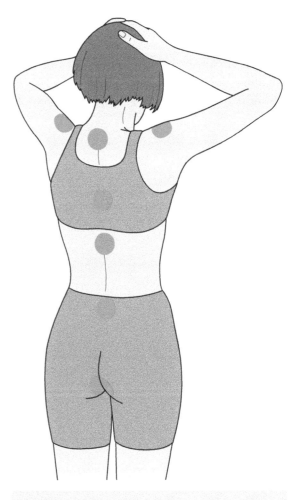

Figure 14.8
Map of "energy (or chakra) fields" of spinal region.

Try to formulate a sense of the difference in *feel* between normal and abnormal, balanced and disturbed energy regions.

When the opportunity arises, compare what you feel/sense in the various chakra positions when assessing/scanning "normal" healthy energetic individuals and those who are unwell or fatigued. See whether particular forms of ill health relate to particular patterns of energy fluctuation.

Note and record your findings.

Exercise 14.9 *Palpating the Tissues Over the Energy Vortex of a Chakra*

Time suggested 4–7 minutes

Notes

Chakra concepts are also discussed later in this chapter in relation to Therapeutic Touch, and also briefly in Chapter 15, which evaluates palpation in relation to emotional and anxiety states.

Your palpation partner should be supine (or seated).

Place one hand beneath (behind) and one above (in front of) the chakra center as described above (see Fig. 14.8), resting your hands on the tissues.

As you palpate the chakras, do you sense any surge, vibration, churning, fluctuation of motion under or between your hands?

This is an exercise to repeat after completing some of the work suggested in the exercises below, if the chakra concept interests you.

Restricted energy flow: the Varma and Upledger models

Both Traditional Chinese Medicine and Ayurvedic medicine suggest that there are channels over the surface of the body, and within it, which are conduits for the flow of energy. If these are blocked or altered, the result is dysfunction or disease.

It may be useful to consider a similarity in the ideas of different clinicians, separated by time and culture, whose concepts were very close, if not identical.

Stanley Lief, the developer of neuromuscular technique (see Chapter 5) was greatly influenced by Dr Dewanchand Varma, an Ayurvedic practitioner working in Paris in the early 1930s, whose method of treatment of energy imbalances utilized an early form of NMT, which he called "pranotherapy."

Varma (1935) discussed the ways in which "electromagnetic currents" derived from the atmosphere (at the chakras) were capable of becoming obstructed "by certain adhesions, in which the muscular fibres harden together so that the nervous currents can no longer pass through them." Varma mentions changes in the skin when such obstructions occur, saying: "If the skin becomes attached to the underlying muscle, the current cannot pass, the part loses its sensibility." This is remarkably close to Lewit's description of hyperalgesic skin zones (see Chapter 4).

Varma's pranotherapy method, a form of manual soft tissue manipulation designed to release these palpable obstructions, was incorporated by Lief into what became NMT (see Chapter 5). He also profoundly influenced Randolph Stone, the developer of Polarity Therapy. For a history of Varma and his work see *Pranotherapy* (Young 2011).

How were obstructions and adhesions dealt with?

Varma suggested a two-stage treatment which, as in NMT, is actually an assessment during which treatment can be imparted. The first part of the assessment/treatment involved the tissues being prepared by rubbing with oil. The actual manipulation of the tissues was performed by first "separating" skin from underlying tissue, followed by a gentle "separation" of the muscle fibers, a process which required: "highly sensitive fingers able to distinguish between thick and thin fibres, and ... highly developed consciousness and sensitivity, attained by hours of patient daily practice on the living body."

While these are descriptions of some interest, they fail to describe adequately what Varma actually did to the tissues.

My late uncle, Boris Chaitow (the co-developer of NMT with his cousin Stanley Lief), has commented on Varma's methods, saying that the most valuable essential which he derived from Varma came as a result of having treatment from him, many times (Chaitow 1983, personal communication).

It was during one of these sessions that the "variable pressure" factor become apparent, something that Chaitow believed to be invaluable in both assessment and treatment. This subtle factor, which allows the palpating hand/digit to "meet the tissues," *not overwhelm them*, is a factor which will be seen again when we come to examine Fritz Smith's research work, later in this chapter.

Upldeger's "energy cyst"

John Upledger (1987) has described how his concept of an "energy cyst" developed as he worked with biophysicists, psychologists, biochemists, neurophysiologists and others at the Michigan State University College of Osteopathic Medicine:

> *The energy cyst is a construct of our imagination, which may have objective reality. We believe that it manifests as an obstruction to the efficient conduction of electricity through the body tissues (primarily fascia), where it resides, acts as an irritant contributing to the development of the facilitated segment [see Chapter 5] and as a localised irritable focus.*

Varma had hypothesized his "obstructions" to energy (prana) flow over 60 years before Upledger's development of the "energy cyst" theory, which is quite remarkably similar. (*Note*: There is no suggestion whatever that Upledger or his fellow workers had, or have, any knowledge of Varma and his work, which quite simply vanished, almost without trace, during World War II, leaving behind Lief's NMT.)

Upledger believed that the "cyst" interrupted the flow of "chi," the Chinese term for energy, and that, by palpation, these obstructions can be readily located. They can result, says Upledger (1987), from trauma, infection, physiological dysfunction (see commentary in Chapter 5 as to how soft tissue changes occur and progress), mental or emotional problems, or through disturbance of the chakras. What do "energy cysts" feel like? "The cyst is hotter, more energetic,

less organised and less functional than surrounding tissues" (Upledger 1987).

How does Upledger pinpoint a cyst?

Upledger uses a method that he terms *interference arcing*, in which he "feels" for waves, or arcs, of energy, relating to such dysfunctional centers. The so-called cysts are said to generate interference waves which can be sensed (usually pulsating at a much faster rate than normal tissue) superimposed on the normal rhythms of tissue. If these waves can be imagined as being like ripples on a pond surface, after a pebble has disturbed the surface, it is possible to visualize that the palpating hands could "zero in" on the center of the wave pattern, to locate the source, the cyst.

It would not matter from which direction, in relation to the cyst, the hands were coming in their palpation, for the center would remain constant, as would the wave pattern. Similar concepts will be noted in Zero Balancing and Therapeutic Touch concepts as described below.

Notes

It may also prove useful to compare the image of an energy cyst, as pictured by Upledger, with that of the "eye" of the disturbance, which Becker describes in his work later in this chapter.

Exercise 14.10 *Palpating for an "Energy Cyst"*

Time suggested 10 minutes

Your palpation partner should be lying prone or supine.

Palpate for "energy cysts/arcs" in an area of soft tissue dysfunction, previously identified using the methods of Lewit, Lief or Nimmo (i.e., use a trigger point or other area of reflex activity as your starting point).

Place your finger(s)/hand(s) in touch with the surface being palpated, without force, waiting for a sense of rhythmic patterns present in the tissues.

Try to determine from which direction waves are being sensed.

Reposition your hands whenever you wish, in order to more clearly localize the focal center of any wave-like patterns you may be picking up.

- Can you sense waves?

- Can you localize the center of an area of disturbance?

A brief introduction to zero balancing

Smith (1986) has explained his concepts and methods, which he named "Zero Balancing," and has clarified this as representing a "guide to energy movement and body structure." He describes the following realization, after 10 years of study of both orthodox and traditional (mainly Oriental) medical methods:

> *During this process I came to recognise a specific area in a person where movement and structure are in juxtaposition, similar to the situation in a sailboat where the wind (movement) and the sail (structure) meet. From the explanation of the interface, in 1973, I formulated the structural acupressure system of Zero Balancing, to evaluate and balance the relationship between energy and structure.*

The sailing boat analogy

Imagine, says Smith, that you are on a sailboat. The wind will move the sailboat, and were you on the downwind (leeward) or full side of a sail, as the wind filled it, your hand touching the canvas would register the power and potency of the wind. Hand or finger pressure against the sail could meet and match that force, and as this varied in direction and strength, so would the degree of pressure on the hand/finger, from moment to moment.

You would in reality be in touch with the invisible energy moving the boat. Other invisible influences, such as those from the ocean itself – the waves, the swell, the currents – would also influence its orientation and motion. And the materials, structure, and design of the vessel (and the sail)

would help to determine how efficiently these energetic influences induced efficient motion and outcomes.

Hopefully it should not be too difficult to make the shift from the sailboat to the human body, and from wind and ocean energy to other forms, in this analogy.

Foundations

Smith has examined the relationship between ancient energy concepts and modern medicine, Eastern esoteric anatomy and Western human anatomy, subjective inner experiences and objective observation. His approach is of considerable value and importance to those practitioners who struggle to align the apparent contradictions faced when comparing the variables in theory and methodology that exist between Western and Eastern medicine.

Smith examines what he terms "the foundations for the energetic bridge" and looks at, among other areas, what he terms "foundation joints." These are, he says, the:

- cranial bones of the skull

- sacroiliac articulations

- intercarpal articulations of the hand

- pubic symphysis

- intertarsal articulations of the foot.

These, Smith maintains, transmit and balance the energetic forces of the body, rather than being merely involved in movement and locomotion. They have in common small ranges of motion and little or no voluntary movement potential. In all cases, movement in these structures occurs in response to forces acting upon them, rather than being initiated by the part itself.

Therefore, if there is an imbalance or altered function in any of these joints, the body is obliged to compensate for the problem, rather than being able to resolve the situation through adaptation. Such compensation can be widespread and will often involve other associated structures, commonly becoming "locked into" the body, limiting its ability to function normally.

Smith believes that these joints have the closest relationship with the subtle (energy) body and any limitation in them, he suggests, can be seen as a direct read-out of the energetic component of the body. He reminds us of the basic law of physics (Hooke's law) that states that the effect of stress on any mechanism will spread until it is absorbed or until the mechanism breaks down.

What Smith is pointing to is the fact that stresses will spread into these "foundation areas" and that, because they have no power of voluntary motion, they will absorb the strains until these become locked, or until there is a restoration of normality by outside forces.

Smith further identifies what he terms "semi-foundation" joints, such as the:

- intervertebral articulations
- rib joints (costovertebral, costochondral, costotransversus)
- clavicular articulations with the first rib and sternum.

He describes a variety of assessment methods capable of identifying reductions in the normal energy flow in tissues associated with distressed foundation and semi-foundation joints, and describes methods he uses to restore normal function, when reduced energy flow is perceived. He makes much of the usefulness in assessment of the ability to identify "end of motion range" in joint play (discussed in Special topic 9, relating to joint play and end-feel).

Smith's energy perspective: a possible model?

Fritz Smith (1986) describes a working energy model of the human body as being composed of three functional units:

- the non-organized background field of energy
- the vertical movement of current conducted through the body which orients us to our environment
- the internal flows of the body which are produced because of the body's unique and individualized presence and which organize us into discrete functioning units.

This last pattern – energy flow within the body – is further divided into three levels:

- the deep current through the bone and skeletal system
- the middle currents through the soft tissues of the body
- the superficial level of vibration beneath the skin surface.

It is Smith's aim to make direct contact with these vibrational fields, and he uses his unique "bridging" methods (pressure, traction, bending, twisting, or a non-moving fulcrum), as described below, to achieve this end.

Via these means, Smith assesses the clarity, density, pliability, and other characteristics of energy, as well as the speed with which it responds (as evidenced by changes in rapid eye movement or breathing pattern, for example) to such contact (or to needles if using acupuncture).

Particular areas of energy dysfunction relate, he believes, to specific forms of mento-emotional discord. Thus sexual problems relate to the sacral area, security/insecurity to the pelvic bowl, power to the lumbar area, anger and frustration to the hips and jaw, compassion to the heart, sadness to the chest, creativity to the throat, and intuition to the brow. He suggests use of these generalizations (his word) to help assess the physical–emotional (or energetic) nature of the patient.

Smith's "essential touch" palpation

Smith's work, therefore, seems to be a bridge between the gross methods of Western physiological methodology and the apparently abstract concepts of "energy" medicine. He explains the way he makes contact with the patient, calling it "essential touch," and saying, quite rightly, that it is common in bodywork to be touched only on the physical level, not to have a significant energetic interchange take place. The connection he wants to achieve transcends physical touching and involves an instinctive, intuitive, yet conscious action on the part of the aware therapist.

What should we feel when this is achieved? Smith describes it as follows:

There are a number of sensations, mostly involving the feeling of movement or aliveness, which let us know we are engaging an energy field. We may perceive a fine vibration in the other person's body, or in the aura, a feeling we are making contact with a low voltage current. This may be described as tingling, buzzing, a chill sensation, "goose bumps", as well as a subtle sensation that some people describe as "vibration". We may also perceive a grosser feeling of movement as though the person's body, or our own, were expanding or contracting, even though we see no physical change.

Note the similarity to Frymann's description, earlier in this chapter.

Smith uses the concept of a fulcrum in order to establish his contact, as do other workers in this field, notably Becker and Lief, although in each case the descriptions of what they mean by the word fulcrum, is slightly different.

A fulcrum is defined, says Smith, as a balance point, a position, element, or agency through, around, or by means of which vital powers are exercised. "The simplest fulcrum is created by the direct pressure of one or more fingers into the body, to form a firm support, around which the body can orient."

The fulcrum needs to be "deep" enough into the body, so that the physical slack of the tissue is taken up; this is the point at which any further pressure meets with resistance in the tissue beneath the fingers. Getting "in touch" with the person's energy field is thus achieved by taking up slack from tissues, so that any additional movement on your part will be translated directly into the person's experience.

Compare the similarity between this description and the request, by Lief and Boris Chaitow (Chapter 5), that digital or hand pressure being applied in use of NMT should be "variable," "meeting and matching" that of the tissues it is meeting.

Notes

Smith insists that there should be frequent breaks (he calls these "disconnects") from the patient when energy exercises (or therapy) are being performed. A loss of sensitivity (which he calls "accommodation") otherwise takes place, as well as a draining of the therapist's vital reserves.

Exercise 14.11 *Smith's Balloon And Rubber Band Palpations*

Time suggested **10 minutes**

- Smith suggests we learn to practice this approach using a water-filled balloon, 25 cm (10 inches) or so in diameter.

- Place this on a table and slip your fingers under it.

- Raise your fingers slowly and be sensitive to the pressure on your fingertips.

- As the fingers are raised, slack is taken out of your own tissues – as well as the slack of the balloon.

- As you increase pressure there will come a moment when you "connect" with the mass of water in the balloon, and, at that moment, the fingertips are acting as a fulcrum for the balloon.

- At any fulcrum – or balance point – there is solid contact with the material.

- In this instance the mass orients around the finger, and any further pressure will affect the energy.

- When you are performing this exercise on the partially water-filled balloon, can you sense the moment when your contact stops removing slack and becomes a fulcrum?

Or:

Other ways of creating a fulcrum, apart from direct pressure with finger or hand, can involve stretching, twisting, bending, or sliding contacts.

- For example, Smith suggests you take a rubber band and stretch it, taking out the slack.

- At that point he likens what you have done to "making contact" when subtly palpating a patient.

- Any further movement, or stretch, will involve the rubber itself.

Exercise 14.12 *Palpation Using Half-Moon Vector*

Time suggested **10 minutes**

- Your palpation partner should lie prone.

- With the experiences of the rubber band and the balloon fresh in your mind, make contact by placing a hand onto soft tissues and lightly pull the hand towards yourself, and when the slack has been removed in that direction, slightly "lift" your hand from the tissues, without actually losing contact.

Smith describes this as a "half-moon" vector, since it combines both lifting and pulling motions which translate into a curved pull, which is the key to what he seeks.

Exercise 14.12 *continued*

Once you have taken out the physical slack and established an interface (fulcrum) with the tissues, any additional movement on your part will be felt by the person being touched, and any movement in the person's body (even very subtle ones) should be perceived by you.

At this point Smith suggests, you are in touch at the energy level.

- Can you feel it?
- Stay with the contact for some time and assess what you feel.
- Record your description of the sensations you are feeling.

Fine-tuning

It is with such a contact (described as a "half-moon vector"), Smith states, that you should feel minute vibrations and currents, and by adding minimal degrees of extra movement you can judge how the tissue (or the patient as a whole) responds.

To *fine-tune* the fulcrum contact he asks himself "How does this feel to the patient?" or "How would this feel if it were done to me?" The response helps Smith decide whether to pull slightly harder, or more gently, to twist more or less.

He also asks the patient how it feels to them, suggesting that with a straight pressure fulcrum a "nice hurt" is what is desirable.

Personal note

Long before I was aware of Smith's work (but possibly after reading Becker's ideas?), I came to use a contact which achieves very similar results to that described by Smith.

I would make a hand contact, mainly involving the palmar surface, with fingers lightly touching but not usually involved. I tried to think of the palm as though I were applying a suction pad to glass, lifting and slightly turning the cupped contact until there is a feel of "suction" between my hand and the patient. Writhing, pulsating, or flickering sensations are commonly noticed almost immediately.

Whether these sensations represent contact with an "energy field" is open to debate. And whether what is being felt is deriving from the tissues being touched, or via intrinsic neurologically mediated influences in the palpating hand itself, is also an open question.

Try this approach yourself, and see what you feel.

Compare it to the "half-moon vector" contact described above (Exercise 14.12).

Is it the same?

Smith suggests the following exercises to help in assessment of bone status.

See "Interpretation" notes below, relating to Smith's explanation of the meaning of what may be felt during these exercises.

Exercise 14.13 *Palpating an Energy Interface in the Forearm*

Time suggested 7–10 minutes

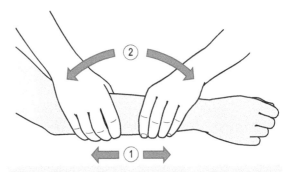

Figure 14.9
Smith's palpation exercise to assess the interface between the physical and the "energetic" structures of the arm.

- Take hold of your palpation partner's forearm, above the wrist and below the elbow.
- Take out the slack by "pulling" your hands apart, until the point is reached where you have created a fulcrum.

After taking up the slack of the physical body, and the soft tissues, by pulling your hands apart (see Special topic 9 notes on end-feel), the resistance of the bone itself will be encountered.

Any additional movement, from this interface position, will be felt by both the person being palpated and yourself.

- Now *gently* put a bend or "bow" into the arm to the point of elastic resistance.

- Try making this "bowing" motion in one direction, just as far as the tissues will allow, and then gently release the tension, before making a bowing motion in the opposite direction (Fig. 14.9).

Try this several times, both with your eyes open and with eyes closed.

Repeat the exercise on the person's other forearm, and compare the findings.

Record your findings.

How much force?

CAUTION: I suggest that when you are trying to introduce twisting, bowing, or any other direction of motion to bony structures or soft tissues you do not try to produce this effect by means of force from your hands alone. Having made the initial contact and allowed time for a melding of the contours of your hands with the tissues, use your arms – rather than the hands – to take out the slack, or to introduce a direction of motion.

It might be helpful to consider the hands to be the means of contact only, with the motive force coming from the shoulders and arms.

Imagine trying to use a spanner to free a tight nut. You would not use the strength of the hands alone, but would introduce the effort through the whole arm.

In a far more subtle manner, the motion or direction of effort in this sort of exercise is best achieved by very fine, whole-arm movements rather than just the hands trying to achieve the desired objective. Anyone who has performed work on the cranium (after suitable instruction) will know that hand contact is introduced, in a similar manner, far more effectively and with less chance of discomfort if leverage is applied by subtle use of arm muscles to guide the hand, rather than letting the hands act alone.

Interpretation of Exercise 14.13

Smith states clearly that this is not an exercise in judging whether things are "good or bad", but is designed to help you to become sensitive to motions and energies not previously registered. He states that if the arm is normal, not injured, it may *bow* more easily in one direction than the other; a bow in one direction may feel obstructed, or it may suggest a twisting distortion, or have the feel of a steel bar, or be more rubbery. Great variations exist, and it is up to each of us to establish what "normal" feels like, to become aware of what is acceptable, and what needs working on.

Smith then suggests a similar exercise involving the long bones of the lower leg. These are probably a better testing ground for practice than the forearm, which has a natural rotational tendency anyway, potentially confusing assessment.

Exercise 14.14 *Palpating an Energy Interface in the Lower Leg*

Time suggested **2–4 minutes**

Place one hand just above the ankle and the other below the knee of one leg.

Take up slack in the soft tissue (pulling the hands apart) and *gently* twist, with your hands going in opposite directions, feeling the bony resistance, as if gently wringing a fragile sweater.

Repeat this in the other direction.

- What do you feel?

Smith says:

> Because the bones are denser in the leg than the forearm, and because the muscles are heavier, it takes a moment longer to perceive the energy currents interacting in the twisting motion. It is an exaggeration to say that energy on this level moves with the speed of molasses, but the principle is true.

Repetition and comparison

As with most exercises in this text, these previous two exercises should be performed on several people, within a short space of time, making comparisons easier. By sharing experiences with others it is possible to validate the subtle perceptions derived from these palpation experiences. If it is possible to palpate limbs which have previously been fractured and which have healed, energy variations may become very instructive. Smith tells us: "Energy fields across a fracture may feel heavy and dense, have low vitality, or be disorganised and chaotic. These qualities relate to the process of reconnecting or bridging the energy fields across the damaged bone."

Can the palpated patterns be altered? Yes, says Smith. He takes a forearm, for example, which has an old fracture, grasping it as in Exercise 14.14. He takes out the slack by stretching apart his hands:

> Holding this, I might add a further stretching force, and then, in addition, a bowing or twisting force. I hold this configuration, being sensitive to the resilience of the bone, for a brief period, possibly 15 to 20 seconds, and then gently release.

On re-evaluation he would expect a lessening of the asymmetry of the original force fields, a greater freedom of energetic movement through the long bone. He says that he allows three such attempts in order to create the greatest degree of "shift" at any one session.

Soft tissue palpation using Smith's methods

Where energy motion in soft tissues is concerned, Smith explains, taking out the slack in pliable tissues is far less easily accomplished, making the reading of *energy currents* and movements in soft tissues more difficult. He suggests that a good way to start is to make two energetic contacts with the fingers, and to "read" the current as if flows from one point to the other.

Exercise 14.15 *Two-Finger Energy Palpation*

Time suggested 3–4 minutes

Make skin contact with one finger pad on the soft tissue below someone's elbow.

Place a finger of the other hand at wrist level of that arm.

Does there seem to be a sense of linkage between these contacts? This may be noted as a pulsation, subtle movement, a "buzzing" or just a sense of "connectedness."

Both the time taken for this connection to happen and the strength and quality of the sensation should be noted and recorded.

Repeat this using different digital palpation sites.

See Smith's thoughts, below, which introduce Traditional Chinese Medicine concepts into the discussion as to what may be happening during the previous exercises.

The link with Traditional Chinese Medicine

Smith debates whether the right hand receives such impulses or sends them, and states his conclusion that the practitioner's thoughts determine the direction of flow.

Upledger (1987) concurs. *Let both* hands be neutral, is his advice, and allow the patient's body to organize itself around your two contact "poles", allowing these to be *organizational fulcrums*, rather than predetermining the direction in which you want flow to take place.

Smith suggests that Traditional Chinese Medicine (TCM) has long used just such energy readings, most obviously during pulse diagnosis (see Special topic 13) , and that once you have convinced yourself that you can indeed feel energy flows, it is time to start understanding the subtle ways in which you can use this information in evaluating the state of the patient. Therapy using these energy flows is only a small step beyond the palpation stage.

Smith states that evaluation of the superficial level of internal energy flow (known as *protective chi* in TCM) is best achieved using your hands just above the body surface, as in "Therapeutic Touch" (see later in this chapter), as well as scanning/palpating the skin texture and temperature (see Chapter 4). Beyond the energy fields that are thought to relate to the superficial soft tissues and bones lies an energy field he terms "background" energy, on which can be "imprinted" past trauma – chemical, emotional, and psychic, as well as physical.

This brings us close to Becker's concepts involving tissue "memory", which we will examine later.

There is also an interesting resemblance between craniosacral "still point" concepts and something Smith describes in energy work.

Exercise 14.16 *Palpation of the Energy Body*

Time suggested 5–7 minutes

Your palpation partner lies supine with feet extended slightly over the end of the table.

You stand at the foot of the table and with each hand grasp just above the ankle (as in Fig. 14.4). Introduce gentle traction until all the soft tissue slack has been removed.

● Sense the connection with the energy field of the patient.

● Does this seem to "elongate" and eventually try to contract? If so, slowly release the tension in your traction, as though it were an elastic band.

● What do you think was happening during this palpation exercise?

Manipulating energy?

Once you have established the fulcrum between yourself and the patient, as in Exercise 14.16, a number of sensations are possible, Smith explains. As you hold traction in Exercise 14.16, he states, you may sense that the patient's energy body is elongating, "stretching," or "flowing" into your hands, a process which at some point will stop.

If, following this, there is not a feeling of contraction, as though the energy body is returning to its previous state, but rather of a stillness, a resting in the "elongated" state, Smith suggests that you gradually release the traction – and rest the patient's legs on the table.

The patient might then remain in a very deep relaxed state for some moments, before returning to normal (he suggests that you observe eye movements, the patient's color and breathing pattern to assess states of consciousness). However, if, for therapeutic reasons, there is a wish to anchor the energy field as it tries to contract again, you can do so by maintaining traction.

This is very similar to the idea of holding the still point (see Exercise 14.5) as the body tries to normalize ("organize" or "unwind") itself around that fulcrum, in craniosacral methodology or osteopathic functional methodology (see Chapter 11).

If, however, you decide to follow the retraction rather than anchoring it, this would be "like letting a stretched rubber band slowly go back to its slack position."

Were you aware of any of these sensations during Exercise 14.16?

Discussion regarding Exercises 14.6–14.16

In this series of palpation exercises you have been trying to evaluate the presence or otherwise of fluctuating movements which seem to be permeate the soft and hard tissues of the body. The explanations regarding the existence of chakras, and of Smith's and Upledger's concepts of palpable energies, are irrelevant to the reality that "something" can usually be palpated.

What "it" is, what "it" means, and how "it" can be used diagnostically, prognostically and/or therapeutically, must remain a matter for you and your particular understanding of the body, your belief system, and approach to health enhancement. The very fact of being able to sense subtle motions is, at this stage, adequate reward for the time and effort you have put into these exercises.

If, on the other hand, you cannot feel what has been described, then repetition and quiet application of the methods outlined thus far in this section is suggested, before moving on to the remaining exercises in this chapter.

Reflection on Smith's sailboat analogy (see earlier in this chapter) may help you break through any sense of resistance to the idea that it really is possible to palpate energy.

Palption without touch

The field of the Therapeutic Touch, "laying on of hands," "bioenergy," "spiritual healing," intercessory prayer, "absent healing," Qigong, Reiki, "chakra balancing," and various other methods of non-touch treatment, have been researched scientifically for many years. Most recently, an investigation of these phenomena by Oschman (2000) has clarified what was until recently largely anecdotal.

To be sure, anecdotal evidence itself can have weight, if there is enough of it, as demonstrated by the data collected, collated, and discussed by Benor (1992). Benor demonstrated that the results (in many clinical studies) of non-touch healing are impressive in their extent and implications, ranging as they do from beneficial changes in patients with anxiety, pain, and chronic headaches; improvements in hemoglobin and hematocrit levels; the healing of dermal wounds; improved blood pressure levels; significantly reduced complications in patients in a coronary care unit; prevention of stroke in hypertensive patients, to improved myopia.

The fact that such methods are also shown to help recovery of damaged and dysfunctional enzymes, single-celled organisms, fungi, bacteria, plants and animals, as well as humans, should remove most of the "it's all in the mind" suggestion as to their reality or efficacy.

Clearly, anyone holding the hands above the surface of the body is not really palpating or manipulating the physical tissues themselves. However, the boundary between what we take to be the physical and something distinctly palpable above the surface requires investigation.

As we can see from Fritz Smith's work (and that of other "energy" workers discussed in this chapter), it helps if we can "visualize" an energy field/body when working in this as yet ill-defined area.

Oschman (2000) has taken our understanding forward, explaining mechanisms that may be operating when non-touch (and a good deal of hands-on) healing is performed, and his books are recommended for further exploration of the evidence.

Therapeutic Touch

Before investigating the concept of tissue memory, Becker's remarkable palpation methods, and Smith's trauma treatment methodology, it is necessary to explore the work of Delores Krieger (1979) and her system, *Therapeutic Touch*.

Therapeutic Touch (TT) is a modern derivative of the laying on of hands, which involves barely touching the patient's body, or the holding of hands away from the body surface, with an intent to help or heal. This method is now taught to many members of the nursing profession worldwide and recent research has validated its therapeutic value.

A number of research studies have validated the usefulness of TT therapeutically in a range of conditions, including fibromyalgia (Denison 2004), anxiety states (Cox & Hayes 1997; Woods & Diamond 2002), chronic pain (Blankfield et al. 2001; Gordon et al. 1998; Lin & Gill 1999; Philcox et al. 2002), and immune dysfunction (Garrard 1995).

Aghabati et al. (2010) demonstrated, in a controlled and randomized study involving 90 patients, that 30 minutes of TT for 5 days "was more effective in decreasing pain and fatigue of cancer patients undergoing chemotherapy than the usual care group."

Winstead-Fry and Good (2009) have summarized key elements of TT methodology as follows (note particularly the "sensations" referred to in item 2 below):

The four phases of Therapeutic Touch

The Therapeutic Touch process is dynamic, not linear. In the beginning, though, it is easier to understand when explained in phases or steps.

1. *Centering*: The therapist begins by Centering her or himself; that is, the therapist brings body, mind, and emotions to a quiet, focused state of consciousness. Characteristics of this state may include: finding an inner sense of equilibrium, a personal reference of physical, emotional, and intellectual stability; quieting the body, mind, and emotions; connecting with one's inner core of wholeness and stillness; feeling integrated; and, being non-judgmental. The therapist continues through the entire TT interaction in a state of "sustained" centeredness.

2. *Assessment*: The second phase or step is also referred to as "scanning". In the Assessment, the hands are used to determine the nature of the dynamic energy field of the patient. The therapist holds her/his hands two to six inches (5 to 15 cms) away from the patient's body, while moving from the head to the feet in a rhythmic, symmetrical manner. The intent is to observe the nature of the flow of energy throughout the patient's field, based upon the assumption that in health the flow is generally open and balanced. The therapist senses carefully for

any differences in this flow. The sensory cues, which are received intuitively, cognitively, and energetically, vary for each practitioner, but may include sensations of tingling, pulsation, or temperature changes.

3. *Intervention/re-balancing*: The third phase or step, Intervention, is also referred to as balancing or re-balancing. The intention of the therapist is to facilitate the symmetrical and rhythmic flow of energy through the patient's field by using the techniques of unruffling/clearing, directing, and modulating energy based on the cues perceived in the assessment, thereby helping reestablish the symmetrical balance, rhythm, and flow in the field. In using unruffling/clearing, the therapist again moves her/his hands through the patient's field with the intention of facilitating the flow, allowing the field to clear itself of congestion or disruption and so return to a more balanced flow. This is thought to help free non-flowing energy and allows access to underlying imbalances.

In choosing to "direct" and "modulate", the therapist consciously evokes the intention to bring energy through her or himself into the field of the patient, to bring balance to areas of imbalance. Energy may be directed through specific areas of the body based on assessment and re-assessment.

While directing energy, the therapist uses modulation to adjust the flow of energy during the TT intervention. As the therapist maintains the state of sustained centering, s/he does not push, force or constrict the flow, but with gentle awareness allows the recipient's field to draw the needed energy. The therapist also recognizes the need to modulate the flow of energy based upon the recipient's sensitivity to the interaction. Sensitive individuals such as the very ill, elderly, very young, or those with psychological disturbances, appear to require an especially light, gentle flow of energy during modulation.

4. *Evaluation or Closure*: In the final phase or step, Evaluation or Closure, the therapist uses professional, informed, and intuitive judgment to determine when the session has come to a close. Re-assessment is an ongoing process. When evaluation reveals the balanced, symmetrical and rhythmical order within the system, as though the biofield has absorbed all it can during the session, the practitioner ends the session. It is helpful if the patient can rest for a short period.

Notes

Exercises described earlier in this chaper, particularly Exercises 14.6–14.9, reflect some of the skills required to apply Therapeutic Touch (actually "no touch" since in TT application there is usually no physical contact).

We will now move back to physical contact as we begin to explore the fascinating topic of *tissue memory*.

Reading the history of trauma

Smith (1986) suggests that we try to distinguish between palpable energy fields that lie beyond the surface of the body, which may reflect present states of health in body and mind (these vibrations not being "imprinted" on the energy field), and those patterns of energy related to forceful trauma or stimulus of a physical, chemical, emotional, or psychic nature. These latter imbalances exist, he says, as freestanding energy waveforms, abnormal currents, vortices, or an excess or deficiency of energy within the field.

These "imprinted" changes are, Smith suggests, likely to develop in response to trauma of a physical nature interacting with emotional trauma, or when a highly aroused or depressed state existed at the time of trauma. This combination of interacting stress factors disrupts the subtle body.

Smith uses the metaphor of "wrinkled clothing" to describe these changes in the subtle energy fields around us; they may disappear on their own or may require help to "iron them out." Compare this with Winstead Fry's mention of "unruffling" the energy field, in her notes on Therapeutic Touch, above.

Assessment of such changes involves two tasks.

1. First, we need to calm the physical body so that we can feel the deeper energy patterns.

2. Second, we have to "take up the slack," a common theme in Smith's work.

We have already noted (Exercise 14.16) that we can achieve this reduction in slack by means of a traction fulcrum, through the legs. Alternatively, for example, we could use a compression fulcrum through the shoulders. Describing the latter Smith says:

> I sit at the head of the table, rest my hands firmly and comfortably over the person's shoulders, and gently press down towards the feet, compressing the body to the point of energetic contact. As I gently push … the body will move beneath my hands until it reaches its compression limit for the amount of pressure I am applying.
>
> In doing this I have taken up the slack.
>
> Having engaged the physical body fully, I add slight pressure, which establishes the connection with the energy fields. When I have made good contact with this I just hold the pressure. If there are abnormal waves in that area, I am able to feel the sensations from the person's body in my hands.

Exercise 14.17 *Palpation of Energy Body via the Shoulders*

Time suggested **5 minutes (reducing to 30 seconds with experience)**

- Sit at the head of the table, with your partner supine, and place your hands over the shoulders. Press toward the feet, taking out slack by compression.

- When this is achieved add just a little more pressure to "engage the energy fields."

- Take your time and see what you (and your partner) feel.

Naturally this requires practice to do well, so practice over and over again.

- Having taken out the slack and applied additional force (slight), allow yourself to be passive when waiting to sense subtle sensations.

Smith states that this particular evaluation takes him anything from 10 to 30 seconds.

This is what you should aim for once you are comfortable with the concepts and your palpatory skills in this area are "literate."

Balancing energy

How does Smith balance any abnormal energy waves he perceives? He could, he says:

- override an abnormal pattern with a stronger, clearer energy field

- introduce a force field which matches the aberrant pattern and by holding it allow the original field to diminish and vanish

- make an "essential connection" with the aberrant pattern and anchor this as the body tries to pull away.

Whichever he chooses, immediate re-evaluation will often show that the aberration is still present. However, reassessment some days, or even weeks, later may show that it has normalized.

This is not dissimilar to many manual treatment results, in which changes at the time of treatment may be apparent but minor, with the majority of change taking place later, as homeostatic mechanisms accomplish their self-regulating tasks.

Example

Smith illustrates his ideas with clinical examples. In one instance he examined a patient who had been in pain since an automobile accident over a year before, in which no significant injury had occurred apart from bruising. Smith was unable to find any cause for the pain until he noted a strong twisting force in the energy field, from the right side of the chest to the left abdomen.

This, he considered, represented the twisting force exerted at the time of the accident.

He used traction on the legs to "engage" this force field (an alternative to the method mentioned above, of pushing down through the shoulders to engage it) and exerted a slightly stronger force field through his body, noting "a sensation of a rebounding effect along the energy imprint itself. By anchoring the new field I allowed the rebound to subside."

A gradual release, initially of the energy body and then the physical body, and a subsequent resting of the legs on the table left the patient with a sense of well-being and quietness.

Two days later, on examination, he was free of pain and there were no twisting currents to be found. A number of zero balancing sessions may be needed if greater degrees of imprinting of forces exist.

Horses and camels

In palpating areas of trauma, Smith (1986) tells us something of variations in patterns we may expect to palpate, depending upon the type of trauma a patient has experienced, specifically detailing ancient Chinese distinctions between "horse kick injury" and "camel kick injury."

1. The first, involving hard *horse hooves*, results in local physical trauma, severe at the onset, with healing after days or weeks.

2. The second, involving softer *camel hooves*, results in mild initial reaction with increasing symptoms as time passes, as the injury "moves deeper." It is as though the "soft" injury fails to stimulate defence mechanisms and therefore disperses through the body/mind/energy fields of the person, with subsequent symptoms emerging.

Focus

Smith makes an important statement when he says: "Energetic connections can be lost if our thoughts drift or we are focused elsewhere. Energy follows thought." Upledger makes very similar pronouncements, as do most workers in the "energy field," and this is something the beginner may find useful. When results don't come, ask yourself where your attention was.

Tissue memory

Upledger (1987) reports evidence showing that decerebrate laboratory rats are able to solve food-oriented maze problems, indicating a "memory" and decision-making facility within the spinal cord. He also reports studies indicating a degree of decision making taking place in the hands of a musician without CNS input. He suggests: "Perhaps these powers develop in these peripheral locations, in response to a person's need to develop certain skills."

Upledger employs techniques such as somatoemotional release in which emotional "scars" are dealt with and he, along with Smith (see above), holds to the concept that palpable changes occur in the energy fields of the body, related to physical, chemical, and emotional trauma.

Is this physiologically possible?

Irvin Korr, a physiologist of international stature, enters this controversial arena, albeit on a neurological rather than an energy level. In an article entitled "Somatic dysfunction, osteopathic manipulative treatment and the nervous system" Korr (1986) states:

> *Spinal reflexes can be conditioned by repetition or prolongation of given stimulus. According to the hypothesis, like the brain, the cord can learn and remember new behaviour patterns. Whether the (memory) once recorded, needs reinforcement by some kind of afferent stimulation is an open question.*

On the influence of somatic changes on the mind he says:

> *Clinical experience indicates that somatic dysfunction (and manipulation) are powerful influences on brain function and on the perceptions and even the personality of the patient. This experience ... raises many fundamental questions and exciting clinical implications.*

So Korr seems to be supporting the ideas of a "memory" independent of the brain as well as of tissue changes (from whatever cause) having a continual impact on "perceptions and personality" factors.

To conclude this survey of opinions, let us look at what Hans Selye, the premier researcher into stress, said on the subject (Selye 1976):

The lasting bodily changes (in structure or chemical composition) which underlie effective adaptation, or the collapse of it, are after-effects of stress; they represent tissue-memories which affect our future somatic behaviour during similar stressful situations. They can be stored.

Speransky (1944), the great Russian researcher, not only hypothesized such a state of affairs, he also proved it and showed how to reverse it. He stated:

Chemical and infectual trauma of nerve structures result in nervous dystrophy, this, in turn, gives the impulses for the development in the tissue of other pathological change, including those of an inflammatory character. Their disposition at the periphery can be predicted by us in advance, and their boundaries remain unchanged often throughout long periods.

Rollin Becker (see below) reports that Speransky changed these imprinted messages by "manually flushing or washing the CNS with the animal's or human's own CSF, and the disabled condition in the peripheral tissues normalised" (Becker 1963).

Becker himself declares:

Memory reactions occur within the CNS system in all traumatic cases ... An area of the body that has been seriously hurt is going to send thousands of sensory messages into the spinal cord segments, and brain areas, that supply that part of the body. If the injury is severe, or long lasting, these messages will be imprinted into the nervous system similar to imprinting a message on a tape recorder.

Thus the tissues and the nervous system "remember" the injury and its pattern of dysfunction long after healing has occurred. It becomes "facilitated" to that pattern, long after the trauma.

Finding the eye of the hurricane, the still point, is the formula which Smith, Upledger, and Becker advocate, if we are to quieten those aberrant patterns of energy which exist after trauma or misuse.

The brilliant research of Bjorn Nordenstrom is outlined later in the chapter. This former Chief of Diagnostic Radiation at the famed Karolinska Institute in Stockholm has shown that there exists a previously unsuspected energy system, which could help to explain the work of researchers such as Smith and Becker. However, before examining his research results we should investigate the dedicated studies, and palpatory techniques, of Rollin Becker (1963, 1964a,b, 1965).

Becker's diagnostic touch

According to osteopathic physician Rollin Becker, when a practitioner is first faced by any patient: "The patient is intelligently guessing as to the diagnosis, the physician is scientifically guessing as to the diagnosis, but the patient's body knows the problem, and is outpicturing it in the tissues." Learning to read what the body has to say is the necessary task of diagnosis and much of this depends upon palpation:

The first step in developing depth of feel and touch is to re-evaluate the patient from the standpoint, just what does the patient's body want to tell you? Having set aside the patient's opinions and your initial diagnosis:

Place your hands and fingers on the patient in the area of his complaint or complaints. Let the feel of the tissues from the inner core of their depths come through to your touch and read, and "listen" to their story. To get this story it is necessary to know something about potency ... and something about the fulcrum.

"Potency" and "fulcrum" are two areas which we must examine closely as we learn of Becker's remarkable palpatory method.

1. **Potency** tells us the degree, the power of strength, of whatever is being discussed. It also, Becker reminds us, speaks to the ability to control or influence something. The diagnostic tool that Becker will teach us to use, as we learn to read and understand potency, is the fulcrum, in which the fingers and hands create a condition in which *potency* becomes apparent.

Becker asks us to acknowledge that:

At the very core of total health there is a potency within the human body manifesting itself in health. At the core of every traumatic or disease condition within the human body is a potency manifesting its interrelationship with the body in trauma and disease. It is up to us to learn to feel this potency.

He likens this concept to the eye of a hurricane, which carries the potency, or power, of the whole storm. In just this way, within each trauma or disease pattern there is an "eye", *"within or without the patient"*, that carries in itself the potency to manifest the condition. This eye is a point of stillness, the existence of which he asks you to accept, as you take the time to develop a sense of touch that can perceive it.

2. The *fulcrum* is a support, or point of support, on which a lever turns when raising or moving something, therefore being a means of exerting pressure or influence.

- Lief used the term "fulcrum" to describe the still resting state of the fingers, as the thumb moved towards them in its searching mode, *meeting and matching tissue tension*, in NMT methodology (see Chapter 5).

- Smith uses the term "fulcrum" to describe a "balance" point, via which the therapist "gets in touch" with the energy body. It is established once the "slack has been taken out" of the tissues and an interface created (something Lief also asked for in NMT palpation).

- Becker suggests that his fulcrum should be understood as a "still-leverage" junction, which may be shifted from place to place, all the while retaining its leverage function.

The would-be palpator achieves this by placing her hand(s) near the site complained of by the patient. A fulcrum is then established using the elbow, forearm, crossed legs or other convenient area as a supporting point (the fulcrum), allowing the contacting fingers/hand(s) to be gently yet firmly molded to the tissues. The fulcrum provides the working point, free to move if needed, yet stable as the palpation proceeds.

Example of Becker's fulcrum

An example is given in which a supine patient with a low back problem is to be examined.

The practitioner sits beside the patient, placing a hand under the sacrum, fingers extended cephalad, and the elbow of that hand supported either on the table or on the practitioner's own knees.

"By leaning comfortably on his/her elbow, the physician establishes a fulcrum from which to read the changes taking place in the back." It is the elbow that is the fulcrum (see Figs 14.10–14.13).

By applying increased pressure at the fulcrum, causing a slight degree of compression at the sacrum, the practitioner will "initiate a kinetic energy that will allow the structure-function of the stress area to begin its pattern to be reflected back to his/her touch" (Becker 1963).

If the other hand were similarly placed under the low back, the fulcrum could be the edge of the table against which the forearm rests (or the elbow could rest on the knee) (Fig. 14.10).

Either or both fulcrums may be employed, to feel "the tug of the tissues deep within".

The practitioner will also become aware, says Becker, of "a quiet point, a still-point, an area of stillness within the stress pattern, that is the point of potency of that particular strain".

Becker makes it clear that he is discussing the kinetics of the energy fields that make up the stress pattern, and not anatomical/physiological units of tissue, when he describes the point of potency.

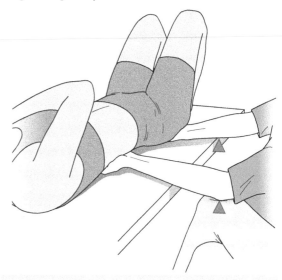

Figure 14.10
Low back palpation. Hands under the sacrum and low back apply no pressure – contact only. Forearm resting on the edge of the table acts as Becker's fulcrum. Increased pressure downwards at the fulcrum enhances the palpator's awareness of tissue status.

Exercise 14.18 *Palpation Using Becker's Fulcrum*

Time suggested **5 minutes**

Palpate a sacrum using Becker's fulcrum, as described above.

Compare this with the sensations noted when using Upledger's sacral assessment, in Exercise 14.2 (Fig. 14.3).

Also compare these results with those you will obtain when you perform Exercise 14.20, later in this chapter.

What are we palpating?

What is the form of energy being assessed here? Becker does not know, and says we do not need to know, any more than we need to know the nature of electricity before being able to use it safely. This thought has been deeply satisfying to those practitioners, aware of the effectiveness of these ideas and methods, who find it difficult intellectually to accept the Upledger/Smith/Krieger (and others) prana/chakra/chi/acupuncture, models of "energy."

Is there any other model?

We have seen that Oschman's perspective (earlier in this chapter) offers explanations that emerge from the world of quantum physics.

It would be appropriate at this point to bring in Nordenstrom's research results, since they may answer the question as to what the form of energy being palpated represents.

Nordenstrom, formerly chair of the Karolinska Nobel Assembly, which selects Nobel prize winners in medicine, is hardly a rebel or maverick. His discoveries are, however, revolutionary. He described his results in his book *Biologically Closed Electric Circuits* (Nordenstrom 1983). It was when using a small spot X-ray technique, in order to define breast and lung tumors, that he first noted an unusual zone around some tumors.

He called this a "corona" and decided to investigate the phenomenon, as there was no histological evidence of change in these tissues. By inserting fine needles into these tissues he demonstrated an electrical flow.

He continued his research on humans and animals, alive and dead, before developing a series of principles.

- The first was that energy conversion in tissues over a biologically closed electric circuit can be defined as a fluctuation in electrical potential in a limited area, resulting from injury, tumor and healing. He found that there was an electrical flow in tissues which followed selected pathways and that large blood vessels function as insulated electricity conducting cables (as described by Oschman earlier in his text on *Energy Medicine*).

- He also demonstrated that biologically closed electric circuits produce magnetic changes around an area that can be measured from a distance.

- Nordenstrom also discovered that biological factors that cause cancer, of a chemical or physical nature, have the ability to polarize tissues, and that therefore "inactivated biologically closed electric circuits" may represent a common factor in carcinogenesis. He was able to show that there exist differences in electrical potential, over an area of a few millimetres, around injured (or malignant) tissues.

- Is this electricity the energy Smith and Becker are feeling?

- Are polarizations and fluctuations what is being palpated in an energy cyst?

What Nordenstrom has demonstrated is that there is another circulation in the body, that of electricity (or energy), and that it changes measurably in response to disease or injury. It can be assessed by machine and possibly, therefore, by palpation.

The following exercise, which Rollin Becker describes (1963, 1964a), is well worth attempting several times until the principles he is teaching become clear.

Exercise 14.19 *Becker's Palpation of Tissue Status: From the Knee*

Time suggested **5–7 minutes for each stage**

Stage 1: First sit facing a patient/model who is seated on the edge of a treatment table.

Chapter 14

Exercise 14.19 *continued*

Place your hands around the knee, fingers interlocked in the popliteal space.

Try to sense as much as you can about the knee, applying a compression force towards the hip to see what you can tell about that area.

You may get some information, but not much.

Stage 2: Now adopt the same contact with the knee but this time rest your own elbows on your knees as you do so.

Apply the same compression towards the hips and assess what you feel, using the fulcrum points.

Becker describes what you might feel this time:

> *Feel how the innate natural forces within the thigh and pelvis want to turn the acetabulum either into an internal rotation or an external rotation position.*
>
> *Note the quality and quantity of that turning. Note that if you lean lightly on your elbow fulcrum points you get a more superficial reading from the tissues under your hands even though your hands and interlaced fingers remain light in their control.*

Note that when you then lean more firmly onto your elbow fulcrum points, you get a deeper and deeper impression from the tissues under examination.

Depth of perception

The depth of perception is dependent on the firmness of the fulcrum contacts, *not on the firmness of the examining finger contacts.*

If there exists a deep strain in the tissues, it is the fulcrum pressure that needs to be increased in order to reach these tissues and their patterns of dysfunction.

This can be done anywhere on the body surface by the simple expedient of creating a contact under the tissues to be examined, establishing a fulcrum point and "tuning in" to the information waiting to be uncovered.

There are two important riders to this, though, says Becker.

- You must know your anatomy and physiology in order to make sense of the information.

- You must divorce yourself from any sense of "doing." Just let the story come through. The fulcrum points are listening posts only.

And yet this is not quite the case. For Becker does suggest the introduction of a slight compression force, or traction, not in order to actively test the tissues, but to *"activate already existing forces within the patient's body".*

The example of the pressure towards the acetabulum, in the previous exercise, is useful as having applied this, it would be the innate tendency of the tissues to externally and internally rotate, which would then be palpated.

Becker is asking for contact with the "interface," which Smith described, and the "still point," which Upledger described, in different terms perhaps, but in essence in much the same manner. What he adds is the concept of being able to gain deeper perception of, and access to, tissue (or energy) states by means of the fulcrum.

Becker calls this diagnostic touch:

> It is a form of palpation that one might call an alert observational type of awareness for the functions and dysfunctions from within the patient, utilizing the motive deep energy, deep within the tissues themselves. It is not the patient voluntarily turning the acetabulum but his tissues within the acetabulum turning it for you to observe.

What should you feel as the body's forces play around the fulcrum?

To the outside observer, watching your work, your hands would apparently be lying quietly on the patient, but the motion, the mobility, the motility you sense from within the patient may be considerable, depending on the problem. There is a deliberate pattern that the tissues go through in demonstrating the strain that is within them. Kinetic energy-wise, they work their way through to a point at which all sense of motion or mobility seems to cease. This is the point of stillness. Even though it is still, it is endowed with biodynamic power.

The "potency within the strain" and "interference waves"

This, then, is the point of potency within the strain pattern, the still point in this functioning unit, which changes as the contact is held, following which a new pattern emerges and is felt. Normality has been encouraged or achieved. Upledger describes the "interference waves" that result from restriction lesions or trauma. These waves superimpose on normal physiological body motions. Once you identify where the interference waves are coming from, the source of the problem is found.

Symmetrical placement (gently) of your hands on the head, thoracic outlet, inferior costal margins, pelvis, thighs, and feet of the patient allows your hands to perceive the arcs, or inherent wave patterns. If these are symmetrical all is well. If the arcs are asymmetrical, then you are asked to visualize the radii of these arcs and to determine where they interact. That will be the location of the lesion (restriction or trauma).

You need to place your hands on as many sites as necessary to pick up the information required to make this assessment. It is as if there were an infinite number of concentric globes around the lesion, each vibrating and describing arcs. Where is the center of all the concentric globes?

The closer you get, the smaller are the arcs. Hands may be placed, one on the anterior, one on the posterior surface of the body; both hands may receive the impression of arcs, which you should evaluate in order to find a point of intersection. This gives the depth of the lesion.

This is Upledger's way of finding "the eye of the hurricane." When you have performed a number of Becker's exercises (below) and you come to Exercise 14.23, compare the methods of Upledger and Becker (as well as Smith). One of these may well suit you better than the others, something you can only discover by trying them all. (See also Ford's work in Chapter 15, and Figs 15.1 and 15.2.)

Becker's exercises

Rollin Becker gives a series of examples in which he palpates different body regions, and describes his contact and fulcrum points. It is suggested that all of these be used in any sequence, on appropriate palpation partners, selecting, if possible, areas where there is or has been dysfunction or pathology, so that variations in what is perceived can be observed and learned from.

Take as much time as possible.

Exercise 14.20 *Pelvic Palpation Using Becker's Fulcrum*

Time suggested **5–7 minutes**

To assess the sacrum and pelvis (Fig. 14.11), have your palpation partner supine, knees flexed. Sit on a stool of appropriate height, on your partner's right side facing the head, and place your right hand under the sacrum, fingertips on spinous processes of the fifth lumbar vertebra.

Your right elbow rests on the table as the fulcrum.

Your left hand and arm bridge the anterior superior spines of the ilium, so that either the left hand on the left ASIS, or the left elbow on the right ASIS, can act as fulcrums if pressure is applied through them.

You may alternate the use of one or the other ASIS as a fulcrum point, in examining the opposite ilium in its functioning relationship with the sacrum.

The pelvis and its relationships with the sacrum, lumbar spine, and hips below can all now be assessed. The positioning as described is said to be particularly useful for assessment of sacral involvement in whiplash injuries.

Compare the results of this exercise with those derived from Exercises 14.2 and 14.18.

Exercise 14.20 *continued*

Exercise 14.21 *Palpating The Lower Thorax Using Becker's Fulcrum*

Time suggested **5–7 minutes**

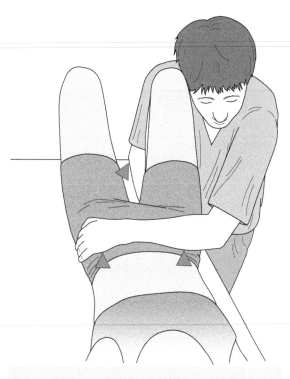

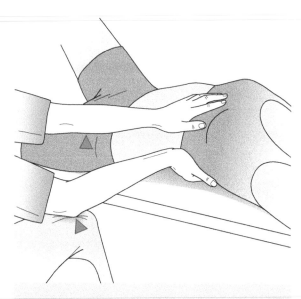

Figure 14.12
Palpation of the ribcage. Becker's fulcrums are on the practitioner's crossed knees and the patient's anterior superior iliac spine (ASIS) (left).

Figure 14.11
Palpation of sacrum and pelvis. Becker's fulcrum points are the right elbow on the table and contacts on the anterior iliac spines with the left hand/arm.

To assess the rib cage, you should sit to the side of the supine patient, one hand lying under the rib cage, with fingertips resting just short of the spinous processes.

The fulcrum point is your elbow resting on your crossed knees.

The other hand rests on the anterior aspects of the same ribs, the fulcrum point being your forearm which rests on the patient's ASIS (Fig. 14.12).

A slight compression at the fulcrum points initiates assessment of motion at the heads of the ribs being examined, allowing strains to be evaluated and possibly treated.

Exercise 14.22 *Cervical Spine Palpation Using Becker's Fulcrum*

Time suggested **5–7 minutes**

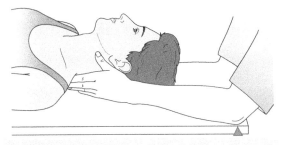

Figure 14.13
Palpation of cervical spine. Becker's fulcrums are forearm and elbow contacts on the table.

Sit at the head of your supine palpation partner, with your hands bilaterally bridging the entire cervical region, from the base of the skull (hypothenar eminence contacts here) to the upper thorax, where the fingertips lie (Fig. 14.13).

The fulcrum points are your forearms, which rest on the table.

General assessment of tissue status may be possible using these contacts.

Individual segments can be localized by finger contact.

Exercise 14.23 *Combined Palpation of Tissue Characteristics*

Time suggested **open-ended depending upon your selection of options, but at least 30 minutes if possible**

Choose an area of dysfunction on your palpation partner and prepare to palpate, incorporating, sequentially – or at the same time – the concepts of Smith and Rollin Becker, as you palpate the intrinsic expressions of function in various areas of your patient/partner.

- Move from the methods of Smith (using a half-moon vector) to those of Becker (using the fulcrum) and back again.

Which gives you the most information? Do the methods confirm each other's findings? Which do you feel more comfortable with?

- Do you now agree that tissue has a memory?
- Are these exercises likely to be of value in a clinical setting?

Discussion regarding exercises in this chapter

Where have we come to by performing the exercises in this chapter? Have we simply acquired a series of experiences which we find hard to use or find relevance for? Or do the subtle skills which these exercises encouraged have a practical value?

Consider the words of one of the leading American osteopathic clinicians and academics, Philip Greenman (1989), who, when discussing myofascial release technique, a subtle yet extremely useful clinical tool, states:

This [myofascial release] is directed towards a biomechanical effect and a neurophysiological effect. Ward has coined a mnemonic: POE(T2). POE stands for point of entry into the musculoskeletal system. Entry may be from the lower extremity, the upper extremity, through the thoracic cage, through the abdomen, or from the cranial cervical junction. The two "Ts" stand for traction and twist. In most of the techniques, traction produces stretch along the long axis of the myofascial elements that are shortened and tightened. The stretch should always be applied in the long axis rather than transversely across myofascial elements. Introduction of a twisting force provides the opportunity to localise the traction, not only at the point of contact with the patient but also at points some distance away.

Greenman suggests that beginners try to develop the ability to sense change in the freedom or restriction of tissues, some distance from the point which is being contacted. Thus, if the ankles are being grasped and traction introduced, an attempt should be made to feel "through the extremities" to the knee, hip, sacroiliac joint, up into the spine itself. Concentration and practice can allow this skill to develop.

In his text Dr Greenman describes exercises which will allow the practitioner to develop the skills necessary to perform myofascial release techniques. These involve palpation of a body area, starting from above the skin, moving to a light contact which attempts "to sense the inherent movement of the patient's tissues under your hand" (an "inherent oscillation") – a concept which we have seen described in other ways, many times, in this chapter. A first step in being able to do this involves the ability to apply pressure or make contact, without movement, followed by being able to palpate the motions that are constantly at work within the tissue, without influencing them. These skills are precisely what the various exercises given in this chapter should allow you to do.

Greenman gives a concluding exercise, palpation of the motion of the sacrum, with the patient first supine and then prone. This you should by now also be able to perform, based on previous exercises. As Greenman says: "When you have been able to identify inherent soft tissue and bony movement you are well on your way to being able to use myofascial release technique."

It is hoped that the methods described above, based on the work of these marvellous researchers into human physiology, will allow greater skill in your diagnostic and therapeutic endeavours.

The next chapter evaluates palpation assessment in relation to emotion.

References

Aghabati N, Mohammadi E and Pour Esmaiel Z (2010) The effect of Therapeutic Touch on pain and fatigue of cancer patients undergoing chemotherapy. Evidence-Based Complementary and Alternative Medicine 7 (3): 375–381.

Bassett C (1978) Pulsing electromagnetic fields, in Buchwald H and Varco R (eds) Metabolic surgery. New York: Grune and Stratton.

Baule G and McFee R (1963) Detection of the magnetic field of the heart. American Heart Journal 66: 95–96.

Becker R (1963) Diagnostic touch (part 1). Newark, OH: Yearbook of the Academy of Applied Osteopathy 63: 32–40.

Becker R (1964a) Diagnostic touch (part 2). Newark, OH: Yearbook of the Academy of Applied Osteopathy 64: 153–160.

Becker R (1964b) Diagnostic touch (part 3). Newark, OH: Yearbook of the Academy of Applied Osteopathy 64: 161–165.

Becker R (1965) Diagnostic touch (part 4). Newark, OH: Yearbook of the Academy of Applied Osteopathy 65 (2): 165–177.

Benor D (1992) Healing research – holistic energy medicine and spirituality, vol 1. Munich: Helix.

Blankfield RP, Sulzmann C, Fradley LG, Tapolyai AA and Zyzanski SJ (2001) Therapeutic touch in the treatment of carpal tunnel syndrome. Journal of the American Board of Family Practice 14: 335–342.

Burr H (1957) Harold Saxton Burr. Yale Journal of Biology and Medicine 30 (3): 161–167.

Burr H (1972) Blueprint for immortality. Saffron Walden: CS Daniel.

Cohen D (1967) Magnetic fields around the torso. Science 156: 652–654.

Cohen D (1972) Magnetoencephalography. Science 175: 664–666.

Cox CL and Hayes JL (1997) Reducing anxiety: The employment of Therapeutic Touch as a nursing intervention. Complementary Therapies in Nursing and Midwifery 3: 163–167.

Denison B (2004) Touch the pain away. New research on Therapeutic Touch and persons with fibromyalgia syndrome. Journal of Holistic Nursing 18: 142–151.

Ford C (1989) Where healing waters meet. New York: Station Hill Press.

Frymann V (1963) Palpation. Yearbook of Selected Osteopathic Papers. Newark, OH: Academy of Applied Osteopathy.

Garrard CT (1995) The effect of Therapeutic Touch on stress reduction and immune function in persons with AIDS. Dissertation Abstracts International 3692B: University Microfilms no 8509162.

Gordon A, Merenstein JH, D'Amico F and Hudgens D (1998) The effects of Therapeutic Touch on patients with osteoarthritis of the knee. Journal of Family Practice 47: 271–277.

Greenman P (1989) Principles of manual medicine. Baltimore: Williams and Wilkins.

Hartman SE and Norton JM (2002) Interexaminer reliability and cranial osteopathy. Scientific Review of Alternative Medicine 6 (1): 23–34.

Josephson B (1965) Supercurrents through barriers. Advances in Physics 14: 419–451.

Iliff JL, Lee H, Yu M, Feng T, Logan J, Nedergaard M and Benveniste H (2013) Brain-wide pathway for waste clearance captured by contrast-enhanced MRI. Journal of Clinical Investigation 123 (3): 1299–1309.

Johanson C, Duncan JA 3rd, Klinge PM, Brinker T, Stopa EG and Silverberg GD (2008) Multiplicity of cerebrospinal fluid functions: New challenges in health and disease. Cerebrospinal Fluid Research 5: 10, DOI:10.1186/1743-8454-5-10.

Korr I (1986) Somatic dysfunction, osteopathic manipulative treatment and the nervous system. Journal of the American Osteopathic Association 76: 9.

Krieger D (1979) The Therapeutic Touch. New York: Prentice Hall.

Lin YS and Gill TA (1999) Effects of Therapeutic Touch in reducing pain and anxiety in an elderly population. Integrated Medicine 1: 155–162.

MacGinitie L (1995) Streaming and piezoelectric potentials in connective tissue, in Blank M (ed) Electromagnetic Fields. Advances in Chemistry Series 250. Washington, DC: American Chemical Society.

Meert GF (2012) Fluid dynamics in fascial tissue, in Schleip R, Findley TW, Chaitow L and Huijing PA, Fascia: The Tensional Network of the Human Body: The Science and Clinical Applications in Manual and Movement Therapy. Edinburgh: Churchill Livingstone, Elsevier, ch 4.5.

Milne H (1995) The heart of listening. Berkeley, CA: North Atlantic Books.

Moskalenko Y and Kravchenko T (2004) Wave phenomena in movements of intracranial liquid media and the primary respiratory mechanism. American Academy of Osteopathy Journal 14: 29–40.

Nelson K, Sergueef N, Lipinski C et al. (2001) The cranial rhythmic impulse related to the Traube-Hering-Mayer oscillation: comparing laser-Doppler flowmetry and palpation. Journal of the American Osteopathic Association 101: 163–173.

Nelson K, Sergueef N and Glonek T (2006) Recording the rate of the cranial rhythmic impulse. Journal of the American Osteopathic Association 106: 337–341.

Nordenstrom B (1983) Biologically closed electric circuits: Clinical, experimental and theoretical evidence for an additional circulatory system. Stockholm: Nordic Medical Publications.

Oschman JL (2000) The electromagnetic environment: Implications for bodywork. Part 2: Biological effects. Journal of Bodywork and Movement Therapies 4 (2): 137–150.

Oschman J (2001) Energy medicine. Edinburgh: Churchill Livingstone.

Philcox P, Rawlins L and Rodgers L (2002) Therapeutic Touch and its effect on phantom limb and stump pain. Journal of the Australian Rehabilitation Nursing Association 5: 17–21.

Pick M (2001) Presentation. "Beyond the neuron." Integrative bodywork – towards unifying principles. Conference, JBMT/University of Westminster, London, October 2001.

Selye H (1976) The stress of life. New York: McGraw-Hill.

Sergueef N, Nelson K and Glonek T (2002) The effect of cranial manipulation upon the Traube Hering Meyer oscillation. Alternative Therapies in Health and Medicine 8: 74–76.

Seto A, Kusaka C and Nakazato S (1992) Detection of extraordinary large biomagnetic field strength from the human hand. Acupuncture and Electro-Therapeutics Research International Journal 17: 75–94.

Smith F (1986) Inner bridges – a guide to energy movement and body structure. New York: Humanics New Age.

Speransky AD (1944) A basis for the theory of medicine. New York: International Publishers.

Upledger J (1987) Craniosacral therapy II: Beyond the dura. Seattle: Eastland Press.

Upledger J and Vredevoogd W (1983) Craniosacral therapy. Seattle: Eastland Press.

Varma D (1935) The human machine and its forces. London: Health for All Publications.

Winstead-Fry P and Good R (2009) Therapeutic Touch, in Chaitow L (ed) Fibromylagia Syndrome 3rd edn. Edinburgh: Churchill Livingstone, Edinburgh.

Woods DL and Diamond M (2002) The effect of Therapeutic Touch on agitated behavior and cortisol in persons with Alzheimer's disease. Biological Research in Nursing 4: 104–114.

Young P (2011) Pranotherapy: The origins of polarity therapy and European neuromuscular technique. USA: Masterworks International.

Zimmerman J (1990) Laying-on-of-hands and Therapeutic Touch: A testable theory. BEMI Currents (Journal of Bio-Electro-Magnetics Institute) 2: 8–17.

Palpation and emotional states

Leon Chaitow

As in Chapter 14, it is suggested that you review Special topic 12 (Synesthesia) and Chapter 13 (Understanding and using intuitive faculties) before you proceed with the exercises in this chapter.

Posture and emotion have long been linked. As far back as the 19th century, Darwin (1899) observed the following in relation to individuals who are depressed: "... the muscles [are] flaccid; the eyelids droop; the head hangs on the contracted chest; the lips, cheeks, and lower jaw all sink downwards from their own weight." In 1937 Sherrington asked: "Can we stress too much that ... any path we trace in the brain leads directly or indirectly to muscle?" And Wilfred Barlow (1959) observed: "There is an intimate relationship between states of anxiety and observable (and therefore palpable) states of muscular tension."

The early user of electromyographic techniques demonstrated a statistical correlation between unconscious hostility and arm tension, as well as leg muscle tension and sexual themes (Malmo and Shagass 1949). Sainsbury (1954) showed that when "*neurotic*" patients complained of feeling tension in the scalp muscles, there was EMG evidence of this.

Wolff (1948), in his famous book *Headache and Other Head Pains*, showed that the majority of patients with headache demonstrated: "Marked contraction in the muscles of the neck ... most commonly due to sustained contractions associated with emotional strain, dissatisfaction, apprehension and anxiety." Even earlier, Jacobson (1930) was able to show that even thinking about activity produces muscular changes: "It is impossible to conceive an activity without causing fine contractions in all those muscles which produce the activity in reality."

Barlow (1959) summed up his views on the emotion/muscle connection thus:

Muscle is not only the vehicle of speech and expressive gesture, but has at least a finger in a number of other emotional pies – for example, breathing regulation, control of excretion, sexual functioning and above all an influence on the body schema through proprioception. Not only are emotional attitudes, say,

of fear, and aggression mirrored immediately in the muscle, but also such moods as depression, excitement and evasion have their characteristic muscular patterns and postures.

More recently, Ford (1989), in his book *Where Healing Waters Meet*, summarized the early, less controversial, work of Wilhelm Reich, who rejected the exclusivity of the concepts that underlying physical conditions created the environment in which psychological dysfunction would occur, or that physical dysfunction was necessarily the result of psychological forces. Rather, he synthesized the two positions, stating that: "Muscular attitudes and character attitudes have the same function ... They can replace one another and be influenced by one another. Basically they cannot be separated."

As Ford puts it:

When [Reich] encountered difficult psychological resistance (character armouring) in a patient, he moved to the corresponding areas of physical tension (muscular armouring) in the body, and used various forms of somatic therapy to correct the underlying physical distortions ... Similarly if he was unable to affect a change in the tension of the patient's body through somatic therapy, he resorted to working with the psychological issues beneath the tension.

Palpation, insofar as it relates to emotional states, therefore requires the ability to observe (patterns of use, posture, attitudes, tics, and habits) and feel for changes in the soft tissues which relate to emotionally charged states, acute or chronic. One of the key elements in this relates to breathing function which is intimately connected with emotion (see Special topic 11).

British osteopath Philip Latey (1980, 1996) has described patterns of distortion that coincide with particular clinical problems. He uses the analogy of "*three fists*" because, he says, the unclenching of a fist correlates with physiological relaxation, while a clenched fist indicates fixity, rigidity, over-contracted muscles, emotional turmoil, withdrawal from communication, and so on:

The lower fist is centred entirely on pelvic function. When I describe the upper fist I include the head, neck, shoulders and arms with the upper chest throat and jaw. The middle fist focuses mainly on the lower chest and upper abdomen.

Current evidence

Is there evidence for these observations, apart from clinical experiences and opinion?

Michalak et al. (2009) have studied associations between depression and gait pattern. They reported that gait characteristics in patients with non-clinical sadness and severe depression include a stronger lateral body sway, vertical movement of the head, and slumped posture when compared to a normal population.

Canales et al. (2010) suggested that, during episodes of depression, individuals with major depressive disorder experience alterations in posture: increased head flexion, thoracic kyphosis, a trend towards left pelvic retroversion, and abduction of the left scapula.

Rosario (2013, 2014, 2016) has analyzed and cataloged links between posture and various emotions, including anger, sadness and depression:

Anger

It was possible to confirm a statistically significant association between postural deviations such as head protrusion, elevation of the shoulders, hyperextended knees, inclination of the shoulders and anger. These results are similar to those of previous studies stating that emotions are related to patterns of contraction of the facial muscles (Ekman et al. 1983) and body posture (Canales et al. 2010). These results demonstrated that there are certain postures adopted by the body in response to the experience of anger. (Rosario et al. 2016)

Sadness

The postural parameter photographed was protraction of the shoulder. The degree of sadness was rated by analog scales representing current and usual sadness. The results indicated that a relationship exists between protraction of the shoulder and usual sadness (p = 0.05). (Rosario et al. 2013)

Selective motor unit involvement

Waersted et al. (1992, 1993) have shown that selective motor unit involvement results from psychogenic influences on muscles. Researchers at the National Institute of Occupational Health in Oslo, Norway, have demonstrated that a small number of motor units, in particular muscles, may display almost constant or repeated activity when influenced psychogenically. The implications of this information are profound, since it suggests that emotional stress can selectively involve postural fibers of muscles, which shorten over time when stressed (Janda 1983). The possible "metabolic crisis" indicated by this research has strong parallels with the evolution of myofascial trigger points as described by Simons et al. (1999).

If emotional states can create specific and predictable musculoskeletal changes, at least aspects of this should be palpable, and sometimes possibly observable.

Postural interpretation

Latey describes the patient who enters the consulting room as showing an "image posture," which is the impression the patient subconsciously wishes you to gain. If instructed to relax as far as possible, the next image we see is that of "slump posture," in which gravity acts on the body, so that it responds according to its unique attributes, tensions and weakness. Here it is common to observe overactive muscle groups coming into operation; hands, feet, jaw and facial muscles may writhe and clench or twitch.

Finally, when the patient lies down and relaxes, we come to the deeper image we wish to examine, the "residual posture." Here we find the tensions the patient cannot release. It is palpable and, says Latey, leaving aside sweat, skin, and circulation, the deepest "layer of the onion" available to examination.

Contraction patterns

What can be seen when someone is looked at from these perspectives varies from person to person, depending on the state of mind, degree of adaptation to life events and activities, as well as the current level of well-being of the individual.

Apparent is a record, or psychophysical pattern, of the patient's responses, actions, transactions, and interactions with his environment, both historically and currently. The patterns of contraction that are found seem to bear a direct relationship with the patient's unconscious (see Waersted's research discussed above), and provide a reliable avenue for discovery and treatment. They are providing sensory input to the patient, and this is of considerable importance.

One of Latey's concepts involves a mechanism that leads to muscular contraction as a means of disguising a sensory barrage resulting from an emotional state. Thus he describes:

- a sensation which might arise from the pit of the stomach being hidden by contraction of the muscles attached to the lower ribs, upper abdomen, and the junction between the chest and lower spine

- genital and anal sensations that might be drowned out by contraction of hip, leg, and low back musculature

- throat sensations that might be concealed, with contraction of the shoulder girdle, neck, arms, and hands.

Emotional contractions

A restrained expression of emotion itself results in suppression of activity and, ultimately, chronic contraction of the muscles that would be used were these emotions expressed, be they rage, fear, anger, joy, frustration, sorrow, or anything else.

Latey points out that all areas of the body producing sensations that arouse emotional excitement may have their blood supply reduced by muscular contraction. Also, sphincters and hollow organs can be held tight until numb. He gives as examples the muscles that surround the genitals and anus, as well as those of the mouth, nose, throat, lungs, stomach, and bowel.

Three fists

As noted above, when assessing these and other patterns of muscular tension in relation to emotional states, Latey divides the body into three regions, which he describes as:

- "lower fist" – (metaphor for a clenched fist) which centers entirely on pelvic function

- "upper fist" – which includes head, neck, shoulders, arms, upper chest, throat, and jaw

- "middle fist" – which focuses mainly on the lower chest and upper abdomen.

Why are Latey's concepts so important? Because he comes close to an explanation of the mechanisms at work in the body–mind problems that are familiar to all who work on the human body with their hands. He avoids more conjectural explanations involving electromagnetic energy, chakras, auras or energy fields or flows (not that such explanations are necessarily any less valid than Latey's, but he provides another way of seeing the problem).

The lower fist

The lower fist describes the muscular function of the pelvis, low back, lower abdomen, hips, legs, and feet, with their mechanical, medical, and psychosomatic significance.

Latey identifies the central component of this region as the pelvic diaphragm, stretching as it does across the pelvic outlet, forming the floor of the abdominal cavity. The perineum allows egress for the bowel, vagina, and urinary tract as well as the blood vessels and nerve supply for the genitalia, each opening being controlled by powerful muscular sphincters which can be compressed by contraction of the muscular sheet.

When our emotions or feelings demand that we need to contract the pelvic outlet, a further group of muscular units comes into play, which increases the pressure on the area from the outside. These are the muscles that adduct the thighs, tilt the pelvis forwards, and rotate the legs inwards, dramatically increasing compressive forces on the perineum, especially if the legs are crossed. The impression this creates is one of "closing in around the genitals" and is observed easily in babies and young children when anxious or in danger of wetting themselves.

You can reproduce these contractions experimentally, as in the following exercise.

Chapter 15

Exercise 15.1 *Sensing Your Own Tensions*

Time suggested **2 minutes**

Stand upright, legs apart a little, and exert maximum pressure and weight through the arches of the feet, trying to flatten them to the floor.

Sustain this effort for at least 2 minutes and sense the changes in your overall posture – feel the details of what is happening in the feet, knees, legs, hips, pelvis, and spine.

Feel the tensions begin to build around the pelvis and upper body parts.

Note where discomfort begins.

Comment

If this sort of contraction is short-lived no damage occurs. If it is prolonged and repetitive, however (weeks rather than days), compensatory, adaptive changes appear, involving those muscles which abduct the legs, rotate them outwards, and pull the pelvis upright (Selye 1956). If this compensatory correction is incomplete the pelvis remains tilted forwards, requiring additional contraction of low back muscles in order to maintain an erect posture.

Buttock muscle tension

Another fairly common pattern involves tension in the muscles of the buttocks, which act to reinforce perineal tension from behind. This tends to compress the anus more than the genitals and produces a different postural picture.

Exercise 15.2 *Self-Evaluation of Postural Effects of Clenched Buttocks*

Time suggested **2–3 minutes**

Demonstrate on yourself the effects of maintaining clenched buttocks for several minutes by standing and squeezing your anus tight, contracting the buttocks really hard, and holding this for 2 or 3 minutes.

Focus on the changes of posture and feelings of tension, strength, and weakness in different parts of your body as time passes.

- What is happening to your low back, your upper back, your hips, knees, and feet?

- What happens to your breathing after a minute or so of this clenching (which directly impacts on the pelvic floor, and therefore the respiratory diaphragm)?

Note the postural and other changes that take place as you stand still for a minute after releasing the clenching action.

Lower fist problems

Problems of a mechanical nature that stem from the lower fist contraction include:

- internally rotated legs and "knock-knees"

- unstable knee joints

- "pigeon-toed" stance, resulting in flattened arches.

Here, then, may lie the onset of symptoms in "knock-kneed, flat-footed children" and here also may reside the answer.

- The main mechanical damage is, however, to the hip joints, due to compression and over-contraction of mutually opposed muscles. The hip is forced into its socket, muscles shorten, and as there is loss of rotation and the ability to separate the legs, backward movement becomes limited.

- Uneven wear commences with obvious long-term end results. If this starts in childhood, damage may include deformity of the ball and socket joint of the hip.

- Low back muscles are also involved, and this may represent the beginning of chronic backache, pelvic dysfunction, coccygeal problems, and disc damage.

- The abdominal muscles are also affected since they are connected to changes in breathing function that result from the inability of the lower diaphragm to relax and allow proper motion to take place.

Medical complications that can result from these muscular changes involve mainly circulatory function, since the circulation to the pelvis is vulnerable to stasis. Hemorrhoids, varicose veins, and urethral constriction all become more likely, as do chances of urethritis and prostatic problems. All forms of gynecological problems are more common and childbirth becomes more difficult.

Exercise 15.3 *Self-Treatment for Chronic "Lower Fist" (Pelvic) Contractions*

Time suggested 3–5 minutes

- Have the person lie face down (or do this on yourself), taking one arm back and down to cup their (your) own perineum.

- Practice feeling at the perineum for the difference between normal motion of the phases of breathing when relaxed and the restricted pattern when the buttocks are clenched.

- By breathing deeply while in this position, with buttocks unclenched, the abdomen is compressed against the floor or table, and perineal motion is forced to occur.

- The person/patient (or you) can learn to increase the excursion by consciously relaxing the muscles of the region.

- This improves further if the tense/shortened pelvic muscles are released by treatment.

- A profound weakness of the legs is often felt as relaxation of these muscles begins, and this may last for hours. As tension goes, so vulnerability increases and reassurance may be required.

- This is only a part of the restoration of normal function, but it is a beginning.

While this is clearly a therapeutic/educational exercise, it has palpation overtones, since normal movements which were previously restricted should improve after inducing relaxation of the perineal area.

The middle fist

When considering this area that he designates the *middle fist*, Latey concentrates his attention on respiratory and diaphragmatic function, and the many emotional inputs that affect this region. He discounts the popular misconception that states that breathing is produced by contraction of the diaphragm and the muscles that raise the rib cage, with exhalation being but a relaxation of these muscles. Instead he asserts:

This is quite untrue. Breathing is produced by an active balance between the muscles mentioned above [the diaphragm and the muscles that raise the rib cage] and the expiratory muscles that draw the rib-cage downwards and pull the ribs together. The even flow of easy breathing should be produced by dynamic interaction of these two sets of muscles.

The muscles that "draw the rib-cage downwards" and so help to produce the active exhalation phase of breathing include the following:

1. *Transversus thoracis*, which lies inside the front of the chest, attaching to the back of the sternum and fanning out inside the rib cage and then continuing to the lower ribs where they separate. This is the inverted "V" below the chest (it is known as transversus abdominis in this region). Latey calls this "probably the most remarkable muscle in the body." It has, he says, direct intrinsic abilities to generate all manner of uniquely powerful sensations, with even light contact sometimes producing reflex contractions of the whole body, or of the abdomen or chest, and feelings of nausea and choking, all types of anxiety, fear, anger, laughter, sadness, weeping, and so on.

The most common sensations described by patients when it is touched include "nausea, weakness, vulnerability and emptiness." He discounts the idea that its sensitivity is related to the "solar plexus," maintaining that its closeness to the internal thoracic artery is probably more significant, since when it is contracted it can exert direct pressure on it.

Latey believes that physiological breathing has as its central event a rhythmical relaxation and contraction of this muscle. Rigidity is often seen in the patient with "middle fist" problems, where "control" dampens the emotions that relate to it.

2. The other main exhalation muscle is *serratus posterior inferior*, which runs from the upper lumbar spine, fanning upwards and outwards over the lower ribs, which it grasps from behind, pulling them down and inwards on exhalation.

These two muscles mirror each other, working together.

Latey comments on the remarkable changes in tone in serratus, relating to speech:

> The tone of this muscle varies with the emotional content of the patient's speech, especially when the emotions are highly labile and thinly veiled near the surface. With the patients lying on their front the whole dorsolumbar region may be seen to ripple in ridge-shaped patterns as they talk. As their words become progressively more "loaded" the patterns become more emphatic. However, it is more usual to find a static overcontracture of this muscle, with the underlying back muscles in a state of fibrous shortening and degeneration, reflecting the fixity of the transversus, and the extent of the emotional blockage.

Middle fist functions

Laughing, weeping, and vomiting are three *"safety valve"* functions of middle fist function that Latey is interested in. These are used by the body to help resolve internal imbalance. Anything stored internally, and which cannot be contained, emerges explosively via this route. In all three functions transversus alternates between full contraction and relaxation.

In laughing and weeping there is a definite rhythm of contraction/relaxation of transversus, whereas in vomiting it remains in total contraction throughout each eliminative wave. Between waves of vomiting the breathing remains in the inspiratory phase, with upper chest panting. Transversus is slack in this phase.

Latey suggests that often it is only muscle fatigue that breaks cycles of laughter/weeping/vomiting, and he reminds us of phrases such as: "I wept/laughed until my sides ached." Nausea and vomiting are often associated with feelings such as: "I swallowed my pride" and "stomaching an insult." He suggests seeking early feelings of hunger, need, fullness, emptiness, overfulness, nausea, rejection, expulsion, and so on when working in this area, if we wish to uncover basic emotional links.

While Latey delves into areas that are clearly within the realm of psychotherapy, the form of bodywork he espouses, which seeks to understand and, where appropriate, to modify the adaptive changes in the soft tissues, can be seen to be potentially important in this field.

Exercise 15.4 *Exploring the "Middle Fist"*
Time suggested **5–10 minutes**

Latey suggests that:

> The feelings of the middle fist disturbance surface most readily with the patient lying on their back. With one hand resting below the sternum (assessing transversus movement) the practitioner's other hand can feel the upper or lower fist movement. Nausea is often felt strongly in this position.

What might you notice in the person as you hold this muscle?

If they are feeling nauseous you might see a sudden pallor, sweat, and protrusion of the chin followed by retching and gagging. A receptacle should be on hand and you should ask "do you want to be sick?" After that you could ask "what was stopping you?" for insights into underlying emotions.

If laughter is going to emerge this may be preceded by a squirming movement, a sideways look of "naughtiness," superficial guilt, shame, or embarrassment. A slight snort, snigger, or grunt can lead to the main explosive laughter release. A comment such as "It's ridiculous, isn't it?" can help.

Before weeping starts the eyes become moist, the mouth quivers, a catch is heard in the voice. There is an expectation of encouragement and of comfort being offered.

These emotions are interchangeable, and one may lead into another, since these safety valves may be releasing feelings from quite different sources at the same time.

If panic starts it is characterized by a fluttering of the transversus and is unmistakable. This can build into a shaking of the whole body, with breathing and chest movements becoming jerky and tremulous. Limbs twitch and eyes open wide. This sort of emotional explosion can have roots in very early experiences.

Latey pays great attention to the transversus muscle during this exploration of the middle fist. He says: "A feeling of tightness behind or below the breastbone marks the beginning of a cycle of emotion linked to this muscle (recrimination, pity, disgust, etc.). Is heartache an overtightness of the transversus muscle!"

As outlined above, he encourages movement of the middle fist components (via breathing and bodywork) and while doing so registers feelings of unease in the patient:

> Panic starts as a very definite fluttering of the transversus muscle itself and is quite unmistakable. Given full play it rapidly builds into a shaking of the whole body. The chest movements and breathing are jerky and tremulous: the limbs are twitchy: the eyes wide and staring in alarm. I have to look elsewhere for the meaning of panic: the chains of investigation are tortuous and difficult – invariably when fully exposed they lead back to earliest feelings.

If any such emotions manifest, use the strategies described by Latey and evaluate their value, as well as recording for future use the knowledge gained from this exploration of emotion and the body.

Exercise 15.4 is an exercise in which you are palpating tissues that are intimately connected to basic emotions, while at the same time you are trying to become aware of subtle changes (breathing pattern, facial expression, voice pitch, muscular tone, etc.), all or any of which may be precursors to an emotional release.

See the notes immediately below for further exploration of this theme.

Middle fist problems

The clinical problems associated with middle fist dysfunction relate to resulting distortions of blood vessels, internal organs, autonomic nervous system involvement, and alteration in neuroendocrine balance. Diarrhea, constipation, or colitis may be involved but more direct results relate to lung and stomach problems. Thus bronchial asthma is an obvious example of middle fist fixation.

There is a typical associated posture, with the shoulder girdle raised and expanded as if any letting go would precipitate a crisis. Compensatory changes usually include very taut deep neck and shoulder muscles. In treating such a problem Latey starts by encouraging function of the middle fist itself, then extending into the neck and shoulder muscles, encouraging them to relax and drop. He then goes back to the middle fist.

Dramatic expressions of alarm, unease, and panic may be seen. The patient, on discussing what they feel, might report sensations of being smothered, drowned, choked, engulfed, crushed, obliterated. These may relate to early life panic sensations and may go to the person's very core.

When middle fist dysfunction involves digestive function this can be associated with postural alterations and emotional conflicts common in adolescents, says Latey:

> The lower end of the oesophagus passes through the muscular part of the diaphragm before joining the stomach. There is an intriguing mechanism which allows for the passage of food, or regurgitation of vomit, between the chest and the abdomen. When the diaphragm is contracted the muscular opening is constricted. In order to allow free flow it must be relaxed (full expiration) with the lower ribs pulled slightly together (transversus contraction). This device frequently fails when there is a chronic disturbance of the middle fist – the "lower end of swallowing" is not happening properly. This may merely lead to wind, burping or fullness. However, when the neuroendocrine/smooth muscle activity is also disturbed the consequences may be more severe. Peptic ulcers, heartburn, reflux oesophagitis, hiatus hernia and so on are all medical conditions associated with middle fist problems. Here the filling and emptying of the stomach and duodenum, with their internal secretions, have become chronically disordered.

We discussed briefly (Exercise 15.4) Latey's methods for the holding and releasing of the middle fist and he suggests that this can lead to total or partial resolution of such dysfunction:

> However, most patients only achieve partial resolution: when the middle fist disturbance begins to resolve the conflict is transferred to the mouth, neck and throat. Even though severe gastrointestinal symptoms may have dissipated, we may still be left with a more complex problem involving the upper fist (the first part of swallowing).

If patients begin to weep, stopping and starting this process of release, Latey suggests the safety valve is only slightly open. He sees the pelvic and middle fist rhythms as coordinated but the head, neck, and shoulders may seem rigid, fighting the movement. In such cases he has found that the situation can change dramatically by laying one's hands across the front of the patient's throat, a very light but firm touch which seems to affect sensitivity in the sternocleidomastoid muscles.

In such cases weeping may become full-bodied, giving a total expression of grief with an orgasmic rhythm. Wailing and high-pitched crying may follow with expressions of complete misery and dejection, even leading to screams of terror. Unfettered rage, snapping, and even biting are possible as the upper fist releases its pent-up tensions and expresses itself for the first time in years.

Patently this is an area where many may not wish to venture. It is powerful and requires nerves of steel on the part of the practitioner; however, it is in such catharsis that the healing of pains and hurts buried for decades may occur.

The upper fist

The metaphor of the clenched fist, which Latey has used to describe regions of the body associated with chronic, often emotionally based contractions, is a powerful image. We have looked at the middle fist (diaphragm, respiratory muscles, abdomen) and also the lower fist which, not unnaturally, focused on the pelvic region (as well as low back and lower abdomen, hips, legs, and feet).

The upper fist involves muscles that extend from the thorax to the back of the head, where the skull and spine join, extending sideways to include the muscles of the shoulder girdle. These muscles therefore set the relative positions of the head, neck, jaw, shoulders, and upper chest, and to a large extent the rest of the body follows this lead (it was FM Alexander (1931) who showed that the head–neck relationship is the primary postural control mechanism).

This region, says Latey, almost with relish, is: "the centre, par excellence, of anxieties, tensions and other amorphous expressions of unease." In chronic states of disturbed upper fist function, he asserts, the main physical impression is one of restrained, over-controlled, damped-down expression. The feeling of the muscles is that they are controlling an "explosion of affect." In contrast to the lower fist, which impresses us with its grip on sensual functions, the upper fist has contracted in response to, or to restrain response to, the outer world.

Just what it is that is being restrained is never obvious from the muscles themselves, but interpreting facial muscles may give a clue. Far more important, though, than the expressions on the face are those that have been withheld. Those experiences that are not allowed free play on the face are expressed in the muscles of the skull and the base of the skull. This, Latey believes, is of central importance in problems of headache, especially migraine. Says Latey: "I have never seen a migraine sufferer who has not lost complete ranges of facial expression, at least temporarily."

Effects of upper fist patterns

The mechanical consequences of upper fist fixations are many and varied, ranging from stiff neck to compression factors leading to disc degeneration and facet wear. Swallowing and speech difficulties are common, as are shoulder dysfunctions including brachial neuritis, Reynaud's syndrome, and carpal tunnel problems.

Latey states:

> The medical significance of upper fist contracture is mainly circulatory. Just as lower fist contraction contributes to circulatory stasis in the legs, pelvis, perineum and lower abdomen; so may upper fist contracture have an even more profound effect. The blood supply to the head, face, special sense, the mucosa of the nose, mouth, upper respiratory tract, the heart itself and the main blood vessels are controlled by the sympathetic nervous system and its main "junction boxes" (ganglia) lie just to the front of the vertebrae at the base of the neck.

Thus headaches, eye pain, ear, nose and throat problems, as well as many cardiovascular troubles may contain strong mechanical elements relating to upper fist muscle contractions.

Latey reminds us that it is not uncommon for cardiovascular problems to manifest at the same time as chronic muscular shoulder pain (avascular necrosis of the rotator cuff tendons) and that the longus colli muscles are often centrally involved in such states.

He looks to the nose, mouth, lips, tongue, teeth, jaws, and throat for evidence of functional change related to upper fist dysfunction, with relatively simple psychosomatic disturbances underlying these. Sniffing, sucking, biting, chewing, tearing, swallowing, gulping, spitting, dribbling, burping, vomiting, sound making and so on, are all significant functions that might be disturbed, acutely or chronically.

And as with middle and lower fist dysfunction, these can all be approached via breathing function.

When all the components of the upper fist are relaxed, the act of expiration produces a noticeable rhythmical movement. The neck lengthens, the jaw rises slightly (rocking the whole head), the face fills out, the upper chest drops. When the patient is in difficulty I may try to encourage these movements by manual work on the muscles and gentle direction to assist relaxed expiration. Again, by asking the patient to let go and let feelings happen, I encourage resolution. Specific elements often emerge quite readily, especially those mentioned with the middle fist, the need to vomit, cry, scream, etc.

In relation to headache Latey observes:

We can often see the headache to be a more general avoidance mechanism. The way in which the generalized focus of pain occupies attention is significant. It clouds and limits concept formation and observation. There is always a deadening and coarsening of sensation and expressiveness. It seems as though the patient uses the headache to hold some perturbation at bay until it can be coped with more responsively, or disappears.

With more severe migraines, with disturbances of vision and nausea, it is often necessary to work through feelings of disgust in considerable detail. Fear of poisoning may be a strong component of nausea, and usually dates back to earliest disturbances of feeling.

Latey also spends time analyzing shock and withdrawal, possibly experienced in the early months of life, as life's realities are recoiled from. This leads, he believes, to our failing to learn from experience as we flinch from emotionally unpleasant episodes. Withdrawal characteristics determine many of Latey's clinical perspectives. Superficially, at any rate, they are easy to recognize:

The dull lifeless tone of the flesh; lifeless flaccidity of larger surface muscle (or spastic rigidity); lifeless hard fibrous state of deep residual postural muscles (with the possible exception of the head and neck muscles); the over-investment of the person in his eyes and ears – hearing and seeing.

More profound pointers to withdrawal are more subtle:

The ritualized expression of any "emotion" in a depersonalized and unspontaneous fashion; the use of language that denies the central presence and unity of self, wards off threats (from outside or inside temptation perhaps) and grasps hold of common insanities of our civilization. These insanities are greatly worsened by social/family mystification.

Exercise 15.5 *Palpating Emotional Effects*

Time suggested **10–15 minutes**

Patiently and slowly examine someone with known emotional stress symptoms, and see whether you can identify patterns of muscular change, as outlined above in the discussion of Latey's "clenched fist" model, seeking tissues that correspond with descriptors such as "dull lifeless," "lifeless flaccidity," "spastic rigidity," "lifeless hard fibrous," and so on.

Also seek evidence of associated breathing pattern dysfunction, as described in Chapter 12.

Additionally look for:

- "ritualized expression of emotion"
- "use of language that denies central presence and unity of self, wards off threats"
- lack of facial expression (which ones are missing?)
- statements about bodily feelings that seem unusual.

What have you noticed that correlates with Latey's words?

Ford's variations on the same theme

Latey suggests that we consider these three "fists," or regions, of abnormal tension, contraction and restriction as we try to look and feel for the physical manifestations of emotional turmoil.

A variation on precisely this same theme is found in the methods grouped together as "somatosynthesis". This is described quite beautifully by Ford (1989):

> There is a close relationship between the diagnostic and therapeutic uses of touch. When touch is involved (palpation), it is not uncommon to hear of the diagnosis turning into therapy without the awareness of the therapist or the patient.

Ford continues:

> My approach to therapeutic touch has always been to keep it simple, getting maximal results from minimal number of techniques and procedures.

Which areas does Ford suggest working on in dealing with emotional problems?

> I might begin by working with the four major areas of cross-restriction in the body; the base of the pelvis [Latey's lower fist], the base of the rib cage [Latey's middle fist], the base of the neck and the base of the skull [together these are Latey's upper fist]. (Fig. 15.1)

It is in these regions, Ford asserts, that the usual vertical orientation of soft tissues is different, as they become horizontally directed:

> Usually the horizontal tissue cross-restricts the vertical tissue of the body, thereby hampering normal muscle movement, fluid flow and nerve transmission. The practical result is that these areas turn out to be the places that most of us experience and retain stress, tension and pain in our bodies. And they are also the areas often related to the deeper psychological issues beneath our physical signs and symptoms. A simple straightforward approach to working with these cross-restrictions is to gently compress them from front to back.

How does he palpate and treat these (and other) dysfunctions?

Seasoned palpators have long known that the best hand is a light hand. The lighter the touch, the more information can be obtained.

Ford suggests that we "remember that palpation and therapy are happening simultaneously." This message should be

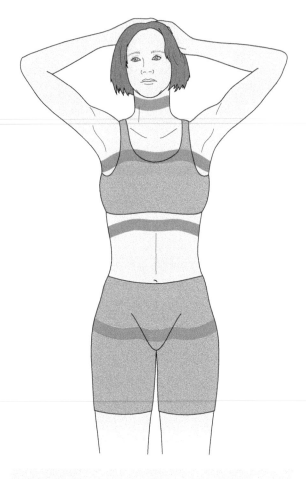

Figure 15.1
Illustration of Ford's cross-restriction areas.

one of our key considerations throughout palpation, particularly as it relates to emotional effects. It is by lightly palpating, projecting the sense of touch, and by being receptive to whatever information radiates into the hand that Ford identifies areas of maximal tension and dysfunction.

> Once I have palpated to determine where to touch (therapeutically), there are three things I take into account: depth, direction and duration. How deep does my touch need to be? Should it be at the level of the energy field where no physical contact is involved, at the skin surface ... or pressing firmly into the (patient's) body.

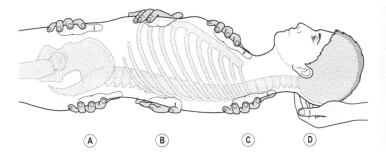

Figure 15.2
The hand positions that would be used in Ford's treatment of horizontal cross-restrictions: (A) pelvic, (B) diaphragmatic, (C) thoracic outlet, and (D) base of skull. By "projecting" his sense of touch he palpates for "depth, direction, and duration" in order to treat these dysfunctions.

He then decides in which direction this hand contact should move: straight down, right, left, pulling, pushing, steady or continuous movement or a combination of these? And finally he allows the tissues themselves to determine how long the force should be held (Fig. 15.2).

We can now see that Latey and Ford approach these problems with slightly different methods, as does Marion Rosen, whose work is considered next.

The Rosen method

Marion Rosen, a brilliant physical therapist, has evolved a method (Mayland 1980) that addresses the same physical manifestations of emotional turmoil as do the approaches of Latey and Ford. The Rosen method is not a mechanical process – it is a journey taken together by client and practitioner towards self-discovery. The practitioner observes the patient's back, as in the following exercises.

Exercise 15.6 *Observation of the Stressed Individual*

Time suggested 10–12 minutes

Have the person lie down prone (if possible the same person, with known emotional stress symptoms, used in Exercise 15.5).

Sit silently and observe to see whether you can identify any of the following.

- Are the muscles tense?
- Where does breath move freely?

- Where is it withheld?
- What statement is the patient making with his body?
- What has to happen so that he can relinquish that contracted space?
- What is the direction in which the muscles are holding?
- Does this holding bear down, hold him together, puff him up or separate the top from the bottom of the body by tightening in the middle (equivalent to Latey's middle fist)?

Compare these observations with the findings you made in Exercise 15.5.

Exercise 15.7 *Palpation of the (Same) Stressed Individual*

Time suggested 12–20 minutes

Lightly palpate the back muscles (ideally of the same person as in the previous exercise – someone with known emotional stress symptoms).

Take your time to locate the most restricted muscular area of the back, where marked tension is palpated and where little or no movement is noted in response to breathing.

"Watch and feel for the place[s] on the back that is [are] most unmoving, held, or not included in his expression of himself. He is unaware that he is holding back."

Hold a flat palpating hand against these tissues, meeting the tension, just taking out the slack.

Exercise 15.7 *continued*

Your other hand may be placed against another similarly tense area, as you patiently and silently wait for a change in the feel of the tissues or for breathing movement to begin to be noted where previously it was not evident.

After the same attention has been given to several tense areas, the hands should be run gently over the back muscles, seeking information, comparing what was initially observed and palpated with what is now being palpated.

- How much has it changed?

Your task is to increase the person's awareness of areas of "restriction and holding" in a non-judgmental manner.

You are also required to follow tense tissues as they release and relax, continuing until all the back is released and breathing function is freely observed in all the tissues.

Try to note:

- what happens to the very tense, unyielding tissues over a period of some minutes, and

- what changes, if any, take place in the breathing pattern itself.

Then attention turns to the diaphragm and the anterior aspect of the body. This major breathing muscle reveals tensions being held, and changes in its function are readily palpated, at the same time as alterations in facial expression are commonly seen.

What may happen?

Compare the description given below, of what might be observed when the Rosen method is used, with the description given by Latey following Exercise 15.4.

> Sometimes as the [Rosen therapy] practitioner works with the muscles that move the diaphragm, a flutter of the diaphragm itself can be seen. Movements in the abdomen might begin as they do when a person is sobbing or crying, although the expression on the face has not changed, leading her [the practitioner] to believe that the sadness that is being expressed in the body is not reaching the face and the consciousness of the client. (Mayland 1980)

What next?

With Rosen therapy, following on from the approach described in the previous exercise, after the back and diaphragm have received attention, other tensions, in the neck or chest perhaps, are then sought which are specifically palpated and worked on in the same manner, until releases occur. The work is accompanied by careful observation and skilled questioning.

As should be clear, the process of palpation is in fact the start of the treatment process (something which can also be said for Lief's neuromuscular technique (Chapter 5)).

The essence of this approach is the identification, via observation and palpation, of restricted areas in which the breathing function fails to manifest itself. Until this is addressed subsequent release is not easily achieved.

As Mayland says:

> All we want is for a person to get connected with what they are holding back. The degree to which they repress, that they will not allow themselves to experience, that they carry around with them ... form a barrier to our living. They are like loads, like rocks in our being.

Pressure during Rosen work

It is perhaps helpful to note that the amount of pressure used on tense "held" areas, when the Rosen method is applied, is very similar to that described by Fritz Smith and Stanley Lief in earlier chapters (Chapters 5 and 14).

The pressure "meets" the muscle, not attempting to overwhelm it or make it do anything. Awareness is the key, with release occurring from the patient's side, not as a forced event.

Rosen's hierarchy of emotions

In the Rosen method, as in Latey's work, there is a hierarchy of emotions, linked to specific areas:

- Deep fear and deep love are associated with the region of the pelvis (or deep in the belly) and where the legs meet the pelvis.

- Repressed anger and sadness are often found in the upper torso or neck.

- Feelings towards others relate to the middle trunk and heart area.

- Fear and anxiety are repressed around the diaphragm.

Anger, sadness and fear are, according to Marion Rosen, easier to release than held emotions associated with love.

The goal of Rosen's method

The Rosen method is characterized by the gentleness of the approach. Emotions are re-experienced, not forced, as the client learns that feelings are just feelings and not the events which precipitated their being locked away. The method leads to self-acceptance and release from long-held tensions, identified by palpation and observation.

Upledger's contribution to emotional release and unwinding

Upledger's somatoemotional release (Upledger 1987) described in earlier chapters (Chapters 3, 14) is worthy of further mention at this point. Using gentle compressive or traction forces, such as:

- slight inferiorly directed compressive force upon the parietals of the seated patient

- compression of the cervical and thoracic vertebrae caudally

- gentle medial compression of the anterior ilia with the patient standing

- grasping of the ankles of the supine patient and introduction of slight compressive or traction force, etc.

Upledger requires the therapist to follow the "unwinding" process which the body may initiate when these (compressive, etc.) forces are applied. Palpatory and proprioceptive skills of a high order are required to achieve this, since not only are the hands required to follow the slow unwinding process, but also to register and prevent any tendency for the unwinding to follow a repetitive pathway.

While this method is used largely to release locked-in, trauma-induced, forces, "repressed emotional components of the somatic injury are frequently and concurrently released." Panic or hysteria related to the trauma may be relived and adaptational energy released.

Upledger warns: "Be alert. Do not inhibit your patient by dragging on their body movements. Try to follow where the patient's body leads you". The patient may finally adopt the position in which the trauma occurred.

While somatoemotional release (as in the Rosen method) seems to describe therapy rather than palpation/ assessment, the distinction is essentially blurred when these approaches are used, as described by their developers.

Palpation skills determine the practitioner's ability to perform these therapeutic methods.

You will probably by now have noted the resemblance that these descriptions have with Smith's work (Chapter 14). Indeed, the overlap between the work of Latey, Rosen, Ford, Upledger, and Smith (and indeed that of Lief and Becker) should not be surprising, since they are all looking at the physical, somatic, manifestations of emotional distress, and are all attempting to both palpate, locate, and initiate or assist in self-generated change in these altered soft tissues.

Cautions and questions

There is justifiably intense debate regarding the question of the induction by bodywork therapists of "emotional release."

If the most appropriate response an individual can make to the turmoil of their life is the "locking away" of these in their musculoskeletal system, we need to ask if it is advisable to unlock the emotions that the tensions and contractions hold.

If there exists no current ability to psychologically process the pain that these somatic areas hold, are they not best left where they are until counseling or psychotherapy or self-awareness leads to the individual's ability to reflect, handle, deal with, and eventually work through the issues and memories?

What is the advantage of triggering a release of emotions, manifested by crying, laughing, vomiting or whatever, as described by Latey and others, if neither the individual nor the manual therapist can then take the process further?

Answers?

The answers to these questions are not readily available, although there are many opinions. However, it is suggested that each patient and each therapist/practitioner should reflect on these issues before removing (however gently and however temporarily) the defensive armoring that life may have obliged vulnerable individuals (i.e., all of us) to erect and maintain.

At the very least, all therapists and practitioners should learn skills which allow the safe handling of "emotional releases" that may occur, with or without deliberate efforts to induce them. Or we should have a referral process in place that leads to the patient having the ability to process, with suitably qualified practitioners, whatever is emerging from these therapeutic endeavors.

Conclusion

The exercises and discussions in this chapter have taken us to the end of this exploration of palpation potentials – but certainly not to the end of the search for optimal palpation skills, which is a perpetual quest.

What should have become evident is the seamless way in which palpation becomes therapy and how manual therapy demands that palpation be continuous during its application.

Another thought is that while the therapist is touching the patient, the patient is also touching the therapist. The brief discussion of the entrainment process (see Chapter 14) might have alerted you to the chance that you are influencing the person you are touching (or perhaps not even touching) in profound ways, and that this can be a two-way process.

The ultimate demand, then, is for the therapist to maintain optimal health, to be focused and centered when working, and to become so practiced in palpation skills that the processes involved are performed with virtually intuitive direction.

I hope you have enjoyed this palpation journey and that this is the start of a never-ending process of exploration.

References

Alexander FM (1931) The use of the self. London: Methuen.

Barlow W (1959) Anxiety and muscle tension pain. British Journal of Clinical Practice 13 (5): 339–350.

Canales JZ, Cordás TA, Fiquer JT, Cavalcante AF and Moreno RA (2010) Posture and body image in individuals with major depressive disorder: A controlled study. Revista Brasileira de Psiquiatria 32 (4): 375–380.

Darwin C (1872, 1899) The expression of emotion in man and animals. London: John Murray.

Ekman P, Levenson RW and Friesen WV (1983) Autonomic nervous system activity distinguishes between emotions. Science 221: 1208–1210.

Ford C (1989) Where healing waters meet. New York: Station Hill Press.

Jacobson E (1930) Electrical measurements of neuromuscular states during mental activities. 1. Imagination of movement involving skeletal muscle. American Journal of Physiology 91: 567–608.

Janda V (1983) Muscle function testing. Butterworths, London.

Latey P (1980) Muscular manifesto. London: Latey.

Latey P (1996) Feelings muscles and movement. Journal of Bodywork and Movement Therapies 1 (1): 44–52.

Malmo R and Shagass C (1949) Physiologic studies of reaction to stress in anxiety and early schizophrenia. Psychosomatic Medicine 11: 9–24.

Mayland E (1980) Rosen method. Palo Alto, CA: Mayland.

Michalak J, Troje NF, Fischer J, Vollmar P, Heidenreich T and Schulte D (2009) Embodiment of sadness and depression – gait patterns associated with dysphoric mood. Psychosomatic Medicine 71 (5): 580–587.

Rosário JL, Diógenes MS, Mattei R and Leite JR (2013) Can sadness alter posture? Journal of Bodywork and Movement Therapies 17 (3): 328–331.

Rosario JL, Bezerra Diógenes MS, Mattei R and Leite JR (2014) Differences and similarities in postural alterations caused by sadness and depression. Journal of Bodywork and Movement Therapies 18 (4): 540–544.

Rosário JL, Diógenes MS, Mattei R and Leite JR (2016) Angry posture. Journal of Bodywork and Movement Therapies 20 (3): 457–460.

Sainsbury P and Gibson JG (1954) Symptoms of anxiety and tension and the accompanying physiological changes in the muscular system. Journal of Neurology, Neurosurgery and Psychiatry 17 (3): 216–224.

Selye H (1956) The stress of life. New York: McGraw-Hill.

Sherrington C (1937) Man on his nature. Gifford Lectures on Natural Theology at Edinburgh University 1937–8.

Simons D, Travell J and Simons L (1999) Myofascial pain and dysfunction: the trigger point manual, vol 1: Upper half of body, 2nd edn. Baltimore, MD: Williams and Wilkins.

Upledger J (1987) Craniosacral therapy. Seattle, WA: Eastland Press.

Waersted M, Eken T and Westgaard R (1992) Single motor unit activity in psychogenic trapezius muscle tension. Arbete och Halsa 17: 319–321.

Waersted M, Eken T and Westgaard R (1993) Psychogenic motor unit activity – a possible muscle injury mechanism studied in a healthy subject. Journal of Musculoskeletal Pain 1 (3/4): 185–190.

Wolff H (1948) Headache and other head pains. Oxford: Oxford University Press.

No.	Symptoms/area	Anterior	Figure	Posterior	Figure
1	Conjunctivitis and retinitis	Upper humerus	4.7	Occipital area	4.9
2	Nasal problems	Anterior aspect of first rib close to sternum	4.7	Posterior angle of the jaw on the tip of the transverse process of the first cervical vertebra	4.9
3	Arms (circulation)	Muscular attachments pectoralis minor to third, fourth and fifth ribs	4.7	Superior angle of scapula and superior third of the medial margin of the scapula	4.9
4	Tonsillitis	Between first and second ribs close to sternum	4.7	Midway between spinous process and tip of transverse process of first cervical vertebra	4.11
5	Thyroid	Second intercostal space close to sternum	4.7	Midway between spinous process and tip of transverse process of second thoracic vertebra	4.9
6	Bronchitis	Second intercostal space close to sternum	4.7	Midway between spinous process and tip of transverse process of second thoracic vertebra	4.11
7	Esophagus	As no. 6	4.7	As no. 6	4.11
8	Myocarditis	As no. 6	4.7	Between the second and third thoracic transverse processes. Midway between the spinous process and the tip of the transverse process	4.10
9	Upper lung	Third intercostal space close to the sternum	4.7	As no. 8	4.10
10	Neuritis of upper limb	As no. 9	4.7	Between the third and fourth transverse processes, midway between the spinous process and the tip of the transverse process	4.10
11	Lower lung	Fourth intercostal space, close to sternum	4.7	Between fourth and fifth transverse processes. Midway between the spinous process and the tip of the transverse process	4.10
12	Small intestines	Eighth, ninth and 10th intercostal spaces close to cartilage	4.7	Eighth, ninth and 10th thoracic intertransverse spaces	4.9
13	Gastric hypercongestion	Sixth intercostal space to the left of the sternum	4.7	Sixth thoracic intertransverse space, left side	4.9
14	Gastric hyperacidity	Fifth intercostal space to the left of the sternum	4.7	Fifth thoracic intertransverse space, left side	4.12
15	Cystitis	Around the umbilicus and on the pubic symphysis close to the midline	4.7	Upper edge of the transverse processes of the second lumbar vertebra	4.12
16	Kidneys	Slightly superior to and lateral to the umbilicus	4.7	In the intertransverse space between the 12th thoracic and the first lumbar vertebrae	4.12
17	Atonic constipation	Between the anterior superior spine of the ilium and the trochanter	4.7	11th costal vertebral junction	4.9

No.	Symptoms/area	Anterior	Figure	Posterior	Figure
18	Abdominal tension	Superior border of the pubic bone	4.7	Tip of the transverse process of the second lumbar vertebra	4.10
19	Urethra	Inner edge of pubic ramus near superior aspect of symphysis	4.7	Superior aspect of transverse process of second lumbar vertebra	4.12
20	Dupuytren's contracture, and arm and shoulder pain	None		Anterior aspect of lateral margin of scapulae, inferior to the head of humerus	4.12
21	Cerebral congestion (related to paralysis or paresis)	(On the posterior aspect of the body) Lateral from the spines of the third, fourth and fifth cervical vertebrae	4.7	Between the transverse processes of the first and second cervical vertebrae	4.11
22	Clitoral irritation and vaginismus	Upper medial aspect of the thigh	4.7	Lateral to the junction of the sacrum and the coccyx	4.10
23	Prostate	Lateral aspect of the thigh from the trochanter to just above the knee. Also lateral to symphysis pubis as in uterine conditions (see no. 43)	4.7	Between the posterior superior spine of the ilium and the spinous process of the fifth lumbar vertebra	4.10
24	Spastic constipation or colitis	Within an area 2–5 cm wide extending from the trochanter to within 2.5 cm of the patella	4.7	From the transverse processes of the second, third and fourth lumbar vertebrae to the crest of the ilium	4.9
25	Leukorrhea	Lower medial aspect of thigh, slightly posteriorly (on the posterior aspect of the body)	4.7	Between the posterior/superior spine of the ilium and the spinous process of the fifth lumbar vertebra	4.10
26	Sciatic neuritis	Anterior and posterior to the tibiofibular junction	4.7	1. On the sacroiliac synchondrosis. 2. Between the ischial tuberosity and the acetabulum. 3. Lateral and posterior aspects of the thigh	4.9
27	Torpid liver (nausea, fullness, malaise)	Fifth intercostal space, from the mid-mammillary line to the sternum	4.8	Fifth thoracic intertransverse space on the right side	4.9
28	Cerebellar congestion (memory and concentration lapses)	Tip of coracoid process of scapula	4.8	Just inferior to the base of the skull on the first cervical vertebra	4.11
29	Otitis media	Upper edge of clavicle where it crosses the first rib	4.8	Superior aspect of first cervical transverse process (tip)	4.9
30	Pharyngitis	Anterior aspect of the first rib close to the sternum	4.8	Midway between the spinous process and the tip of the transverse process of the second cervical vertebra	4.11
31	Laryngitis	Upper surface of the second rib, 5–8 cm from the sternum	4.8	Midway between the spinous process and the tip of the second cervical vertebra	4.11
32	Sinusitis	Lateral to the sternum on the superior edge of the second rib in the first intercostal space	4.8	As no. 31	4.11
33	Pyloric stenosis	On the sternum	4.8	Tenth costovertebral junction on the right side	4.12

No.	Symptoms/area	Anterior	Figure	Posterior	Figure
34	Neurasthenia (chronic fatigue)	All the muscular attachments of pectoralis major on the humerus, clavicle, sternum, ribs (especially fourth rib)	4.8	Below the superior medial edge of the scapula on the face of the fourth rib	4.10
35	Wry neck (torticollis)	Medial aspect of upper edge of the humerus	4.8	Transverse processes of the third, fourth, sixth, and seventh cervical vertebrae	4.11
36	Splenitis	Seventh intercostal space close to the cartilaginous junction, on the left	4.8	Seventh intertransverse space on the left	4.9
37	Adrenals (allergies, exhaustion)	Superior and lateral to umbilicus	4.8	In the intertransverse space between the 11th and 12th thoracic vertebrae	4.12
38	Mesoappendix	Superior aspect of the 12th rib, close to the tip, on right	4.8	Lateral aspect of the 11th intercostal space on the right	4.9
39	Pancreas	Seventh intercostal space on the right, close to the cartilage	4.8	Seventh thoracic intertransverse space on the right	4.12
40	Liver and gall bladder congestion	Sixth intercostal space, from the mid-mammillary line to the sternum (right side)	4.7	Sixth thoracic intertransverse space, right side	4.12
41	Salpingitis or vesiculitis	Midway between the acetabulum and the sciatic notch (this is on the posterior aspect of the body)	4.12	Between the posterior superior spine of the ilium and the spinous process of the fifth lumbar vertebra	4.10
42	Ovaries	The round ligaments from the superior border of the pubic bone, inferiorly	4.8	Between the 9th and 10th intertransverse space and the 10th and 11th intertransverse space	4.10
43	Uterus	Anterior aspect of the junction of the ramus of the pubis and the ischium	4.8	Between the posterior superior spine of the ilium and the fifth lumbar spinous process	4.10
44	Uterine fibroma	Lateral to the symphysis, extending diagonally inferiorly	4.8	Between the tip of the transverse process of the fifth lumbar vertebra and the crest of the ilium	4.9
45	Rectum	Just inferior to the lesser trochanter	4.8	On the sacrum close to the ilium at the lower end of the iliosacral synchondrosis	4.12
46	Broad ligament (uterine involvement usual)	Lateral aspect of the thigh from the trochanter to just above the knee	4.8	Between the posterior superior spine of the ilium and the fifth lumbar spinous process	4.10
47	Groin glands (circulation and drainage of legs and pelvic organs)	Lower quarter of the sartorius muscle and its attachment to the tibia	4.8	On the sacrum close to the ilium at the lower end of the iliosacral synchondrosis	4.12
48	Hemorrhoids	Just superior to the ischial tuberosity (these areas are on the posterior surface of the body)	4.10	On the sacrum close to the ilium, at the lower end of the iliosacral synchondrosis	4.10
49	Tongue	Anterior aspect of second rib at the cartilaginous junction with the sternum	4.7	Midway between the spinous process and the tip of the transverse process of the second cervical vertebra	4.11

INDEX

Note: Page number followed by f and t indicates figure and table only.

A

Abdominal assessment, by neuromuscular technique,
115–117, 115f
Abdominal muscles, 295, 296
Abrams, Albert, 192
Accuracy, 15
Acetylcholine, 62
Achilles tendon, 152
Acromioclavicular (AC) dysfunction, assessment of, 224
Active movements, 200–201
Active range of motion (AROM), 237
evaluation, palpation during, 237, 238f, 239–240, 240f
Acupressure, 194
Acupuncture points
and fascia, 91–92
morphology of reflex and, 91
Adipose layer, 147
Ah Shi points, 119
Algometer, 27–28, 28f
American Physical Therapy Association (APTA), 251
Amplification, 41
Anatomical landmark, assessment of, 15–16
Anatomy Trains, 147, 148
Ankle drawer test, 246, 246f
Anterior longitudinal ligament (ALL), 167
Anterior superior iliac spine (ASIS), 139, 139f, 150
Anterior talofibular ligament, damage to, 246
Apley scratch test, 244, 245f
Areolar layer, 147
Arm lines, 156, 158f–159f
Articulation, visceral, 290–291, 291f
ARTT palpation, 40–41, 102–103
asymmetry, 40
exercise, 103
range of motion, 40
tissue tenderness, 40
tissue texture change, 40
ASIS palpation, 215–217, 216f
Asterion, 228
Asymmetry, 40
Atlanto-occipital joint, 278–280
Atrichial sweat glands, 61–62
Auscultatory percussion, 189
Autonomic nervous system, 290

B

Barlow, Wilfred, 357
Barral, Jean- Pierre, 63
Bathroom scales, for pressure evaluation, 27
Beal, Byron, 75
Becker, Rollin, 100, 332, 347
cervical spine, palpation of, 353f
diagnostic touch, 347–349
fulcrum and, 348
low back palpation, 348f
potency and, 347–348
ribcage, palpation of, 352f
sacrum and pelvis, palpation of, 351, 352f
Beighton Joint Mobility Index, 12
Benign joint hypermobility syndrome (BJHS), 12
Bergson, Henri, 309
Bimanual inherent motion palpation 1 (exercise), 47
Bimanual inherent motion palpation 2 (exercise), 47–48
Bindegewebsmassage, 67
Biologically Closed Electric Circuits, 349
Biomechanics, visceral, 290
Black bag/box palpation (exercise), 44
Black line phenomenon, 185
Bones, 148
Breathing. *See also* Respiratory function
function, assessment of, 296–302
muscle and joint activity and, 295–296
muscle pain and, 294–295
pattern disorders, 293, 294
retraining, 285
wave assessment, 221, 221f
Brow chakra, 332
Bullock-Saxton, Joanne, 22
Buttock muscle tension, 360

C

Cancer, 330, 349
Carpal tunnel syndrome, 156
Cerebrospinal fluid (CSF), 323
Chaitow, Boris, 335
Chakra system, 332–334
Chapman's reflex areas/points palpation (exercise), 84

Chest wall tenderness (CWT), and acute coronary syndrome

non-reproducible, 17
reproducible, 17
Chi emission, 330, 330f
Chinese pulse, 317–320. *See also* Traditional Chinese Medicine (TCM)
Clavipectoral fascia, 160
Clinical reasoning, 236
Coin palpation (exercise), 43
Coin through paper palpation (exercise), 43
Combined skin palpation exercise (exercise), 79
Common compensatory pattern (CCP), 230. *See also* Compensatory patterns, assessment of
Compensatory patterns, assessment of, 231
cervicothoracic area, 231, 232f, 233f
lumbosacral area, 232, 233f
occipitoatlantal area, 231, 232f
thoracolumbar area, 231–232, 233f
Compression test, 267
Connective tissue massage (CTM), 67, 69
Contractile tissue, 239, 240
Contraction patterns, 358–359
Convex-concave rule, 197–198, 198f
Cooper, Gerald, 3
Costocoracoid ligament, 160
Cranial rhythmic impulse (CRI), 324
Cranial sutures and landmarks, palpation of, 226–229, 227f–230f
Craniosacral rhythm, 290
Craniosacral rhythmic motion via feet, 327, 328f
Crown chakra, 332
Cruder touch perception, 36
Crural fascia, 147
Cupule phenomenon, 92
Cytoskeleton, tensegrity-based changes in, 31

D

Deep front line, palpation of, 161–168, 164f–165f
abdomen, 166–167
lower leg, 161–162
neck, 168
thigh, 162–163, 166
thorax, 167
De Jarnette, B., 183–184
Depressed ribs, palpation for, 221–222, 222f

Depression, and gait pattern, 358
Dermis, 147
Detection, 41
Diagnostic palpation, 9
Diagnostic touch, 347–350
Diaphragm, 296
Dicke, Elizabeth, 67
Direct palpation for temperature differences (exercise), 67
Discrimination of information palpation (exercise), 48–49
Dominant eye
    identification of, 55
    use of, 55–56
Double crush phenomenon, 173
Double-leg drop vertical jump test, 256–257, 256f
Drag palpation of skin, 75–77
    after physical exercise, 76
    variation of focus, 76
Dupuytren's contracture, 156

E

Ease and bind, concept of, 135
Elbow flexion, 240
Elbow flexion test, 247–248 248f
Electromagnetic currents, 334
Elevated ribs, palpation for, 223
Emotion
    and exercises
        exploring middle fist, 362–363
        palpating emotional effects, 365
        self-evaluation of postural effects of clenched buttocks, 360
        self-treatment for chronic lower fist contractions, 361
        sensing your own tensions, 360
        stressed individual, observation of, 367
        stressed individual, palpation of, 367–368
    Ford approach, 365–367
    and musculoskeletal changes, 357–358
    posture and, 357, 358
        anger, 358
        contraction patterns, 358–359
        depression, 358
        emotional contractions, 359
        postural interpretation, 358
        sadness, 358
    Rosen method, 367–369
    selective motor unit involvement, 358
    three fists analogy, by Latey, 357, 359

lower fist, 359–361
middle fist, 359, 361–364
upper fist, 359, 364–365
Upledger on, 369–370
Empty can test, 242–243, 242f
Encoding-transmission-decoding (communication pattern), 310
End-feel, 197–201. See also Joint play
    normal, 199–200
    during passive evaluation, 238
    pathological, 200
Energy cyst, 332, 335–336
Energy fields, 314
Energy patterns, model of, 332
Entrainment, 52
Epitrichial sweat glands, 61
Erector spinae, 153
Essential touch, 337
Extension-rotation test. See Kemp's test
Extensor retinaculae, 149
Eye
    body position and, 56
    dominant, 55
    peripheral vision, use of, 55
    visual judgment, 56
    visual screening (exercise), 57

F

F-Ab-ER-E test, 213–214, 214f
FABER test, 12
Facilitated segment, 101
    ARTT palpation, 102–103
    Beal's palpation method, 104, 104f
    descriptions of palpatory findings, 105
    identification of, by palpation, 103–104
    palpatory features of, 101–102
    Tilley and Korr on, 101
Fascia, 100, 147. See also Fascial palpation; Muscles
    contractile properties, 239
    density of, 148
    layers, 147, 148f
Fascia lata, 147
Fascial palpation (exercises), 147–168
    deep back arm line, 160
    deep front arm line, 156, 160
    deep front line, 161–168, 164f–165f
    functional lines, 161, 162f–163f
    lateral line, 153–155, 154f
    shoulder and arm lines, 156, 158f–159f
    spiral line, 156, 157f
    superficial back arm line, 156
    superficial back line, 152–153, 152f

superficial front line, 149–151, 149f
Fascia profundis, 147
Fat globules, 80
Feather-edge of barrier, 199
Feather-light touch, 76
Fibromyalgia, 261
    American College of Rheumatology (ACR) criteria for, 261
    points to assess, 262–263, 262f
    tender point assessment (exercise), 263
    tender point palpation protocol, 261
Fibromyalgia syndrome (FMS), and chest pain, 294
Finger stroke, 107, 107f, 109
Forearm layer palpation (exercises)
    active elbow joint, 51
    blood vessels, 50
    deeper fascia, 50
    muscle fibers, 51
    musculotendinous interface, 51
    passive elbow joint, 51–52
    skin, 49–50, 49f
    skin on subcutaneous fascia, 50
Form and force tests, 211–212
    prone active straight leg raising test, 211, 212f
    supine leg raising test for pelvic stability, 211–212, 213f
Foundation joints, 336
Friction, skin, 62
Frymann's forearm palpation for inherent motion (exercise), 46–47
Frymann, Viola, 1, 2, 6, 35, 42, 67, 99, 323
Fulcrum, concept of, 338
Fulcrum palpation technique, 100
Functional diagnosis, 266
Functional movement, 251
Functional palpation, 265–266. See also Functional technique
Functional technique, 265
    Bowles's summary of, 267, 272
    direct and indirect term, 272
    ease/comfort position, 265
    exercise
        Bowles's self-palpation method, 268

combined functional and SCS palpation of atlanto-occipital joint, 278–280
functional spinal palpation, 273, 274f
Greenman's functional literacy palpation, 274–275
Greenman's functional spinal palpation, 275–276
Hoover's clavicle palpation, 276–278, 276f
Hoover's thoracic experiment, 270–271
Stiles and Johnston's sensitivity exercises, 268–269
Hoover's experiments, 270–271
Johnston's protocol, 272
key elements of, 266
listening hand and, 266, 267
palpating contact, 267
spinal application of, 272
terminology, 266–267
Function and structure, changes in, 31–32

G

General adaptation syndrome (GAS), 98
Generalized joint hypermobility (GJH), 12
Gibbons, Peter, 21
Gillet test, 209, 210f
Glabrous skin, 62
Glenoid labrum tear, 17
Glymphatic system, 323
Goossen, Shannon, 21
Gray's Anatomy, 6
Greater trochanteric tenderness, assessment of, 12
Greenman, Philip, 3, 41, 49, 353–354
Greenman's rib palpation method, 223

H

Hair-root plexus, 35
Hair through paper palpation (exercise), 43
Half-moon vector, 100, 338
Hamstring shortness, palpation for lower fibers, 138–139, 138f
upper fibers, 137–138, 138f
Hands, loci of sensitivity in, 38, 39
Hawkins- Kennedy test, 12, 17
Headache and Other Head Pains, 357
Heart chakra, 332
Heat, manual scanning for, 63
High-velocity thrust (HVT), 200

HiLo test, 297, 297f
Hip abduction observation test, 132, 132f
Hip extension test, 131, 131f
Hippocrates, 309
Hoag, Marshall, 183
Holism, 314
Horse hooves, and camel hooves, 346
HSZ. *See* Hyperalgesic skin zones
Hutchinson, Robert, 190
Hyperalgesic skin zones (HSZ), 5, 62, 70–71, 73, 75
Hypermobile joints, 200
Hypermobility of lumbar spine, 205
Hypermobility tests, 245–246
Hypertonicity, 97–98
intrinsic, 97
neuromotor, 97
Hyperventilation, 283–286
and anxiety, 294–295
dealing with, 285
Nijmegen Questionnaire, 284–285, 284 t
symptoms with, 283

I

Iliosacral dysfunction, 207
standing flexion test for, 206–207, 207f
Iliotibial tract (ITT), 148, 154–155
Image posture, 358
Inanimate object discrimination (exercise), 43
Induration technique, 185
Inert tissues, 239
Inguinal ligament, 150
Inter-examiner reliability, 9, 20
Interference arcing, 335
Interference waves, 351
Intermuscular septa, 147
Internal malleoli, palpation of, 215
Interneural fibrosis, 173
Intersegmental mobility, 105
Intervertebral joints, 129
Intra-examiner reliability, 9, 11
Intrinsic hypertonicity, 97
Intuition, 309–315
and analytic method, difference between, 310
conclusion and, 309
exercise related to
developing intuition via sensory awareness Part 1, 311–312
developing intuition via sensory awareness Part 2, 312–313
energy fields and healing Part 1, 313

energy fields and healing Part 2, 314
and instinct, 309
memory and, 310
use of, 310
and visualization, 310–311
Ischial tuberosity height, palpation of, 215

J

Janda, Vladimir, 56
Joint play, 197
active and passive movements, 200–201
barriers, 199–200
convex and concave rule, 197–198, 198f
glide/translation, 197
hypermobile joints, 200
importance of, 198–199
joint separation, 197
at proximal tibiofibular joint, 201
Joints, palpation and assessment of, 203–234
acromioclavicular dysfunction assessment (exercise), 224
ASIS palpation (exercise), 215–217, 216f
body language and, 205
body's compensation potential (Zink and Lawson's method), 229–234, 231f
breathing (exercise), 221
breathing wave assessment, 221, 221f
depressed ribs, palpation for, 221–222, 222f
elevated ribs, palpation for, 223
Greenman's rib palpation method, 223
rib palpation method, 223–224
crest height palpation (exercise), 205–206
F-Ab-ER-E test (exercise), 213–214, 214f
form and force tests (exercise), 211–212, 212f, 213f
prone active straight leg raising test, 211, 212f

supine leg raising test for pelvic stability, 211–212, 213f

internal malleoli, palpation of (exercise), 215

ischial tuberosity height, palpation of (exercise), 215

normal gait, 204

observation of patient (exercise), 204–205

postural observation (exercise)
  posterior and lateral aspects, 205
  and range of spinal motion, 205

prayer test (exercise), 225f, 226

PSIS position, palpation of (exercise), 206

pubic tubercle palpation (exercise), 214

repetitive movements and, 204

restriction barrier and, 203

rotoscoliosis, observation of
  during seated flexion, 209
  during standing flexion, 207–208

seated flexion test (exercise), 208, 208f

shrug test (exercise), 224, 225f

SIJ (sacroiliac joint) dysfunction, 206

skull, palpation of, 226
  cranial sutures and landmarks, 226–229, 227f–230f

spinal dysfunction, 217
  lumbar palpation (exercise), 220
  semantics, 220
  spinal palpation assessment sequence (exercise), 217–218, 219f

standing flexion test (exercise), 206–207, 207f

standing hip extension test (exercise), 210

standing iliosacral stork test (exercise), 209, 210f

symptoms and, 204

Jones, Lawrence, 185

Jones's strain/counterstrain palpation, 119–122

Journal of Bodywork and Movement Therapies (JBMT), 19

Juhan, Deane, 59

K

Kemp's test, 16

Knock-knees, 360

Korr, Irvin, 35, 171–172, 265, 346

Krause's end-bulb, 36

L

Labrum tear, tests for, 17

Lachman's test, 17, 241

Lambdoidal sutures, 228

Lamont, Keith, 185

Lateral line, palpation of, 154f
  foot and lower leg, 153–154
  neck, 155
  thigh and pelvis, 154–155
  trunk, 155

Lateral raphe, 153

Latey, Philip, 357

Laughing and weeping, 362

Layer palpation using inanimate materials (exercise), 44

Lee, Diane, 20–21, 22

Leg length symmetry assessment, reliability of, 12

Lewit, Karel, 1, 3, 20, 62, 70, 78
  hyperalgesic skin zones (HSZ), 70–71
  skin-stretch methods, 72–74
  sustained skin stretch of HSZs (exercise), 74

Liebenson, Craig, 20

Lief, Stanley, 106, 334

Ligamentous laxity, 245

Light touch, 35–36

Linea alba, palpation of, 118

Linguistic armament, 267

Liver motility, palpation for, 292, 293f

Living bone palpation (exercise), 45–46

Local adaptation syndrome (LAS), 98–99

Locomotor soft tissues, 235, 236

Log roll test, 12

Long dorsal sacroiliac ligament (LDSIL), 210, 211f

Lumbar pain, 94

M

Magnetoencephalogram, 330

Manual resistive tests (MRT), 237, 238, 240, 240f
  grading scale, 238f
  recognizing muscle resistance in, 238–239

McMurray test, 17

Mechanical interface (MI), 173

Mechanical tension in neural structures, abnormal, assessment of, 171–181
  base tests, 172–173
  mechanical interface, 173

neural transportation and, 171–172

neurodynamic stretching and slider exercises, 179–181, 179f, 180f

passive neck flexion (PNF), 177

precautions and contraindications, 174

prone knee bending (PKB), 175

slump test, 176–177, 178f

straight leg raising (SLR), 175

tension points and test descriptions, 174

upper limb tension tests (ULTT), 177–178

variations of passive motion of nervous system, 174

Mechanoreceptors, 35

Mechanotransduction, 31

Medial collateral ligament (MCL), 246

Meissner's corpuscle, 35

Meniscal tears, diagnosis of, 17

Merkel's disc, 35

Mesenteric ligaments, 291, 291f

Mirror-touch synesthesia, 307

Mitchell, Frederick, 2, 3, 56

Mobility, 291
  evaluation of, 292

Modified Thomas test, 244, 244f

Morrison ligament, 150

Motility, 291
  evaluation of, 292

Motive hand, 267

Motor control impairment (MCI), 252

Movement evaluation, 252–253
  exercises
    double-leg drop vertical jump test, 256–257, 256f
    prone knee bend test, 254–255, 255f
    standing bow test, 255–256, 256f
  therapist skills and, 254
  use of findings, in treatment, 252–253

Movement health, 251–252

MRT. *See* Manual resistive tests

MSDs. *See* Musculoskeletal disorders

Murphy, Donald R., 21, 22

Muscle energy technique (MET), 200

Muscles, 97, 148
  altered muscle function, 130–134
  facilitated segment, 101
    ARTT palpation, 102–103
    Beal's palpation method, 104, 104f
    descriptions of palpatory findings, 105
    identification of, by palpation, 103–104
    palpatory features of, 101–102
    Tilley and Korr on, 101
  and facilitation, 105
  hypertonicity, 97–98
  intersegmental, 105
  Jones's strain/counterstrain palpation,

119–122
Jones's tender point palpation, 120–122, 120f
local adaptation syndrome, 98–99
neuromuscular technique, 105–119
abdominal assessment, 115–117, 115f
anterior thoracic and abdominal NMT palpation (exercise), 116
application in assessment mode (exercise), 111–112, 112f–115f
assessment palpation by, 109
comprehensive NMT evaluation (exercise), 119
control and delicacy of touch, 108
finger and thumb NMT strokes (exercise), 111
finger, use of, 107, 107f, 109
intelligent quality, addition of, 108
lateral rectus sheath, palpation of, 118
Lief's methods, 106–107, 107f
linea alba, palpation of, 118
Nimmo's contribution, 106
for particular areas, 109–111
point systems, 106
practitioner's posture and positioning, 107–108
pulsating mass and caution, 117
rectal sheath, palpation of, 117–118
relaxed working arm in, 108
symphysis pubis, palpation of, 118
thumb, use of, 106, 107f, 108
umbilicus region, palpation in, 118
variable pressure and, 108
overuse, misuse and abuse of, 97–99
palpation
and assessment of structure, 100–101
light and variable touch, 99
skill status, 142–143
solutions of problem, 100
tasks, 97–99
periosteal pain points, 129–130
shortness, evaluation of, 134–142
trigger point palpation, 122–128
Musculoskeletal disorders (MSDs), 235
clinical reasoning
in action, 248
and evaluation process, 235–236
exercises
ankle drawer test, 246, 246f
Apley scratch test, 244, 245f
AROM, PROM, and MRT evaluations, 241
elbow flexion test, 247–248 248f
empty can test, 242–243, 242f
modified Thomas test, 244, 244f
recognizing muscle resistance in MRTs,

238–239
straight leg raise, 247, 247f
tennis elbow test, 243–244, 243f
valgus stress test, 245–246, 245f
HOPRS assessment protocol, 236–237
history, 237
observation, 237
palpation, 237
range of motion and resistance testing, 237–241
special tests, 241–248
hypermobility tests, 245–246
locomotor soft tissues and, 235, 236
neurodynamic tests, 246–248
orthopedic assessment, 236
pain provocation tests, 242–244
positional or postural tests, 244
Myers, Tom, 5
Myofascial pain index (MPI), 28
Myofascial trigger points, 12

N

Nausea and vomiting, 362
Navel chakra, 332
Neer impingement test, 241
Neer test, 12, 17
Neural transportation, 171–172
negative influences on, 172
Neurodynamic sliding, 179–181, 180f
Neurodynamic stretching, 179, 179f
Neurodynamic tests, 246–248
Neurological lens, 101
Neurolymphatic reflex points, 79–84
anterior surface, 81f, 82f
clinical value of, 81–83
exercise, 84
location of, 81
palpation sequence, 83–84
posterior cervical surface, 83f
posterior surface, 82f, 83f, 84f
validating study, 80
Neuromotor hypertonicity, 97
Neuromuscular technique (NMT), 105–119
abdominal assessment, 115–117, 115f
anterior thoracic and abdominal NMT palpation (exercise), 116
application in assessment mode (exercise), 111–112, 112f–115f
assessment palpation by, 109
comprehensive NMT evaluation (exercise), 119
control and delicacy of touch, 108

finger and thumb NMT strokes (exercise), 111
finger, use of, 107, 107f, 109
intelligent quality, addition of, 108
lateral rectus sheath, palpation of, 118
Lief's methods, 106–107, 107f
linea alba, palpation of, 118
Nimmo's contribution, 106
for particular areas, 109–111
point systems, 106
practitioner's posture and positioning, 107–108
pulsating mass and caution, 117
rectal sheath, palpation of, 117–118
relaxed working arm in, 108
symphysis pubis, palpation of, 118
thumb, use of, 106, 107f, 108
umbilicus region, palpation in, 118
variable pressure and, 108
NMT. *See* Neuromuscular technique
Nociceptors, 35, 36
Non-specific chronic low back pain (NSCLBP), 252, 254
Nordenstrom, Bjorn, 347, 349
Normal motion demand, 267
Noxious points, 124

O

Observation, soft-tissue injury and, 237
Orthopedic assessment, 236
Overbreathing, 283
Overuse syndrome, 178

P

Pacinian corpuscles, 36
Pain
anterior thorax and, 88–89
central, 88
changes in motor recruitment in, 252
chronicity of, 252
compression test, 93–94
Cyriax's strength tests, 93
evaluating soft tissue and joint involvement (exercise), 94–95
local, 88
muscle or joint problem, 93, 94
referred, 87
resisted tests, 93
source of, 87–88
visceral factors and imposter symptoms, 88

Index

Painful arc, 200
Pain provocation, 11, 16
  digital, 16
  tests, 242–244
Paired descriptors, 42
Palmar surface of hand, 36
Palpating for inherent motion
(exercise), 46
Palpation, 1–2, 39
  and amplification, 41
  of bone, real and plastic (exercise), 45
  comparative descriptors and exercises,
    41–52
  and description of feel, 6
  and detection, 41
  diagnostic, 13
  by feeling, 4
  as fifth dimension, 6
  fundamentals of, 35–52
  interdisciplinary views, 6–7
  interpretation, 41
  mistake in, 41
  objectives of, 3
  and observation, 32
  structural alterations and functional
    change, 32
  subtle (see Subtle palpation)
  variations, 4–5
  without touch, 342–343
Palpatory sensitivity, 35
Palpatory test
  reliability of, 9, 19
  validity of, 13, 19
Paracelsus, 314
Paradoxical breathing, 297–298
Paravertebral muscle assessment, 139–140,
  140f
Passive accessory intervertebral motion
tests (PAIVMs), 16
Passive movements, 201
Passive neck flexion (PNF) test, 177
Passive physiological intervertebral motion
tests (PPIVMs), 16
Passive range of motion (PROM), 237
  evaluation, palpation during, 238–240,
    240f
Pectus excavatum, 167
Pelvic tilt, 209
Percussion, 189–195
  abdominal, 191
  auscultatory, 189
  cardinal rules, 191
  of chest, 303
  immediate/direct, 189
  mediate/indirect, 189
  method, 191
  orthopedic/neurological, 192

palpatory, 189
  and sounds, 190, 190f
  spinal, 193
  therapeutic, 192
  upper and lower borders of liver by
    (exercise), 191–192
  validity of method, 189–190
Periosteal pain points (PPPs), 129–130
  palpation for (exercise), 130
  sites and significance, 129–130
Periosteum, 147, 148
Peripheral vision, use of, 55
Phalen's test, 241
Physical examination
  deeper palpation and, 41
  superficial palpation and, 41
  visual assessment in, 56–57
Piaget, Jean, 309
Pick's palpation guidelines, 28–29
Piriformis, shortness of, 139
Plantar fascia, 152
Pleximeter, 189
Positional/postural tests, 244
Positional release technique, 72
Positional Release Techniques, 119
Posterior drawer test, for posterior cruciate
ligament tear, 17
Posterior superior iliac spine (PSIS), 139,
139f, 206
Postural muscles, 130–131
Postural muscle shortening, tests for,
134–142
Postural screening (exercise), 57
Potency within strain pattern, 351
PPPs. See Periosteal pain points
Pragmatic criteria, 14
Pranayama breathing, 285–286
Pranotherapy, 334
Prayer test, 225f, 226
Precision, 9
Pre-season screening, in sport, 253
Pressure
  algometer, 27–28, 28f
  at rejection level, 28, 29
  at surface level, 28, 29
  threshold, 27
  use of, 27
  at working level, 28, 29
Principles of Manual Medicine (Philip
Greenman), 3
Projected pain, 88
Prone hip extension test, 131, 131f
Prone knee bend (PKB) test, 175, 254–255,
255f
Proprioception, 35
Proprioceptive receptors, 38
Protective chi, 341

Proximal tibiofibular joint, 201
Pseudoradicular syndromes, 59
Pubic tubercle palpation, 214
Pulse taking, Frymann's views on, 48
Pulsing electromagnetic field therapy (PEMF),
330

Q

Quadrant test. See Kemp's test
Quantum tunnelling, 330

R

Radial pulse assessment (exercise), 48
Radicular syndrome, 87
Range of motion, alteration in, 40
Rapidly firing receptors, 38
Receptive field, 36
Receptor adaptation, 38
Receptor-tonus technique, 106, 124
Rectal sheath, palpation of, 117–118
Rectus abdominis, 151
Rectus femoris, 148
Red reflex, 183–185
Red reflex assessment (exercise), 186–187
Reference standard, 13–14
Referred pain, 87–88
Reflex Pain, 183
Reich, Wilhelm, 357
Rejection level, concept of, 28, 29, 29f
Reliability, 9
  determination of, 10–11, 10t
  experts opinions and recommendations
    on, 19–22
  importance of, 10
  inter-examiner, 9
  intra-examiner, 9
  kappa values, 10, 10t
  of manual diagnostic procedures, 11
    hand, 12
    hip, 12
    knee, 12
    leg length, 12
    myofascial trigger points, 12
    primary respiratory mechanism, 12
    sacroiliac (SI) joint, 12
    shoulder, 12
    spine, 11–12
  of palpatory test, 9
    improvement in, 19
  variables affecting, 10t
Residual posture, 358
Resisted tests, 93

Respiratory diseases, 293
Respiratory dysfunction. *See also*
Respiratory function
    breathing
        and muscle and joint activity, 295–296
        and muscle pain, 294–295
    palpation and observation for, 293
    structural considerations and, 293–294
Respiratory function
    assessment of (exercise), 297–299
    comprehensive respiratory assessment
        (exercise), 302
    cross-referral to other palpatory findings,
        299–300
    observation, 300–301
    results of assessment, 300, 301
Retrograde transportation, 171
Reversed double crush, 173
Rib palpation method, 223
Rolf, Ida, 5, 32
Rolfing, 5
Rollgliding, 197
Root chakra, 332
Rotator cuff-related shoulder pain (RCRSP),
    256
Rotator cuff tear, full-thickness, diagnosis
    of, 17
Rotoscoliosis
    during seated flexion, 209
    during standing flexion, 207–208
Ruffini's ending, 36

S

Sacroiliac (SI) joint
    dysfunction, 94, 206
        seated flexion test for, 208, 208f
    force closure, 210–211, 211f
    form closure, 210, 211f
    long dorsal, 210, 211f
    palpatory tests for
        reliability of, 12
        validity of, 17–18
Sacro-occipital technique (SOT), 183–184
Sacrotuberous ligament, 153
Scalene muscles, 168
Scapulohumeral rhythm test,
    133–134, 134f
Scapulothoracic joint, 160
Scar, 78
    abdominal, and back pain, 78
    deep palpation for pain spots near, 78
    focus of disturbance, 78
    palpation (exercise), 79
    saboteurs, 78
Schultz band, 151

Seated flexion test, 208, 208f
Segmentally related sympatheticotonia, 184
Selected Writings of Beryl Arbuckle, 80
Selective tissue tension paradigm, 239
Selye, Hans, 346
Semi-foundation joints, 337
Sensitivity, 15, 241
Sensory literacy, 39, 56
Serratus posterior inferior, 361–362
Shock-absorber, 198
Shoulder impingement syndrome,
    12, 17
Shoulder symptom modification procedure,
    256, 256f
Shrug test, 224, 225f
Simons, David G., 21–22
Simultaneous palpation of normal and
    abnormal tissues (exercise), 46
Skeletal muscles, 97
Skin
    atrichial glands activity, influence of, on
        palpation, 61–62
    changes to be read by palpator, 59
    Chapman's neurolymphatic reflex points,
        79–84
    drag palpation of, 75–77
        after physical exercise, 76
        variation of focus, 76
    drag phenomenon, 62–63
    epitrichial and atrichial sweat
        glands, 61
    exercises
        Chapman's reflex areas/points palpation,
            84
        combined skin palpation
            exercise, 79
        direct palpation for temperature
            differences, 67
        evaluating skin on fascia resistance,
            67–72
        Lewit's large skin area assessment/
            palpation, 74
        Lewit's skin-stretching palpation (A),
            72–73
        Lewit's skin-stretching palpation (B), 73
        Lewit's skin-stretching palpation (C), 73
        Lewit's sustained skin stretch of HSZs,
            74
        off-body scanning for temperature
            differences, 66–67
        scar palpation, 79
        skin drag palpation, 75–76, 76f
        skin drag (watch strap) palpation, 77
        temperature discrimination, 63–64
        temperature discrimination using
            inanimate objects, 63–64
        testing different regions for thermal

sensitivity, 65
    thermal conductivity and influence of
        moisture, 64–65
    glabrous and non-glabrous, 62
    hyperalgesic skin zones, 62
    importance of, 59
    as monitor of reflexive behavior, 59–60
    palpation and assessment of, 59–84
    palpation findings, 77–78
    physiology of, 59–63
    scars, 78–79
    sensory receptors in, 61
    superficial palpation, and changes to be
        noted, 75
    temperature and skin variations, palpation
        for, 66–75
    temperature measurement, by touch,
        63–66
    thermography in bodywork, 62
Skin drag palpation (exercise),
    75–76, 76f
Skin drag (watch strap) palpation (exercise),
    77
Skin elasticity, 32
Skinfolds, lifting of, 69, 69f
Skin friction, 62
    variations in, 76, 76f
Skin rolling, 70
Skin stretching, 70
Slump posture, 358
Slump test, 176–177
Smith, Fritz, 100, 324, 332, 336–342
Smith's energy model of human
    body, 337
Soft tissue and joint involvement, evaluation
    of, 94–95
Soft tissue palpation, and exercises, 97, 100.
See also Muscles
    anterior thoracic and abdominal NMT
        palpation (exercise), 116
    application in assessment mode (exercise),
        111–112, 112f–115f
    ARTT palpation, 103
    Beal's compression palpation, 104
    combined viscerosomatic reflex palpation,
        104
    comprehensive NMT evaluation (exercise),
        119
    finger and thumb NMT strokes (exercise),
        111
    Goodridge's ease and bind palpation,
        136–137, 136f
    hamstring shortness, palpation for
        lower fibers, 138–139, 138f
        upper fibers, 137–138, 138f
    hip abduction firing sequence test,
        132–133

hip extension firing sequence, 131–132

Jones's tender point palpation, 120–122, 120f

palpating for feather-edge barrier in muscle shortness, 135–136, 136f

palpation for trigger points using Nimmo's guidelines, 128

paravertebral muscle assessment, 139–140, 140f

periosteal pain points, palpation for, 130

piriformis shortness, palpation for, 139

scapulohumeral rhythm assessment, 134

trigger point palpation, 124

upper trapezius shortness, palpation for, 141–142, 141f, 142f

Somatic nervous system, 290

Somatosynthesis, 366

Specificity, 15, 241

Spinal mechanics of respiration, 295–296

Spinal motion, palpatory tests for, 16

Spinal palpatory procedures, reliability of, 11–12

Spinal percussion, 193

Spinal splinting, 102

segmental facilitation and, 102

Spine

digital palpation of, 101

flat areas of, 140

Spiral line, 156, 157f

Spleen chakra, 332

Spondylogenic reflexes, 89

Spondylotherapy, 192–193

Spray and stretch methods, 194

SQUID (Superconducting Quantum Interference Device), 330

Standing bow test, 255–256, 256f

Standing flexion test, 206–207, 207f

Standing hip extension test, 210

Standing iliosacral stork test, 209, 210f

Sternoclaviclar restriction, 224–225

Sternocleidomastoid (SCM), 151, 155

Still point, 329

Stone, Randolph, 334

Straight leg raising (SLR) test, 175, 247, 247f

Strain/counterstrain (SCS), 119–122

Stress, and functional/structural change, 32

Structure and function, interdependence of, 31–32

Subclavius, 160

Subpatellar tendon, 150

Subtle palpation, 323

altered energy flow and, 334

Upldeger's energy cyst, 335–336

Varma model, 334–335

cerebrospinal fluid and glymphatic motion, 323

cranial rhythmic impulse and, 324

craniosacral connection and, 326, 327f

depth of perception, 350

energy dense areas (chakras) and, 332–334

of energy flow, 329–330

exercises

Becker's palpation of tissue status: from knee, 349–350

cervical spine palpation using Becker's fulcrum, 353, 353f

chakra scanning, 333–334

combined palpation of tissue characteristics, 353

cranial motion from legs, 327

cranial rhythmic impulse (CRI) palpation, 324–326, 325f

energy body, palpation of, 342

energy body via shoulders, 345

energy cyst, 335–336

energy interface in forearm, 339–340

energy interface in lower leg, 340

half-moon vector, palpation by, 338–339

learning to palpate energy, 331–332, 331f

lower thorax palpation using Becker's fulcrum, 352, 352f

palpating tissues over energy vortex of chakra, 334

palpation using Becker's fulcrum, 349

pelvic palpation using Becker's fulcrum, 351, 352f

scanning someone's energy field, 333

Smith's balloon and rubber band palpations, 338

sphenoidal decompression layer palpation, 327–328

still point, creation of, 329

synchrony between occiput and sacrum, 327, 328f

two-finger energy palpation, 341

inherent motion and, 323–324

soft tissue palpation by Smith's methods, 341

still point and, 328–329

zero balancing, 336

Superficial back line, palpation of, 152f

back, 153

foot and lower leg, 152

head, 153

thigh, 153

Superficial fascia, 91, 100

Superficial front line, palpation of, 149f

abdomen, 150–151

anterior rib cage, 151

foot and lower leg, 149–150

neck, 151

thigh, 150

Surface level, 28, 29

Sutherland, W.G., 4

Symphysis pubis, palpation of, 118

Synesthesia, 305–307

bodywork implications, 306–307

color-auditory, 305

color-graphemic, 305

mirror-touch, 307

strong, 305

weak, 305

T

Tactile discrimination, 36, 37f

TCM. See Traditional Chinese Medicine

Tehan, Philip, 21

Temperature discrimination (exercise), 63–64

Temperature discrimination using inanimate objects (exercise), 63–64

Tender points, 261

Tennis elbow test, 243–244, 243f

Tension in nervous system, abnormal, assessment of, 171–181

Tension point, 175, 181

Therapeutic percussion, 192

Therapeutic Touch (TT), 330, 341, 343–344

assessment in, 343–344

centering in, 343

evaluation/closure in, 344

intervention in, 344

Thermal conducting coefficient (TCC), 64

Thermal conductivity and influence of moisture (exercise), 64–65

Thermal perception, variables affecting, 66, 66f

Thermal properties, of exchanging surfaces, 64

Thermal sensitivity, testing different regions for (exercise), 65

Thermographic hot-spots, 63

Thermography, in bodywork, 62

Thermoreceptors, 35, 36, 64–66, 66f

Thoracolumbar fascia (TLF), 153

Three fists analogy, by Latey, 357, 359

lower fist, 359–361

middle fist, 359, 361–364

Index

upper fist, 359, 364–365
Throat chakra, 332
Thumb stroke, 106, 107f, 108
Tilley, McFarlane, 102
Tissue density, 44
Tissue memory, 3, 5, 346–347
Tissue mobility, testing of, by bilaterally
pushing skin with fingerpads,
68, 68f
Tissue tenderness, 40
Tissue texture, change in, 40
Touch, physiology of, 35
  ARTT model, 40–41
    asymmetry and, 40
    range of motion and, 40
    tissue tenderness and, 40
    tissue texture change and, 40
    validity of, 40
  filtering of information, 38
  localizing dysfunction, 40
  palpation of movement, 39
  receptor adaptation, 38
  receptors and perception, 35–36
  sensitivity of different parts of hand, 36,
    38
  two-point discrimination test, 36, 37f
  variations in sensitivity, 36–37
Traditional Chinese Medicine (TCM), 91, 317,
341
  palpating water flow through a tube
    (exercise), 318
  pulse palpation on self and others
    (exercise), 318–319
  pulses, 317–320, 319f
Transversus thoracis, 361
Trapezius, upper, assessment of shortness
in, 141–142, 141f, 142f
Trauma, and energy changes, 344–345
  balancing energy, 345–346
  Smith on, 344–346
Trigger point (TP), 122
  central, 123
  compression guidelines,
    123–124, 123f
  definition of, 106
  exercise, 124
  flat palpation, 123
  Lewit's view of, 128
  Nimmo's perspective on, 123–128
  palpation, 122–128
  pincer compression, 123, 123f
  potential, 106
  symptoms, 123
Trigger point percussion technique, 193–195
Turner, Roger Newman, 185
Two-point discrimination test, 36, 37f

U

Ulnar collateral ligaments, 160
Umbilicus region, palpation in, 118
Upledger, John, 4, 75, 335
Upper limb tension tests
  ULTT 1, 177–178
  ULTT 2, 178, 178f

V

Valgus stress test, 245–246, 245f
Validity, 13
  determination of, 15
  of diagnostic palpation
    cervical spine, 18–19
    cranial motion palpation, 19
    knee, 17
    lumbar spine, 18
    sacroiliac joint, 17–18
    shoulder, 17
  importance of, in palpatory diagnosis,
    14–15
  of manual diagnostic procedures, 15
    anatomical landmark assessment,
      15–16
    pain provocation, 16
    palpatory tests for spinal motion, 16
  reference standard for, 13–14
Valsalva maneuver, 296
Van Allen, Paul, 5, 6, 44
Variable pressure, 100, 108, 335
Varma, Dewanchand, 334
Vastus intermedius, 148
Vault hold, 324, 325f
Visceral and Obstetric Osteopathy, 289
Visceral Manipulation, 289
Visceral motility and mobility, 289–290. See
also Visceral palpation
Visceral palpation, 289. See also Respiratory
function
  elements, 291
  embryological influences, 290
  exercises
    palpation for liver motility, 292, 293f
  importance of, 289
  inspir and expir and, 290
  mobility and motility, 291–292
  muscular influences, 291
  visceral articulation, 290–291, 291f
  visceral motion and, 289–290
Viscerosomatic reflex, 101
Visual analog pain scale, 14
Visual assessment, in physical examination,
56–5
Visual literacy, 2, 56
Vocal fremitus, palpation of, 303
Vomiting, 362

W

Walton, William, 217
Weakness, muscle, 238
Webster, George, 3
Weight transference, 107
Where Healing Waters Meet, 357
Whole systems theory, 310
Wood density palpation (exercise), 44
Working level, concept of, 28, 29, 29f
Wrist flexion, 240–241

Z

Zero Balancing, 5, 324, 332, 336
Zink and Lawson's hypothesis,
229–234, 231f